David J. Goldberg

Facial Rejuvenation

David J. Goldberg (Ed.)

Facial Rejuvenation

A Total Approach

With 215 Figures and 30 Tables

Springer

David J. Goldberg
Skin Laser and Surgery Specialists
of New York and New Jersey,
UMDN-New Jersey Medical School, Newark,
New Jersey, USA,
and Mount Sinai School of Medicine,
New York, New York, USA

ISBN-13 978-3-540-69517-2
Springer Berlin Heidelberg NewYork

Library of Congress Control Number: 2007923872

Springer is a part of Springer Science+Business Media
springer.com

Editor: Marion Philipp, Heidelberg, Germany
Desk Editor: Ellen Blasig, Heidelberg, Germany
Production: LE-TEX, Jelonek, Schmidt & Vöckler GbR, Leipzig, Germany
Typsetting and reproduction of the figures:
Satz-Druck-Service (SDS), Leimen, Germany

Printed on acid-free paper
24/3180/YL - 5 4 3 2 1 0

Preface

Facial rejuvenation, once almost solely a surgical technique for the treatment of aging skin, has increasingly become a discipline involving the synergistic use of noninvasive approaches. Today, the nonsurgical approach to facial rejuvenation involves the use of a combination of lasers and laser-like technologies, used in conjunction with fillers and botulinum toxins. Nonsurgical laser and light-based treatment of the skin now also encompasses subcategories of treatment such as photodynamic photorejuvenation and photomodulation with light emitting diodes (LEDs). The esthetic physician may also use a variety of peels, mesotherapy, and topical cosmecueticals to optimize the process of facial rejuvenation.

This book is divided into eight chapters, each written by an international expert in his or her respective field. All chapters, where appropriate, have a unifying theme. Chapters start with bulleted "Core Messages". This is then followed with chapter sections taking a look at currently available technologies, advantages, disadvantages, indications, contraindications, patient's informed consent, author's personal approach, postoperative care and complications, results and photographs and finally the author's look to the future with respect to each treatment approach to facial rejuvenation.

Facial Rejuvenation is meant as a primer for any physician interested in the total approach to the noninvasive treatment of aging skin.

David J. Goldberg

Contents

Chapter 5
Dermal Fillers
Derek Jones

Chapter 6
Chemical Peeling
Ross M. Campbell and Gary D. Monheit

Chapter 7
Mesotherapy and Injectable Lipolysis
Adam M. Rotunda

Chapter 8
Cosmeceuticals
Zoe Diana Draelos

List of Contributors

Kenneth Beer
Palm Beach Esthetic Center,
University of Miami
Department of Dermatology,
Miami, Florida, USA

Ross M. Campbell
Total Skin and Beauty Dermatology Center,
P.C.,
Department of Dermatology,
University of Alabama at Birmingham,
Birmingham, Alabama, USA

Joel L. Cohen
AboutSkin Dermatology and DermSurgery,
University of Colorado
Department of Dermatology,
Denver, Colorado, USA

Zoe Diana Draelos
Department of Dermatology,
Wake Forest University School of Medicine,
Winston-Salem, North Carolina, USA

Michael Gold
Gold Skin Care Center, Vanderbilt
University,
Nashville, Tennessee, USA

David J. Goldberg
Skin Laser and Surgery Specialists
of New York and New Jersey,
UMDN-New Jersey Medical School,
Newark, New Jersey, USA,
and Mount Sinai School of Medicine,
New York, USA

Greg J. Goodman
Skin and Cancer Foundation of Victoria,
Monash University,
Toorak, Victoria, Australia

Derek Jones
Dermatology, UCLA,
Los Angeles, California, USA

Gary D. Monheit
Total Skin and Beauty Dermatology Center,
P.C.,
Department of Dermatology,
University of Alabama at Birmingham,
Birmingham, Alabama, USA

Adam M. Rotunda
Dermatology, UCLA,
Los Angeles, California, USA

Robert A. Weiss
Maryland Laser, Skin and Vein Institute,
Johns Hopkins University School
of Medicine,
Baltimore, Maryland, USA

Chapter 1

Lasers and Lights

Greg J. Goodman

1

Core Messages

- Laser facial rejuvenation is often required to improve environmental- and disease-related skin damage.
- A variety of laser- and light-based therapies are now used for facial rejuvenation. An understanding of basic laser physics is required to fully evaluate light-based technologies.
- Ablative lasers such as carbon dioxide and erbium:yttrium aluminum garnet lasers improve skin surface texture and problems of skin topography (wrinkles, scars, sun damage, benign skin appendages, and rhinophyma). Such lasers can be associated with significant morbidity.
- Lasers and light sources with minimal morbidity and some degree of efficacy have often replaced techniques requiring significant healing, down time, and risk.
- Many light-based technologies can now deliver multiple wavelengths and/or have special hand pieces allowing them to target pigmented and vascular targets.

History of Lasers

The history of lasers had its beginnings in the 19th and 20th centuries. Descriptions of wave theory by Maxwell in 1864 set the scene for a very productive period of nuclear physics. In 1905, Max Planck suggested that electromagnetic radiation can exist in small packets (quanta). The energy was related to the wavelength by the now very famous equation of $E=h\nu$ where E is the energy, ν is the frequency of the electromagnetic wave and h is Planck's constant. These quanta of energy have now become known as photons.

Soon Neils Bohr noted that atoms, when irradiated with white light, would absorb only certain spectral components of that light that were unique for that atom. Based on these observations he proposed the theory that electrons surrounded a nucleus of an atom in defined orbits and that these electrons could make transitions between these orbits, with characteristic energy emissions when they did so. These characteristic energy emissions were the photons suggested by Planck. Spontaneous transitions between these orbital electrons lead to spontaneous emissions of photons with characteristic wavelengths. Adding energy such as light to the atoms may lead to absorption of this energy by electrons in a lower level orbit, raising its energy to a higher level (Fig. 1.1), and then by relaxation back down to the lower level emitting similar characteristic photons as occurring spontaneously.

In 1917 Albert Einstein theorized that in addition to the emissions of photons by spontaneous and absorbed energies, a further mechanism of photon production was likely and this was termed "stimulated emission": "A splendid light has dawned on me about the absorption and emission of radiation..." [1].

Stimulated emission begins with an atom with an electron in an excited state occupying

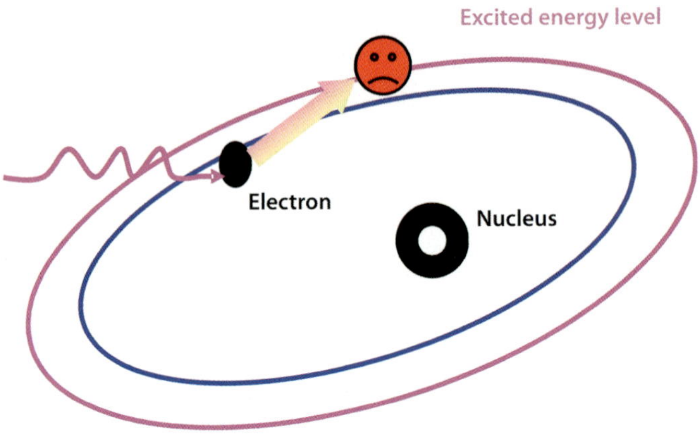

Fig. 1.1. Incoming photons excite the electrons raising them to their next energy level. When the majority of atoms in the lasing or gain medium become "excited," population inversion is said to occur

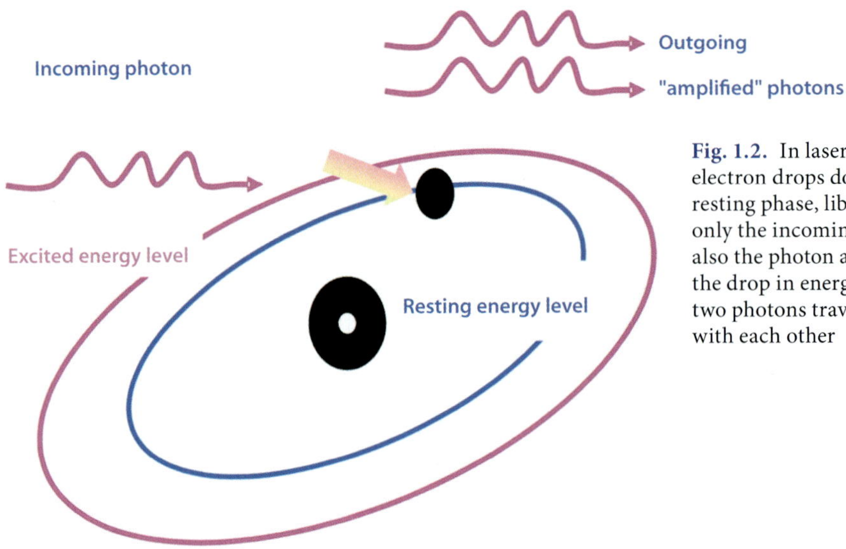

Fig. 1.2. In lasers, an excited electron drops down to its resting phase, liberating not only the incoming photon, but also the photon associated with the drop in energy level. These two photons travel off in phase with each other

a high orbit. If this electron was to spontaneously decay to a lower-energy orbit it would elaborate a photon of characteristic energy as described above. If this electron (whilst still excited) is targeted by a photon matching the photon that would be elaborated spontaneously it will result in the ejection of two photons, the incoming one, and a forcible expulsion of the photon from the excited electron with a return of this electron to its resting state (Fig. 1.2).

Over the ensuing decades other investigators not only corroborated this theory of stimulated emission, but also showed that the incoming photon and the expelled photon were identical in phase, direction, wavelength, and frequency. Initially masers (microwave amplification for the stimulated emission of radiation), which were designed by Gordon in 1955, made use of this theory, followed by the first laser in 1960 when Maiman demonstrated the production of stimulated emission via a ruby crystal.

What followed in the 1960s was an explosion in the literature of descriptions of many of the lasers that we currently employ today.

In 1961, Javan described the helium neon laser (He-Ne) and, within the next few years, Q-switched lasers and the neodymium (Nd): yttrium aluminum garnet (YAG), argon, carbon dioxide (CO_2), and pulsed-dye lasers were described.

Currently Available Technologies

Making the Laser Light

Lasers are simplistically thought of as comprising of three essential components – an outside energy source that can transfer energy to the system, the lasing or gain medium, and the resonating tube to keep the process active (Fig. 1.3).

The outside energy source may be an electrical current as in the miniature diode lasers, radiofrequency as in some CO_2 lasers, or a chemical reaction as in the case of the hydrogen fluoride laser. Lasers may also be used to pump or provide energy to another laser, such as the argon-ion laser pumped-dye laser used for vascular lesions. The remaining common method of energizing a laser system is by the use of a flashlamp like that of a camera flash. This type of stimulation is used commonly in lasers such as ruby, Nd:YAG, and erbium:YAG lasers.

The lasing medium contains the substance that most often lends its name to the ensuing laser beam and denotes its intrinsic wavelength and characteristics. The laser medium may be gaseous, liquid, or solid. Examples of gases include CO_2, argon, krypton, copper vapor, and gold vapor. Liquid lasing mediums use fluorescent liquid dyes and solvents to give rise to the various pulsed-dye lasers. Solid-state lasers are designed around crystals to which impurities are added, such as Nd being added as an impurity to the YAG crystal to give the characteristic Nd:YAG laser. Other impurities may be added to this useful crystal, such as potassium tritanyl phosphate (KTP) and erbium, to render resultant wavelengths with very different interactions in skin.

Within the lasing medium, most atoms are in their resting state with their electrons occupying a low-energy orbit close to the nucleus. When energy is added to this system the atoms become excited as their electrons are induced to move to a higher orbit or energy level. As the electrons relax back to their more desired resting orbital level, the shift from the higher energy orbit to the lower one is accompanied by the "spontaneous" emission of a photon. This photon is a discrete bundle of energy and is characteristic of the atom in the lasing medium, or more specifically the energy difference between the electron's excited and resting orbital levels. This photon has a characteristic wavelength and it is this wavelength that largely characterizes the laser's interaction with tissue.

When the outside energy has been in action for some time, most of the atoms will become excited, causing what is known as "population inversion." When this state is achieved

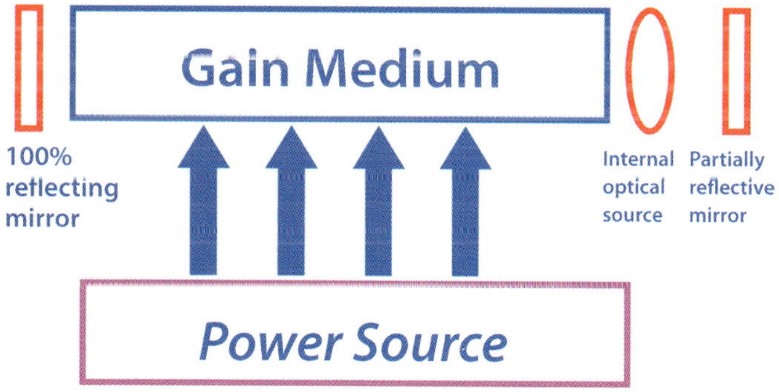

Fig. 1.3. The basic elements of all lasers include the lasing or gain medium, power source, and resonating tube, which often contains a mirror system to reflect and amplify the laser energy produced in the lasing medium. The output laser beam emerges through the partially reflective mirror and sometimes an internal optical element

then another phenomenon, stimulated emission, occurs. Stimulated emission is the central occurrence that allows lasers to be what they are. In fact lasers are an acronym that stands for "light amplification by the stimulated emission of radiation."

As discussed earlier in this chapter, stimulated emission is produced when a photon that is the same characteristic wavelength and energy as the difference between the energy levels of the material in the lasing medium approaches an already excited atom with its electron in its higher orbital plane (Fig. 1.2). When this photon interacts with the excited atom, not only does it come away unchanged from the collision, but it also takes with it another photon of exactly the same characteristics as the excited atom as this atom relaxes back to its resting state. The peculiarity is that the incident photon and the resultant photon not only have the same wavelength and energy characteristics, but also are perfectly in phase with each other, the two photons going off in the same direction like two synchronized swimming tadpoles. Thus it appears that one incident photon has produced two exiting photons that are capable of similar exchanges with other pre-excited atoms in the lasing medium. Thus it takes little time for the lasing medium to build up a head of steam with lots of photons of the same characteristics being released.

The resonating tube housing this process often has mirrors at either end, the function of which it is to amplify and direct this rising tide of laser light. By bouncing these back and forth only the laser light traveling in the one desired direction is utilized, the rest being absorbed by the sidewalls of the chamber. At one end the mirror is totally reflective, at the other it is 99% reflective. The output beam is eventually allowed out of the partially reflective end and becomes the utilizable laser beam.

The Characteristics of the Laser Beam

Laser light is different to ambient light in that it is coherent, collimated, monochromatic, and able to be pulsed (Table 1.1).

Spatial and Temporal Coherence

The light waves in laser light are "in step," traveling in exactly the same direction with very little beam divergence.

Collimation

This refers to a laser beam's ability to retain its intensity over a long distance with low diffusion of light compared to a torch or other light source. These two factors allow a laser's beam to be tightly focused to a point of maximum energy as necessary. This point may be used to cut tissue or just be a maximum point of energy for high-energy interaction with a target in the tissue termed a chromophore.

Monochromicity

The third important characteristic of lasers is that the light is of the same single wavelength, that is, it is monochromatic. This allows the laser to interact with certain structures in the

Table 1.1. Characteristics of Lasers and IPLs.

Characteristic	Lasers	IPL
Spatial and temporal coherence	Yes	No
Collimation	Possible	Not possible
Monochromicity	Yes	No
Ability to be pulsed	Yes	Yes

skin that are able to absorb that wavelength better than its neighboring structures.

Pulsing

The fourth characteristic of laser beams is their ability to be pulsed. Although occasionally lasers are used in continuous mode, most are used in a pulsed fashion. This allows the pulse to impact the target in tissue just long enough to damage it without damaging the surrounding structures to any degree. The duration of the pulse required is proportional to the size of the target.

Intense Pulsed Light

Intense pulsed light makes use of an incoherent high-output flashlamp to produce a multiwavelength output. This uses the additive effects of bands of wavelengths rather than a single wavelength to exert a tissue effect. Thus, it does not rely on monochromicity, collimation, or spatial and temporal coherence, and cannot be focused, but simply adds the effect of a little light in each of many wavelengths to exert a powerful absorption by the target chromophore. This technology relies on the fact that chromophores absorb energy over a broad spectrum of light wavelengths and do not have to be targeted by just the most highly absorbed peak of that absorptive band.

Types of Laser–Tissue Interaction

Once the laser has generated the laser beam it must then be pointed at someone or something and be absorbed by that body. Its passage in skin, for example, is a series of scattering and absorption as obstacles are encountered. The absorbing targets or chromophores are few in number (Table 1.2).

The uses of lasers in dermatology span the visible light lasers from about 300 nm through to the mid-infrared (Fig. 1.4). These wavelengths are able to locate specific chromophores or targets in the skin. Endogenous targets in the skin include hemoglobin (oxygenated and deoxygenated), melanin, and water. Sometimes exogenous chemicals may find their way into the skin such as implanted tattoos or other foreign materials allowing us another target. Other times we may add or augment an existing target to the skin by applying, implanting, or ingesting a sensitizing material to an area and then shining light or laser, as is done with photodynamic therapy (PDT).

The finding of these targets has allowed the selective targeting and destruction of

Table 1.2. Chromophores for cutaneous laser therapy. *YAG* Yttrium-aluminum-garnet, *KTP* potassium tritanyl phosphate, *PDT* photodynamic therapy

Intrinsic	Example	Extrinsic	Example
Water	Infrared lasers – CO2, erbium, 1320 nm, 1450 nm, 1540 nm lasers (including fractionated photothermolysis)	Tattoo pigment	Q-switched YAG, ruby, alexandrite
Melanin	Argon, KTP	Porphyrins	PDT (Blue, yellow, green, red light or laser sources)
Oxy and deoxy-hemoglobin	KTP, flashlamp pumped-dye laser, near-infrared lasers (755, 810, 940, 980, 1064 nm)		

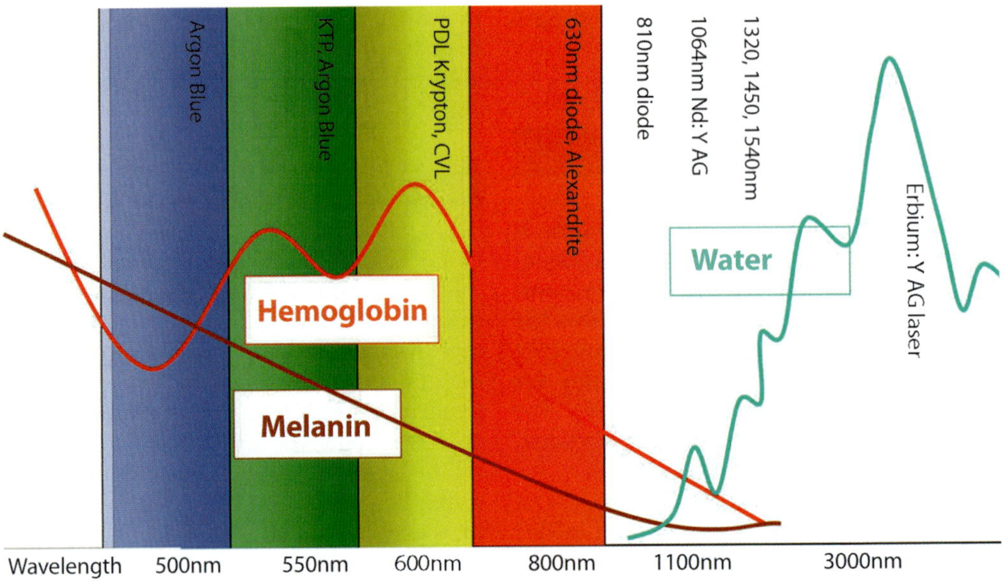

Fig. 1.4. Absorption curve of major skin pigments and the lasers and lights that take advantage of this absorption. *KTP* Potassium tritanyl phosphate, *PDL* pulsed-dye laser, *CVL* copper vapor laser, *Nd* Neodymium-doped, *YAG* yttrium-aluminum-garnet

Table 1.3. Types of laser or light tissue interaction. *LEDs* Light-emitting diodes

Interaction	Examples
Photomechanical	Q-switched lasers for tattoos and dermal and epidermal pigment
Photothermolysis	Visible light and near infrared lasers
Photoablation	Resurfacing with CO_2 and erbium lasers
Photochemical	PDT, excimer laser
Photomodulation	LEDs

cellular and subcellular structures. However, appropriate wavelength selection is not enough to ensure selective damaging of that target. Damage by mechanisms such as heating must be localized to the target. Supplying the correct wavelength energy continuously allows that target to become excessively hot and radiate that energy to the surrounding tissues. This will in turn produce secondary damage to nearby structures, thereby greatly increasing complication rates. These secondary problems are minimized by shortening of the heating phase to confine the heat to the immediate vicinity of this intended target. Each target is a different size and needs heating for a different time period. Small structures such as single melanocytes and tattoo granules are best destroyed by short-duration, high-energy pulses, whilst larger structures such as blood vessels and hair follicles require longer, slower, less peak-power pulsing.

The interaction of the laser beam with tissue may be any of five varieties (Table 1.3). Most injury to tissues from lasers and lights requires heating and selective destruction of the target. The speed of heating the target may lead to a variety of effects. First there may be mechanical injury to tissues from rapid heating by very high-energy, short-duration laser pulses. This is important with small targets such as pigment in tattoos and melanocytes in pigmented lesions. This produces very-high-pressure waves and rapid thermal expansion, literally shattering the target apart, and has been termed a photoacoustic effect.

The most common mechanism that is used by lasers is selective-photothermolysis-induced thermal injury, denaturing and coagulating target cells. The concept of selective photothermolysis stresses selective absorption by colored targets such as blood vessels, pigmented cells of appropriately pulsed laser light [2]. This tenet has revolutionized the safety and efficacy of laser therapy, ensuring that thermal injury is specifically confined to the intended target, leaving the rest of the skin relatively unaffected.

Another mechanism of laser interaction also involves the heating of tissues but in a slightly different way. When a laser has water as its prime target, the beam becomes relatively nonselective, as all skin contains this chromophore. However, the laser may be made capable of limiting the damage to the intended target. The laser is deigned to produce a high-energy, short-duration pulse that is capable of superheating the water in the cells, vaporizing this water, and producing a smoke or plume containing steam and cellular contents. If the energy, pulse duration and choice of laser are appropriate, relatively little thermal injury is left in the tissue. In this way, selectivity of ablation occurs and unintended targets are spared. Ablation as a form of laser–tissue interaction is seen with CO_2 and erbium laser resurfacing.

The fourth mechanism of interaction is a photochemical interaction. Photochemistry exists all around us with photosynthesis in plants, ultraviolet photochemotherapy for the treatment of psoriasis and eczema, some photosensitive skin disorders, vitamin D production, and the act of vision being examples. The excimer laser (308 nm) used in the treatment of hypopigmented disorders and psoriasis [3,4], cutaneous T cell lymphoma [5], atopic dermatitis [6], and many other dermatologic disease states is an example of a photochemical reaction inducing apoptosis of target cells including T lymphocytes [7]. PDT involves the use of a long-wavelength, deeply penetrating laser or light to activate porphyrin-labeled tissues such as skin cancers and precancerous lesions, or shorter wavelengths to target more superficial diseases [8]. Porphyrins, which may be injected or applied selectively, target certain rapidly dividing tissues such as tumors, and after being activated by red laser light they produce singlet oxygen and free radicals, which are terminally damaging to the cells that house these chemicals.

Photomodulation is a different process again, attempting to make use of nonthermal light–tissue interactions usually by banks of narrow-band light-emitting diodes (LEDs). This is presumed to work at the cellular and subcellular level to change the regulation of protein synthesis. LEDs emit low-intensity light ranging from ultraviolet to visible to infrared. LED devices may be arranged in quite large panels so that large surface areas can be treated. LEDs in the 590-nm range have produced clinical improvement [9–11].

Currently Used Facial Rejuvenation Systems

There are systems designed for facial rejuvenation that take advantage of all the above discussion of laser tissue interaction. Ablative systems that remove epidermal and dermal targets will be discussed first, followed by nonablative technologies. Nonablative technologies may work through the use of colored chromophores with or without the protection of the epidermis, or via the use of selective dermal heating, usually using water as a chromophore with epidermal protection. PDT utilizing porphyrins as its chromophore and photomodulation will be dealt by other authors in this text and will only be explored in connection with augmenting lights and lasers used in facial rejuvenation techniques.

Ablative Infrared Resurfacing Laser Systems

Descriptions of Available Infrared Systems

In the early 1990s these lasers largely replaced dermabrasion and stronger chemical peeling as the treatment of choice for general facial resurfacing, especially for photodamage, wrinkles, and atrophic scarring.

CO_2 Lasers

CO_2 lasers still have a role in facial rejuvenation, but it is diminishing with (or maybe being enhanced by) the rise of nonablative and safer ablative technologies. However, it is probably reasonable to suggest that few existing technologies rival the efficacy of CO_2 lasers in many of its applications. The advent of the high-energy short-pulse CO_2 laser and very clever scanning technologies have provided the first safe reproducible laser therapies for facial rejuvenation. Collected patient data show a relatively successful technique with a satisfactory complication profile.

The CO_2 laser operates in the far-infrared wavelength (10,600 nm) and is absorbed by water. The laser will thus ablate all tissue in its path to an even depth. Energy at this wavelength is rapidly absorbed and dissipated in a very short distance of tissue [12].

Modern CO_2 Lasers

Many advances have been made in the use of CO_2 lasers for treating the surface of the skin (skin resurfacing). Improved technology has decreased the dependence on the skill of the operator, thus improving reproducibility of results. CO_2 lasers are able to ablate a relatively thin layer (20–50 μm) due to the rapid extinction of the beam in tissue. For successful char-free laser therapy system must deliver enough energy to vaporize the tissue (5 J/cm^2) in a time shorter than the thermal relaxation time of the skin (1 ms) [13]. Two approaches have satisfactorily provided the required scenario of epidermal vaporization with minimal thermal damage to the papillary dermis: high-energy, short-pulsed defocused CO_2 lasers and short-dwell-time scanning focused CO_2 lasers.

■ **High-Energy, Short-Pulsed, Defocused CO_2 Lasers.** The first approach involves very high energy, short-pulsed, defocused CO_2 lasers [14,15]. The Ultrapulse laser (Lumenis lasers, Yokneam, Israel) utilizes a laser tube that is pumped electronically to produce high-powered short (well under 1 ms) pulses. This pulse vaporizes tissue rapidly, removing it as steam (plume) so that less heat is left in the tissue to allow transmission of heat to nontarget tissues.

Scanning devices are now commonplace for CO_2 lasers, thus further standardizing the procedure. It places pulses in patterns of different size, shape, and area of overlap, enabling uniform application of laser energy to the skin and precise reproducibility between operators. The device also collimates the beam (keeping the beam defocused and the waves parallel to each other), enabling the operator to work at a distance from the skin.

■ **Short Dwell-time, Scanning, Focused CO_2 Lasers.** In a different approach, the Silk-touch and Feather-touch lasers (Lumenis lasers, Yokneam, Israel) utilize an optomechanical flash scanner that scans the laser beam in a spiral pattern for short exposure times (dwelling time < 1 ms). This produces char-free ablation by sharply focusing the beam, thus allowing high energies to be applied from a comparatively low-energy laser system. A scanner rapidly moves a continuous focused beam in a spiral, keeping the dwell time at any particular point on the spiral below 1 ms [16,17].

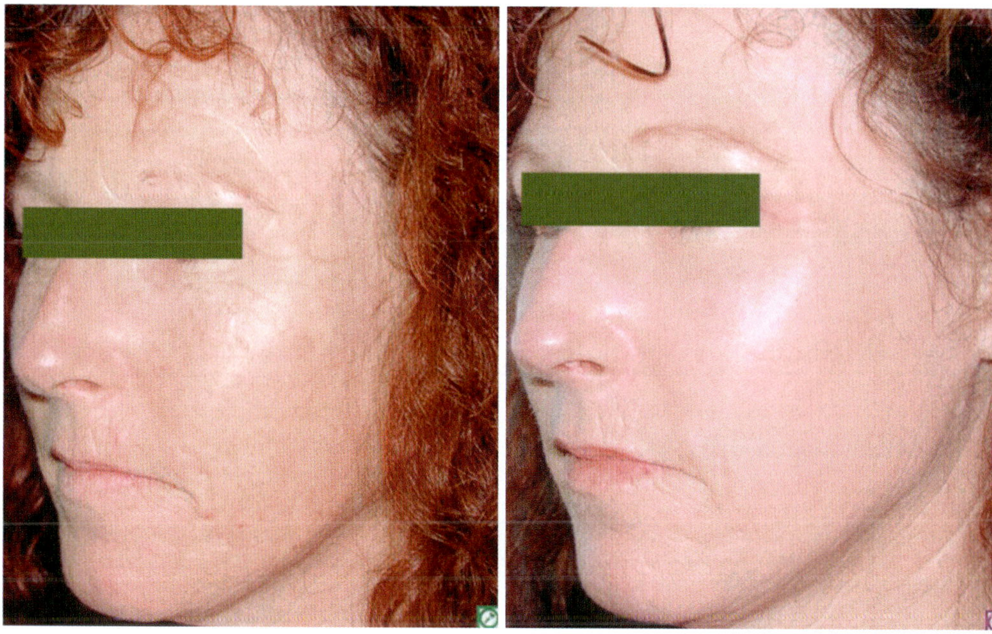

Fig. 1.5. Before (*left*) and 3 months after (*right*) CO_2 laser resurfacing

Both these types of CO_2 lasers achieve superficial ablation by delivering their energy within the ideal short heating time of skin (less than 1 ms). It is important to deliver enough energy to the tissue in this short time period to rapidly vaporize this tissue rather than delivering it slowly and boiling it. A characteristic brown char was associated with earlier CO_2 lasers. This char correlates with a slow boiling of tissue and indicates heat transmission outside the intended target. The char is virtually absent with these highly ablative lasers. This results in faster healing with fewer complications.

The requirement for char-free ablation is to keep the dwell time on tissue down to below 1 ms. This may be achieved by either of these methods (by dwelling on it for a short period or by means of a rapid pulse the result will permit selective tissue ablation). CO_2 lasers may be used as an isolated procedure or in combination with blepharoplasties, fat transfer, and in a limited way with rhytidectomy (Figs. 1.5–1.7).

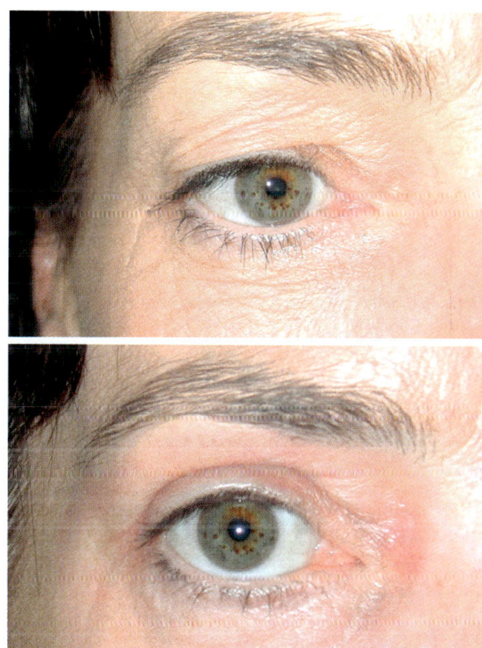

Fig. 1.6. Before (*top*) and 3 months after (*bottom*) CO_2-laser-assisted upper-lid blepharoplasty in combination with periorbital CO_2 laser resurfacing

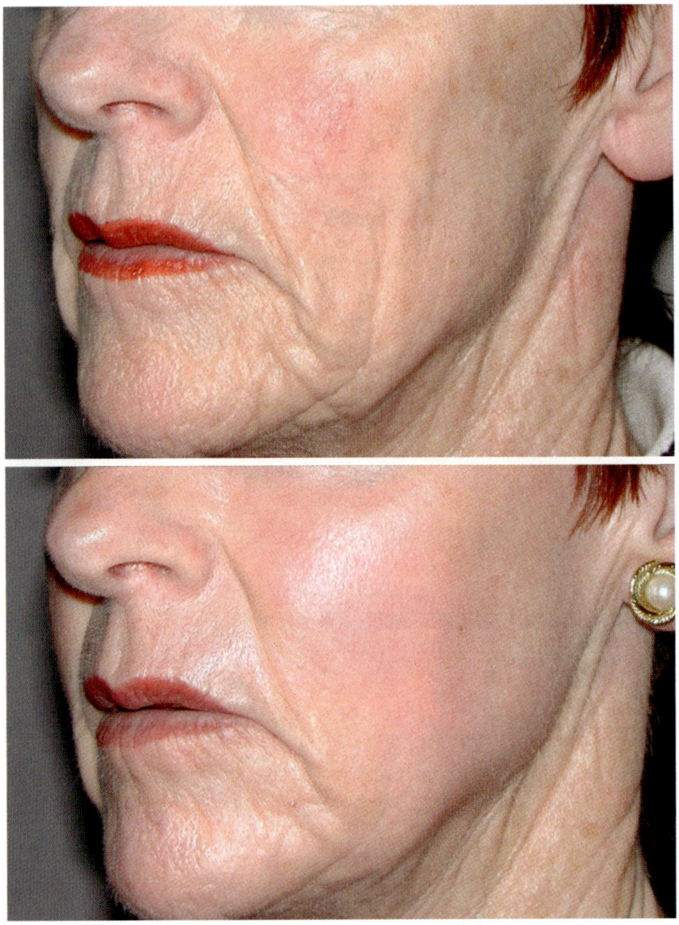

Fig. 1.7. Before (*top*) and 3 months after (*bottom*) CO_2 laser resurfacing and fat transfer

Erbium: YAG Laser

Despite the quite impressive advances represented by the CO_2 laser, inherent problems of this laser system were apparent. These include their somewhat delayed healing due to a protracted inflammatory or "lag" phase. This phase describes the removal of heat damage in the base of the wound before the phase of reepithelialization. Although much improved over previous laser systems, the new CO_2 lasers still left some necrotic thermally damaged tissues at the base of the wound that must be removed before epidermal regrowth can ensue. There were also reports of delayed appearance of alabaster (white) skin some months to years after CO_2 laser resurfacing alone [18,19].

Recently, an option has become available utilizing ablative resurfacing and autologous epidermal cell suspensions. An interesting commercial kit has been developed that allows the operator to efficiently harvest a small donor site of skin and change this into a cell suspension with trypsin digestion of the donor skin. This suspension may be sprayed or drizzled on the resurfaced recipient site of hypopigmented skin or normal skin in a high-risk patient or in a high-risk area.

This cell suspension will contain a mixture of cells including keratinocytes, melanocytes,

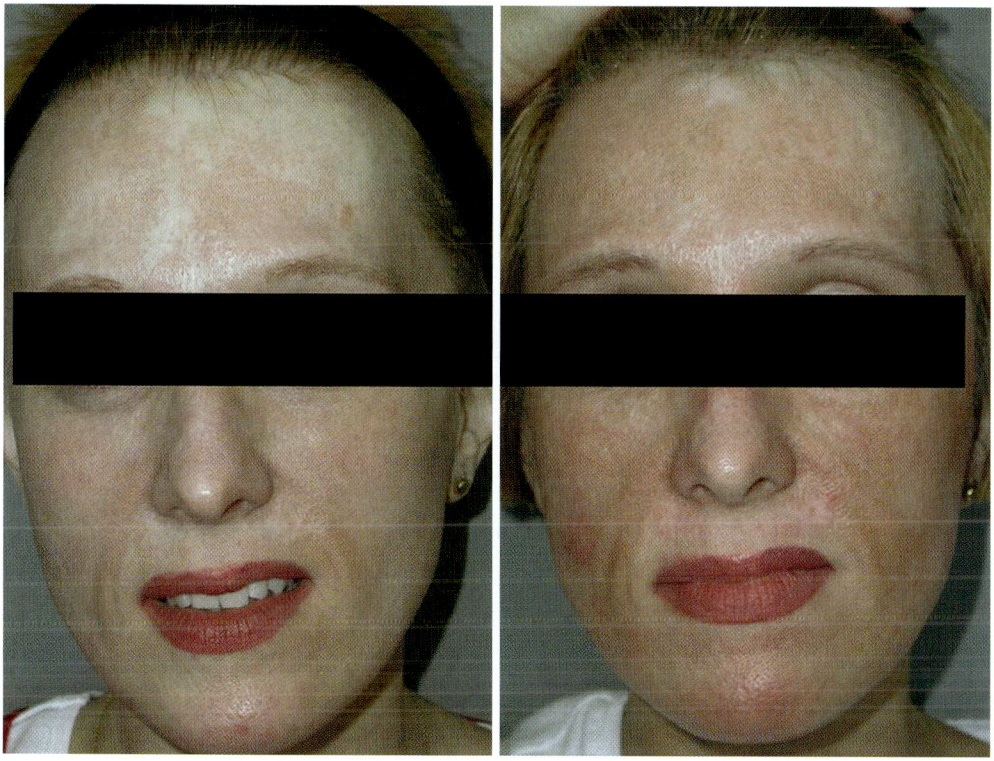

Fig. 1.8. Before (*left*) and 5 months after (*right*) erbium laser resurfacing and application of autologous epidermal cell suspension (ReCell) for iatrogenic hypopigmentation. Most of the hypopigmentation is reversed

and fibroblasts amongst others. Theoretical implications may be an improvement in the speed of wound healing, as well as an improvement in the pigmentation of the skin. Previous work has shown that both autologous cultured and noncultured cell preparations are able to repigment vitiliginous areas [20,21]. Figure 1.8 shows a patient who had undergone numerous resurfacing procedures for iatrogenic scarring but had never achieved repigmentation of hypopigmented, scarred areas. Almost complete repigmentation is shown after a single session of this transplant technology.

The search for a laser able to minimize this transmitted energy began with still shorter-pulsed CO_2 lasers, but eventually the emphasis turned to a laser with still less thermal tissue residue, the erbium:YAG laser [22].

The erbium laser wavelength is ten times more avidly taken up by water than is the CO_2 wavelength, leading to more complete ablation of tissue and producing only a very fine layer of thermal damage [23,24]. Most investigators suggest that 4–5 µm of tissue is removed per joule of fluence utilized. With an epidermis of 60–100 µm in thickness, somewhere between 15 and 25 J of energy is required for complete epidermal ablation. There is almost a perfectly linear relationship between the energy delivered and the depth of ablation, whether one is in the epidermis or dermis. There is little residual heat damage with this machine, essentially becoming in effect like an ultimately controllable dermabrasion. This makes the erbium laser useful for resurfacing with relatively rapid and predictable healing.

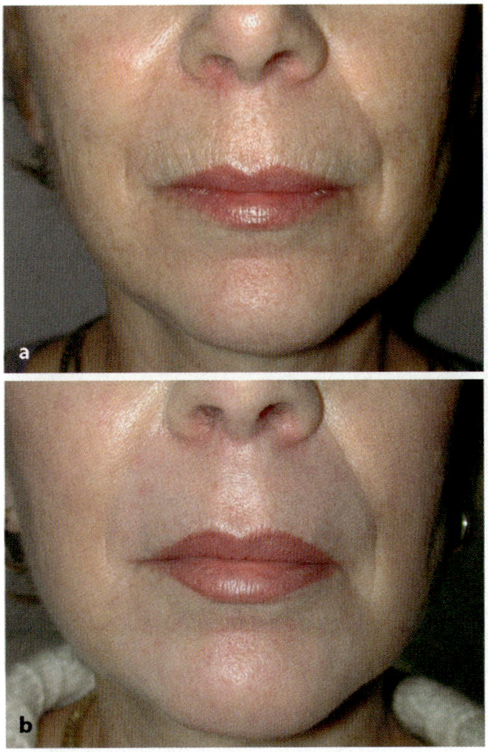

Fig. 1.9. **a** Before and **b** 3 months after erbium laser resurfacing to the upper lip for rhytides

It is able to be used either alone, or with other procedures (Figs. 1.9 and 1.10) and in combination with CO_2 laser resurfacing.

The erbium laser can also be used to treat actinic cheilitis, postoperative scars, and elevated grafts (Figs. 1.11 and 1.12). It also can be effective in the treatment of a variety of epidermal and dermal conditions such as seborrheic keratoses, xanthelasma, and syringomas (Figs. 1.13 and 1.14).

Long-pulse erbium lasers have also been used as a mechanism for providing enhanced hemostasis, allowing a short-pulsed erbium laser to penetrate deeper. This can be useful where the depth of penetration is important, such as the more severe photodamage patient or in conditions such as rhinophyma.

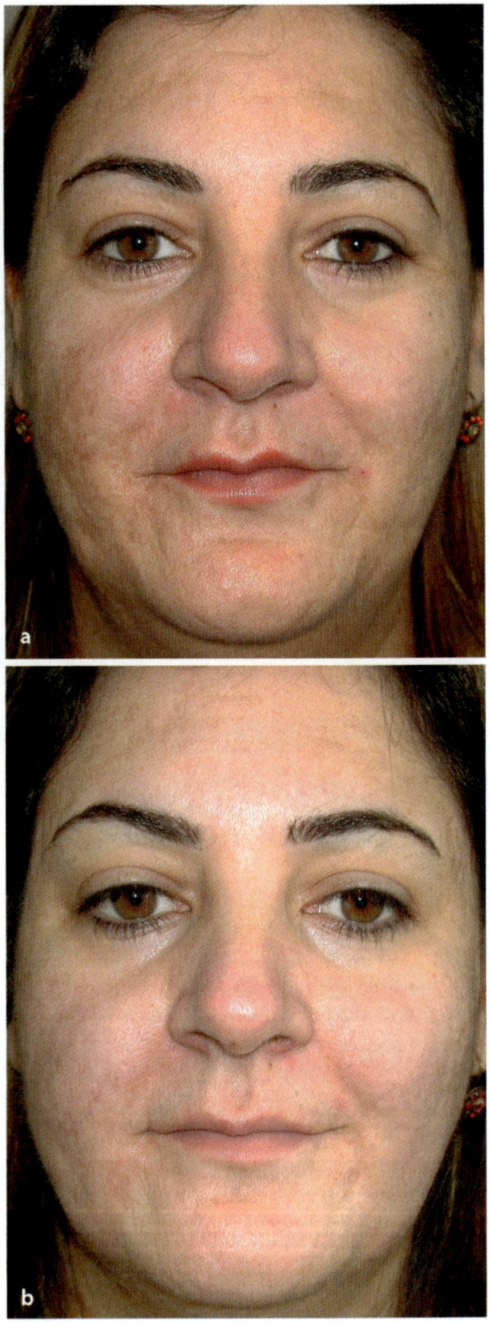

Fig. 1.10. **a** Before and **b** 3 months after full facial erbium laser resurfacing and fat transfer

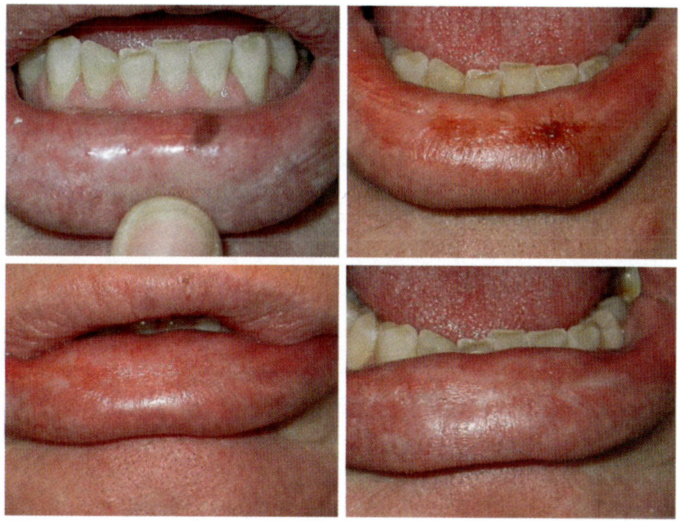

Fig. 1.11. Actinic cheilitis. Patient before (*upper left*), 2 weeks (*upper right*), 6 weeks (*lower left*), and 3 months (*lower right*) after erbium laser resurfacing

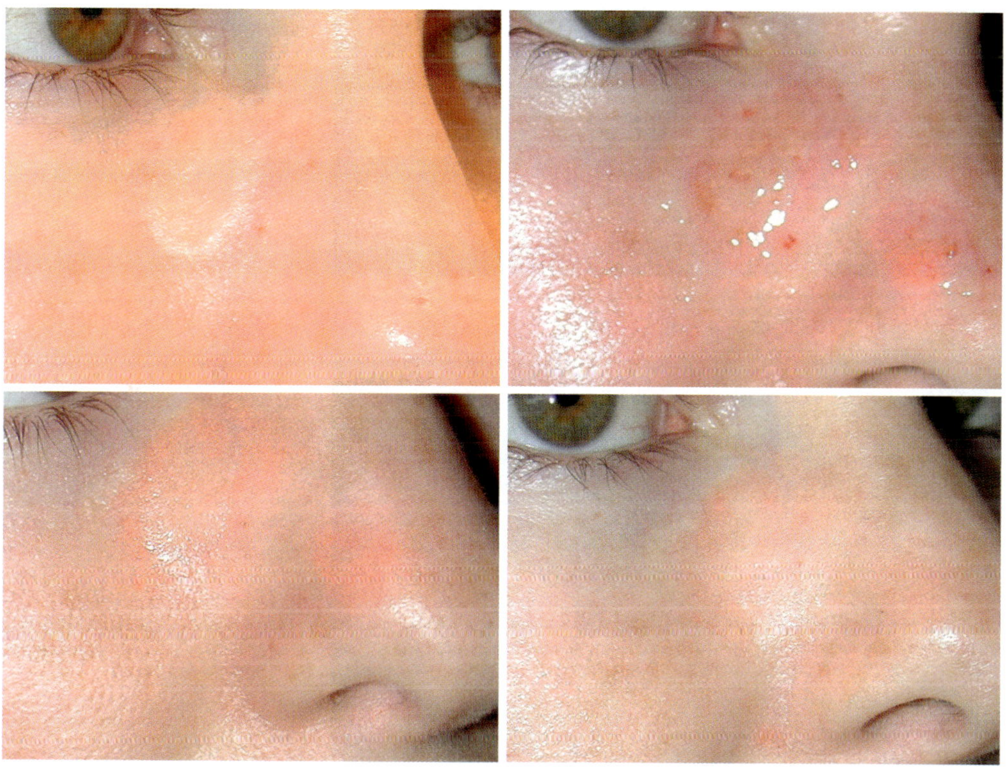

Fig. 1.12. Graft in right nasofacial crease Patient before (*upper left*), and 1 week (*upper right*), 6 weeks (*lower left*), and 3 months (*lower right*) after erbium laser resurfacing

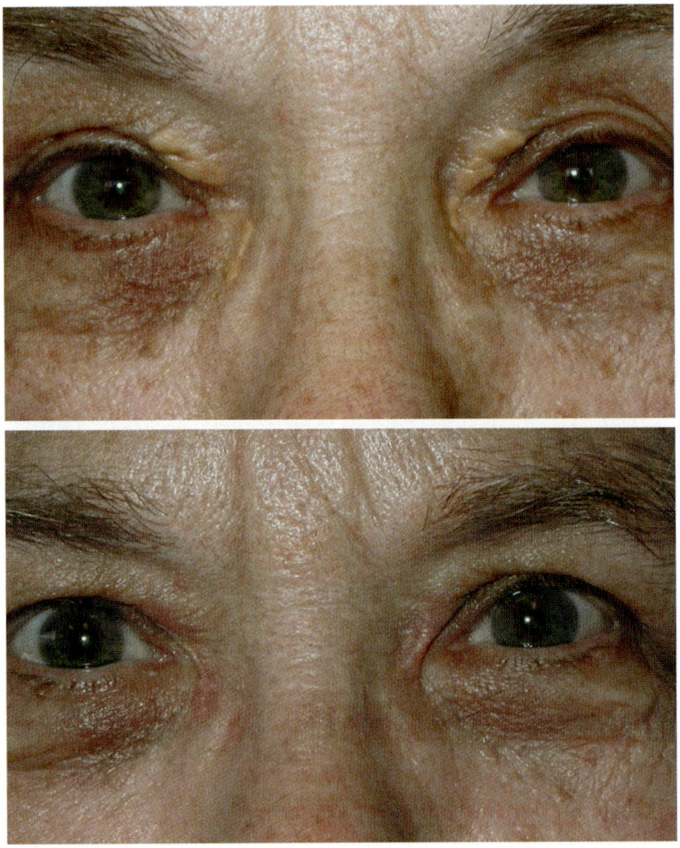

Fig. 1.13. Patient with xanthelasma before (*top*) and 3 months after (*bottom*) erbium laser

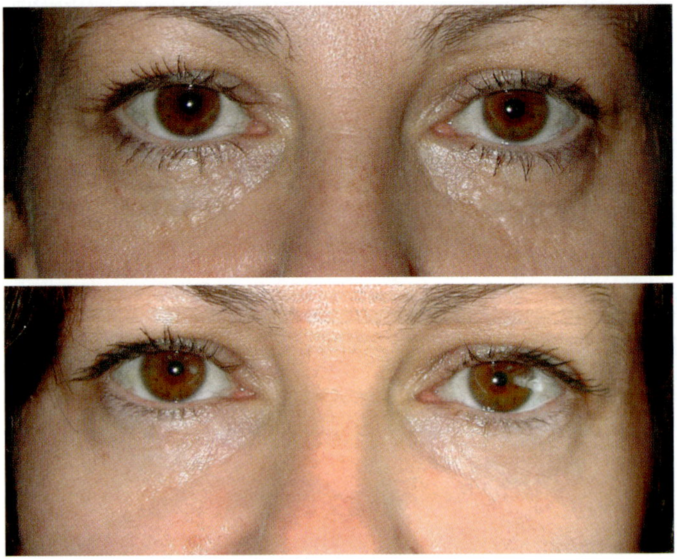

Fig. 1.14. Patient with syringomas before (*top*) and 3 months after (*bottom*) erbium laser treatment

Combined CO_2 and Erbium Laser Resurfacing

Combined CO_2 and erbium laser resurfacing may be delivered either sequentially or at the same time through a machine that can combine the erbium pulse and CO_2 pulse. This seems to produce a more impressive result than erbium laser in many instances of significant photodamage or atrophic acne scarring and with faster healing than with a CO_2 laser alone (Figs. 1.15–1.17) [25–29]. This combination seems to adopt more the healing profile of the erbium laser with an apparent reduced complication risk of long-term pigment change.

Plasma Skin Resurfacing

A new technology utilizes a nonlaser device to generate plasma, a cloud of electrons from nitrogen atoms, and a spark of radiofrequency. This energy is transferred into the skin. Initially the epidermis is left intact, shedding later as healing is completed. The resultant effect may be similar to the rejuvenation effect induced by an erbium laser but

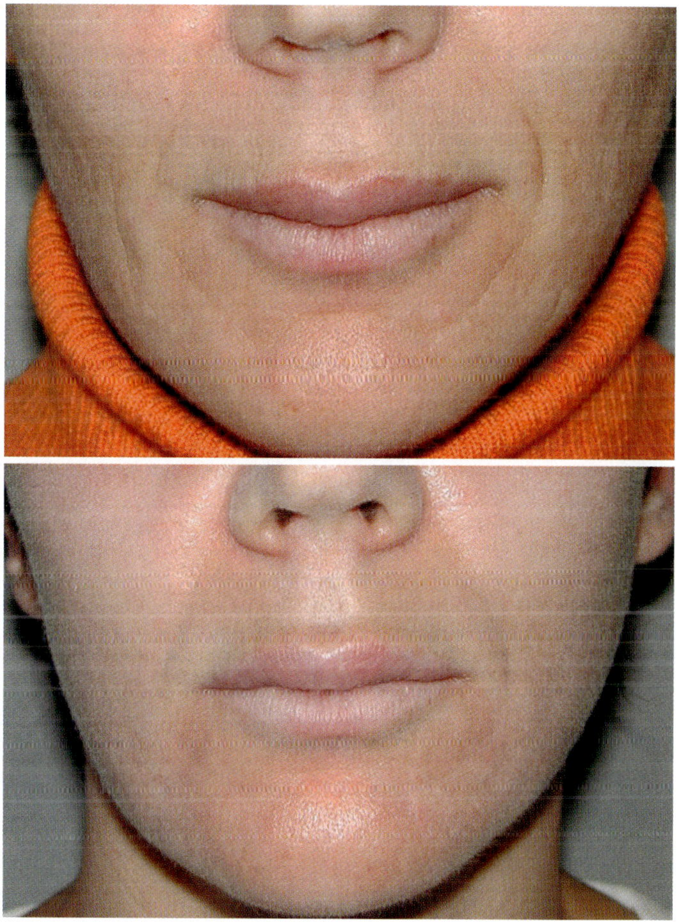

Fig. 1.15. Before (*top*) and 3 months after (*bottom*) combined erbium and CO_2 laser treatments

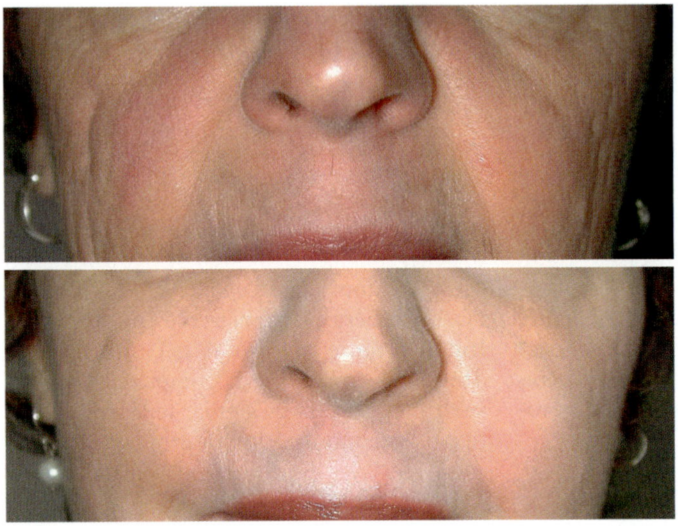

Fig. 1.16. Before (*top*) and 3 months after (*bottom*) treatment with both erbium and CO_2 lasers for a combination of acne scarring and photoaging

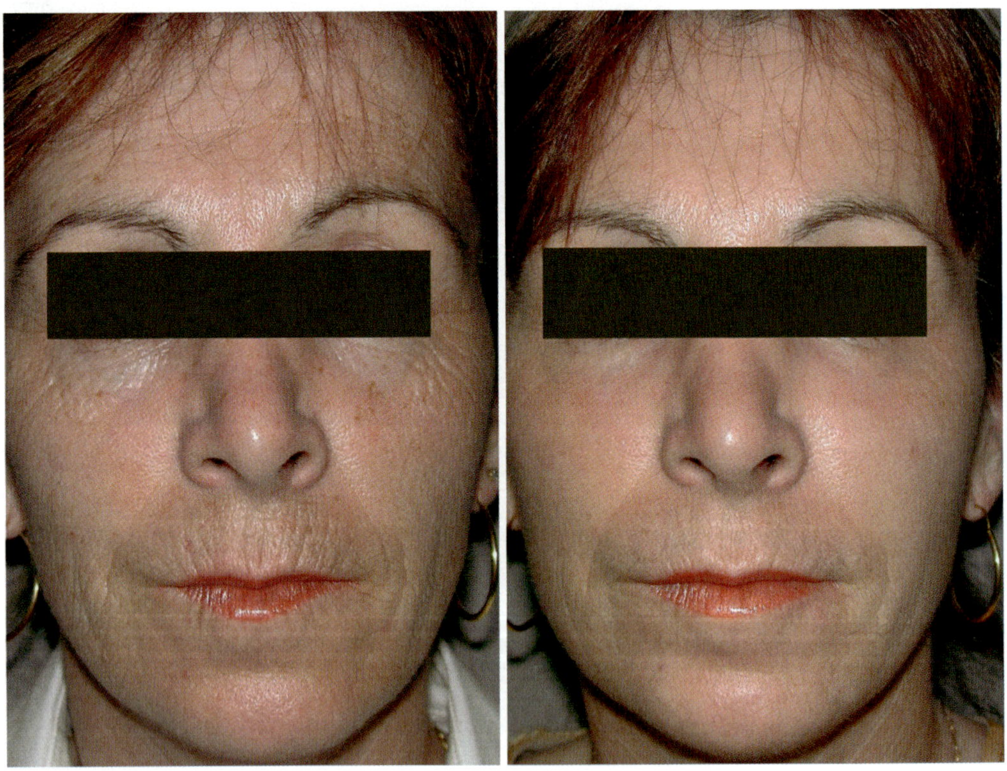

Fig. 1.17. Before (*left*) and 3 months after (*right*) treatment with combined erbium and CO_2 lasers for severe photoaging changes

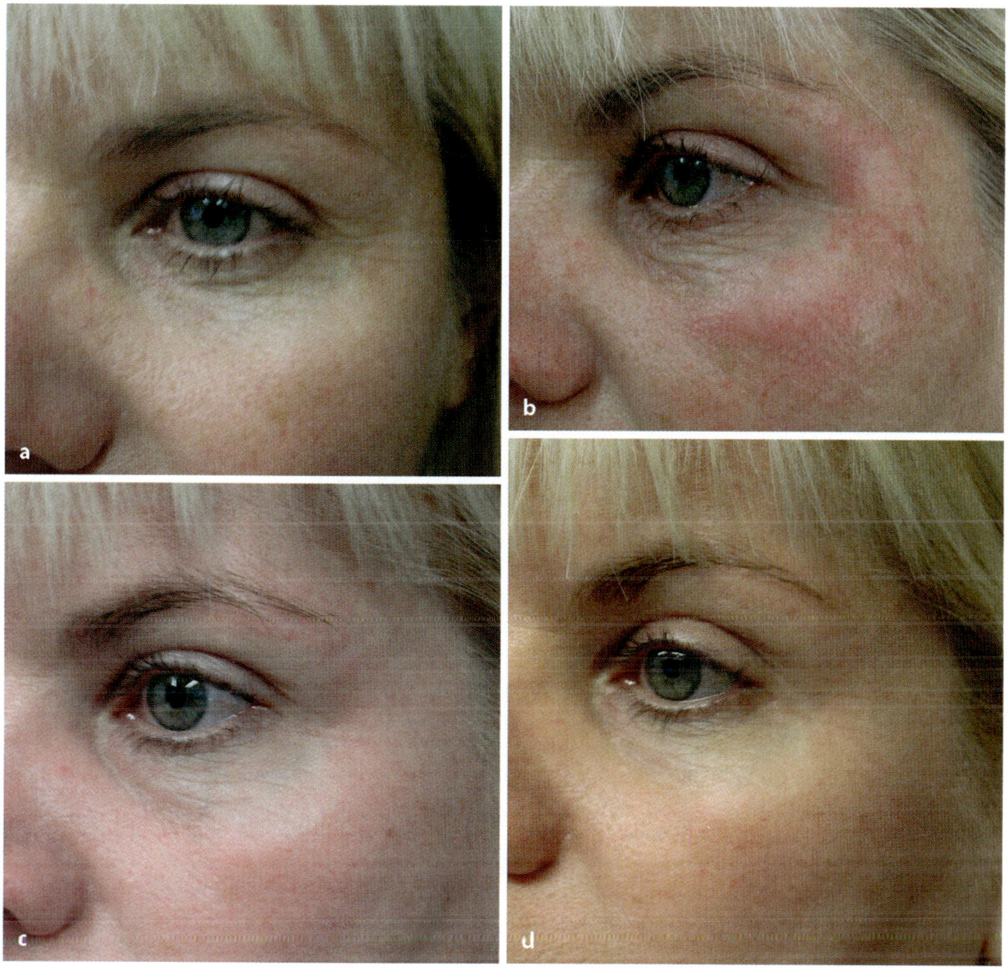

Fig. 1.18 a–d. Patient treated with Portrait plasma skin resurfacing at **a** baseline, **b** 1 week, **c** 6 weeks, and **d** 3 months after the procedure

with perhaps less posttreatment morbidity (Fig. 1.18).

Nonablative Technologies

These technologies may be divided in various ways; a reasonable method of dividing these myriad systems is by the target affected by the lasers (Table 1.4).

Colored chromophores are impacted upon predominantly by visible light lasers and light sources. Such systems deliver a variety of wavelengths such as the frequency doubled Nd:YAG, KTP green light 532 nm, and pulsed-dye yellow light 585–595 nm lasers, broadband flashlamps (intense pulsed light, noncoherent filtered flashlamp light source), or narrowband LED systems

A distinctly different category of nonablative technologies includes near-infrared-wavelength-emitting lasers and other technologies targeting dermal water. All of these systems provide a general heat injury leading to neocollagenesis.

Table 1.4. Nonablative lasers or light sources used for photorejuvenation. *Nd* Neodymium-doped, *RF* radiofrequency

Colored chromophore-seeking lasers and light sources (visible and near-infrared wavelengths)	Water-seeking lasers and other technologies (near- and mid-infrared wavelengths)
Frequency doubled Nd: YAG, KTP (green 532 nm)	Q-switched and millisecond domain Nd:YAG
Pulsed dye (yellow 585–595 nm)	1320 nm Nd:YAG laser
IPL broadband filtered light of various wavelengths.	1450 nm diode laser
LED	1540 nm erbium glass laser
	1550 nm fractional photothermolysis
	RF and combined RF light sources and lasers (RF and IPL, RF and 810 nm laser)

Nonablative Technologies Using Colored Chromophores

There are lasers and light sources that were originally designed for the treatment of vascular and pigmented abnormalities in the skin that have been adapted successfully for the more general "photorejuvenation" of the patient. Many improvements have been made in the delivery of light energy in areas as diverse as energy delivery, spot size, beam profile, pulsing, and protection of the epidermis, and the advent of noncoherent lamps. Higher-powered lasers have allowed for larger treatment spot sizes, allowing for facial, chest, and neck treatment.

Color is an important independent sign of aging and gives the person a somewhat an unkempt appearance. Particular focal signs of photoaging such as telangiectases and pigmented lesions are now particularly well targeted along with the broader problems of diffuse erythema, flushing, and dyschromia. Treatment of these problems produces a significant change that is clearly visible and highly satisfying for the patient and clinician alike.

In 1 study, 170 women (aged 10–70 years) were photographed and all signs of their age (all wrinkles, folds, sagging) were digitally removed. Their skin was then "computer wrapped" around a 20-year-old skull. A total of 430 independent observers were then asked to view the photos and position these morphed images according to their perceived ages. It was possible for these observers to accurately position their ages, albeit with a somewhat decreased span of 20 years (16–36 years instead the original 60 years).

This would appear to show that color alone, without any other signs of aging being visible to an observer, is responsible for up to 20 years of visible aging. Hence, one can see the importance for the patient in removing variation of color from their facial landscape.

Recent Changes in Colored Chromophore Laser and Light Therapy

Vascular Lasers and Light Sources

Appropriate Wavelength

Continuous or quasicontinuous lasers with wavelengths well matched for vascular lesions such as krypton (568 nm), copper vapor (578 nm), argon dye (577 nm), and KTP (532 nm) were introduced in the 1970s and 1980s. Since then, other wavelengths (530-600 nm) have also been used. Although some use has been made of wavelengths between 800 and 900 nm, most attention to longer wavelength devices has been directed toward 1064 nm Nd:YAG lasers, which are used for the treatment of deeper vascular targets

(Fig. 1.4). A recent growing trend has been toward the use of multiwavelength laser machines. Examples include a 532-nm and 1064-nm laser (Gemini, Laserscope, San Jose CA, USA) and a combined 585-nm and 1064-nm laser (Cynergy, Cynosure, Westford, MA, USA). Some laser manufacturers offer combined lasers and light sources with the base unit acting as the powering source and various handpieces clipping into this base unit. Such systems provide either variously filtered wavelengths for intense pulsed light therapy or actual lasers powered by the base light source (StarLux, Palomar Medical, Burlington, MA, USA, or Harmony, Alma Lasers, Fort Lauderdale, FL, USA). One should expect that such multiple-wavelength systems will be used increasingly in the future.

Treatment Issues

Many different laser systems are able to adequately treat general facial telangiectases and benign epidermal pigmented lesions [30–37]. These early lasers, however, were restricted in their ability to treat large areas of the skin. Initially, robotized scanners were used so as to allow a larger area to be treated in a single treatment session [38–43]. However, today's modern lasers rely on large spot sizes and speed to provide adequate area treatment. Current examples include the yellow light, 585–595 nm pulsed-dye laser [44,45] and the long-pulsed green light frequency-doubled Nd:AG laser [46,47].

Dynamic and Static Epidermal Cooling

When the target is in the dermis rather than in the epidermis, it is appropriate to protect the epidermis from inadvertent injury. This may occur either from incident laser light interacting with melanocytes or water in the epidermis, or by reflected or scattered beams secondarily affecting the epidermis after vascular or other dermal chromophore interaction. This may be minimized with the use of either dynamic cooling employing a rapid pulse of a freezing agent timed to coincide with the laser pulse, or static freezing where a cold probe or footplate is utilized continuously to minimize epidermal involvement.

Cooling of the epidermis has also been shown to increase the depth of penetration of thermal-induced coagulation [48–54].

Major Visible Chromophore Laser Systems

Q-Switched and Long-Pulsed Laser Systems

Q-switched lasers are able to deliver pulses of laser light with high peak powers and nanosecond duration. Using wavelengths that are selectively absorbed by pigment granules (melanosomes), such lasers tend to break up pigment particles. Since the duration of the pulse is so short, heat damage to adjacent tissues is minimized.

The Q-switched frequency-doubled Nd:YAG, the Q-switched ruby, and the Q-switched alexandrite lasers are probably equally effective in the treatment of pigmented lesions (Fig. 1.19)

Although Q-switched lasers are the accepted gold standard for dermal melanocytic lesions and tattoos, a recent interest in longer pulsed lasers and light sources (millisecond domain) has resulted in several of these lasers also being used for both the treatment of superficial pigmented lesions and general dyschromia – two major issues in facial rejuvenation. Frequency-doubled KTP:YAG (532 nm), long-pulsed-dye, and alexandrite (755 nm) lasers are among such lasers successfully utilized for photorejuvenation. Intense pulsed light may also be preferable to Q-switched lasers for certain darker skin types because use of such light-based systems may lessen the incidence of treatment-rebound postinflammatory hyperpigmentation [55,56].

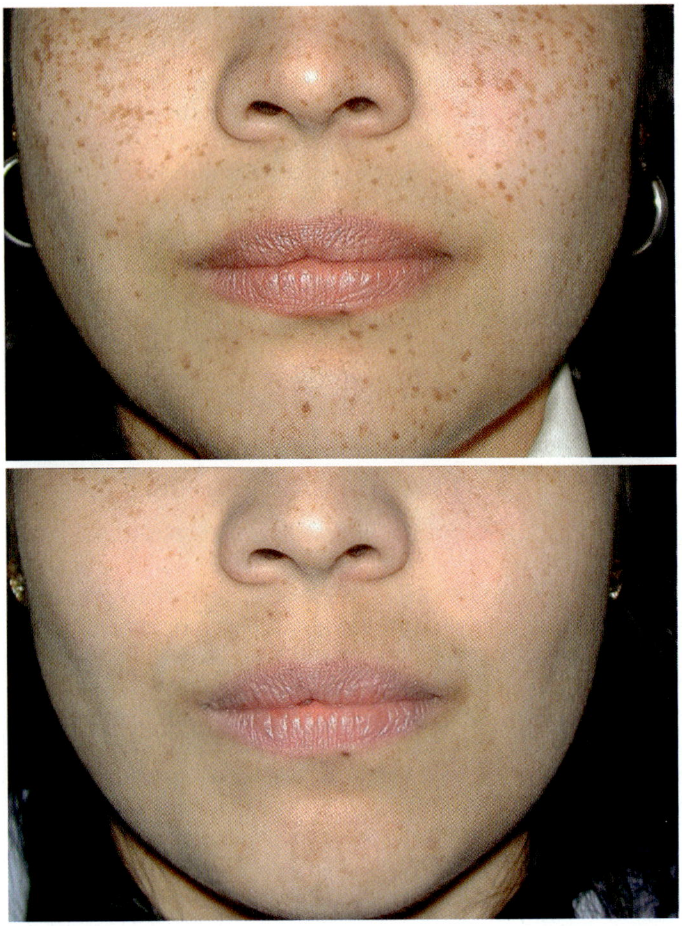

Fig. 1.19. After two treatments of Q-switched 532-nm laser treatment of lentigines and ephelides

Yellow- and Green-Light-Emitting Lasers

The yellow light pulsed-dye laser has always been important for the treatment of a variety of vascular malformations. This laser was initially less popular for the treatment of widespread adult vascular ectasia because of the treatment-induced purpura that was an obligate accompaniment of earlier laser models that emitted short (0.45-ms) pulse durations. In later models (V-Beam, Candela, Weymouth, MA, USA and V-Star, Cynosure, Chelmsford, MA, USA), longer pulsing has enabled mostly nonpurpuric treatments. Pulse durations have been extended up to 40 ms for nasal vascular treatment and usually at 6–10 ms for general facial rejuvenation treatment. Cryogen or forced air cooling limits pain and adverse reactions. Usual fluences will typically vary between 5–10 J/cm^2. Such longer-pulsed systems have found great utility for the treatment of individual telangiectases, angiomas, general facial erythema, and flushing. Pulse stacking (multiple pulsing of the same area) for vascular lesions appears to be relatively safe with these newer pulsed-dye lasers.

Flashlamp pumped-dye lasers appear to have some ability to increase dermal collagen and thus possibly have an impact on the treat-

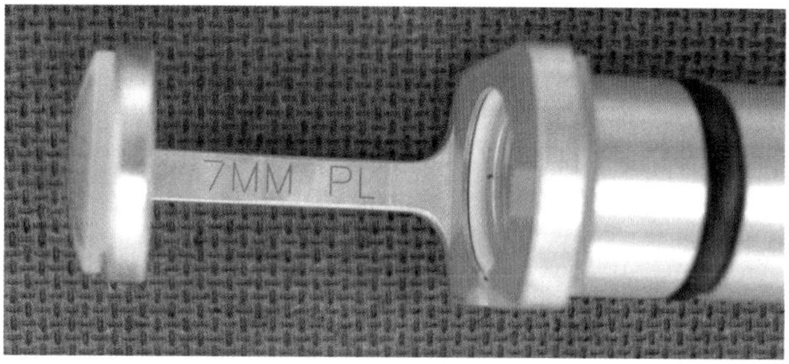

Fig. 1.20. Domed hand piece 595 nm pulsed-dye laser

ment of some dermal signs of photodamage [57]. It has been suggested that they are as effective as the nonablative infrared lasers in inducing new collagen formation [58,59]. This laser-induced neocollagenesis has been presumed to be an effect of the interaction between the laser and the vasculature, inducing the release of inflammatory cytokines and mediators of inflammation. This is then followed by an increase in fibroblastic activity, initiating reparative mechanisms including increased collagen formation [60,61]. Clinically, a decrease in periorbital rhytides has been observed in a split-face study after one or two treatments with a low fluence, 350-ms pulse duration, 585-nm laser [62]. Similarly positive results have been found in another study that also showed electron microscopic ultrastructural changes that were consistent with new collagen formation [63]. The same laser treatment, with similar average settings, seemed to improve atrophic acne scars with a 47% improvement in optical profilometry in the ten patients treated after a single subpurpuric session without cooling [64]. Similar improvements in collagen synthesis have been seen with other pulsed dye lasers [65,66]. According to some investigators, combining treatments with an infrared laser may have benefit in improving the effect on dermal remodeling [67]. A domed pigmented lesion handpiece has become available that acts by diascopy, pushing the blood out of superficial vessels, leaving only the melanin as a target for the yellow light (Fig. 1.20). This seems to be a very effective method of removing pigmented lesions. In one study, such an approach was suggested to be superior to Q-switched laser treatment [68].

The KTP:YAG laser is useful for many rejuvenation purposes. The most recent version of this machine has two handpieces. The first has a variable spot size of between 1 and 5 mm and is useful for individual lesions including vessels, pigmented lesions, and a variety of unusual applications such as sebaceous hyperplasia, syringomas, fibrous papules, seborrheic keratoses (unpublished personal observation), and actinic keratoses (with the prior application of aminolevulinic acid or its esters; Fig. 1.21). Smaller individual targets are usually dealt with first. This is then followed by treatment using a handpiece with a larger spot size. With the 10-mm spot size fixed-diameter handpiece, the 532 nm wavelength can be highly effective in treating broad areas of telangiectases, background erythema, and flushing (Figs. 1.22–1.24). It may also be used to treat pigmented lesions and dyschromia (Figs. 1.25 and 1.26). This laser can also emit a long pulsed emission through the same handpieces. When used with the variable smaller spot size, this 1064-nm laser is useful for venous lakes, periorbital veins, and perialar telangiectases. It has also been suggested that the 10-mm spot size augments the effect of the 532-nm treatment, possibly by impacting on the perivascular edema created by the 532-nm green wavelength.

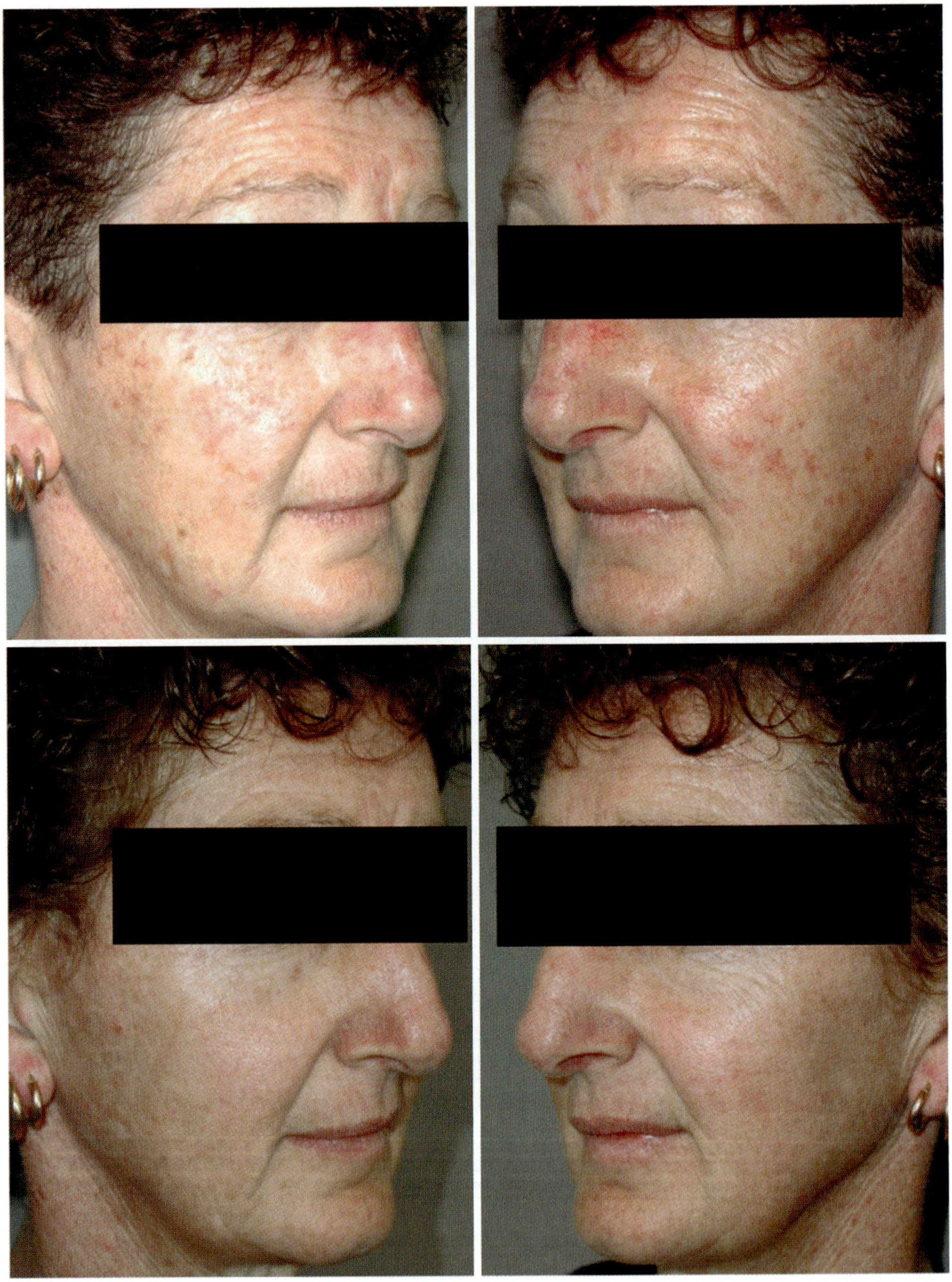

Fig. 1.21. "Photodynamic photorejuvenation" utilizing a 532-nm laser after a 30-min prior application of aminolevulinic acid. Before (*top*) and 3 months after (*bottom*) three treatment sessions

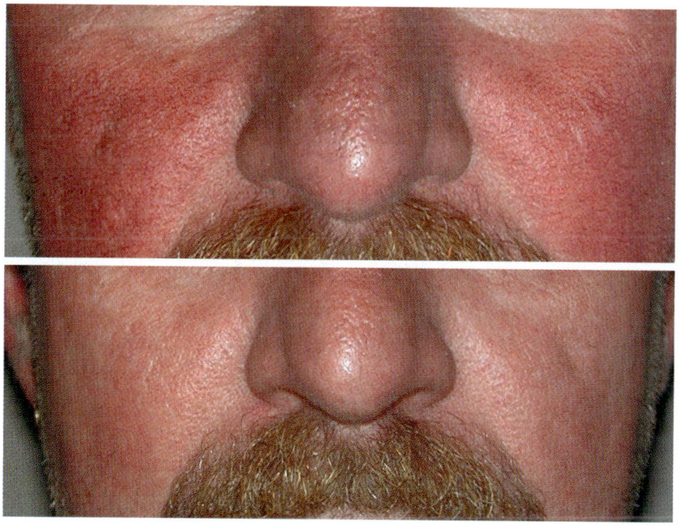

Fig. 1.22. Patient with severe sun damage before (*top*) and after (*bottom*) four vascular laser treatments

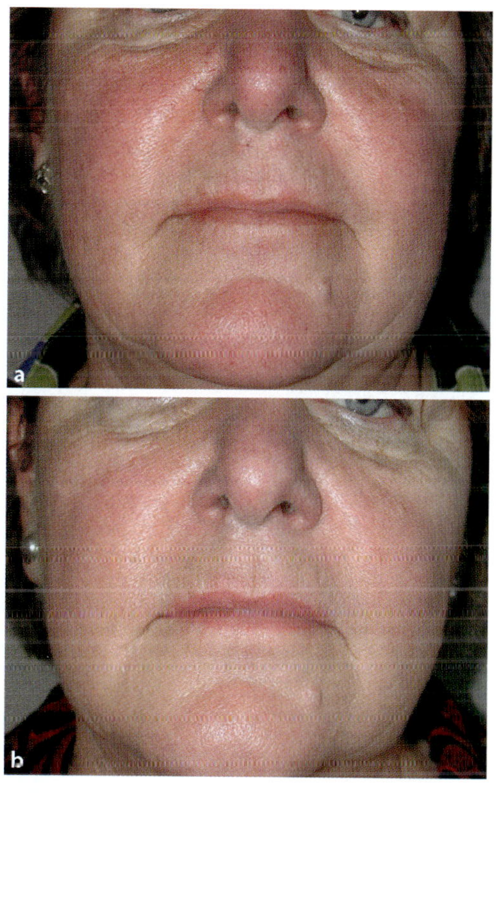

Fig. 1.23. Patient with flushing **a** before and **b** after four treatments of combination 532 nm/1064 nm laser treatment

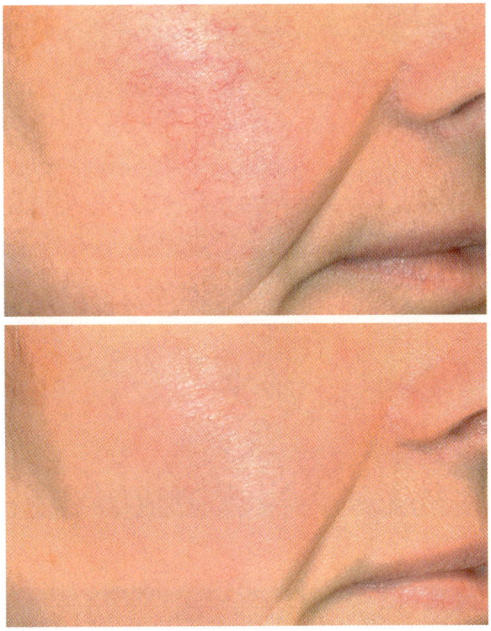

Fig. 1.24. Patient with widespread telangiectases before (*top*) and after (*bottom*) two treatments with a KTP laser

Nonlaser Light Sources

A chromophore, such as hemoglobin in blood vessels or melanin contained within melanocytes, has a characteristic spectrum of absorption over a wide range of wavelengths. Absorption is generally better at some wavelengths than at others. Lasers usually focus on a single wavelength at or near a peak on the absorption spectrum. Another, now highly popular approach, has been to use an intense pulsed light source to emit small amounts of light over a broadband of wavelengths to interact with the target over the extent of the absorption spectrum. When added together, these emitted energies, at all the different wavelengths, equate to a high enough total energy to adequately treat several vascular and epidermal manifestations of photodamage [69–73].

It has been suggested by some that current nonlaser light-based systems will eventually become more popular than lasers because of

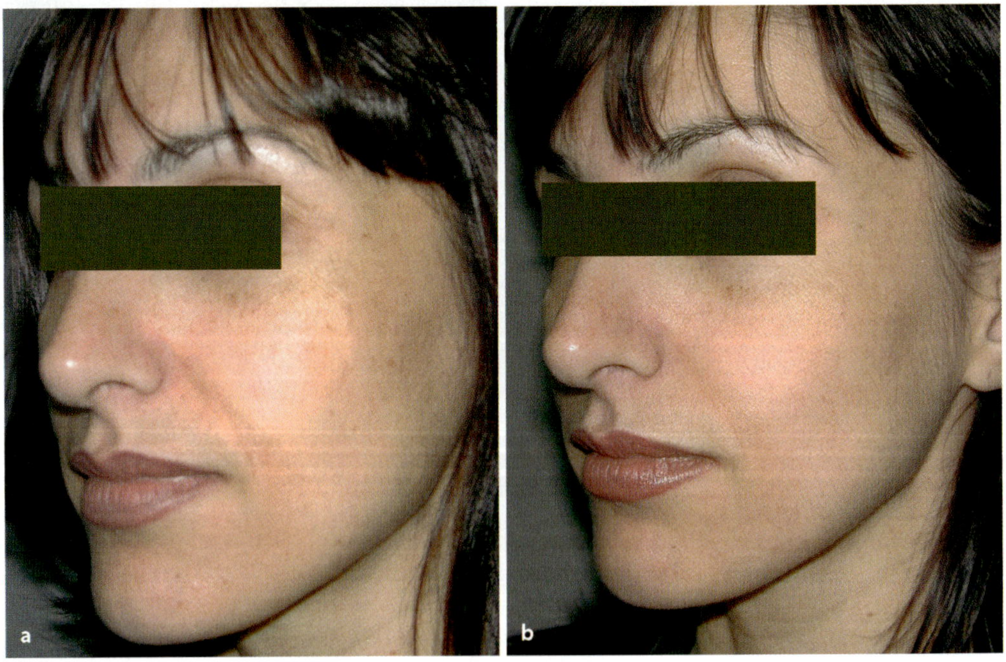

Fig. 1.25 a, b. Patient, with dyschromia **a** before and **b** after three treatments with a KTP:YAG laser

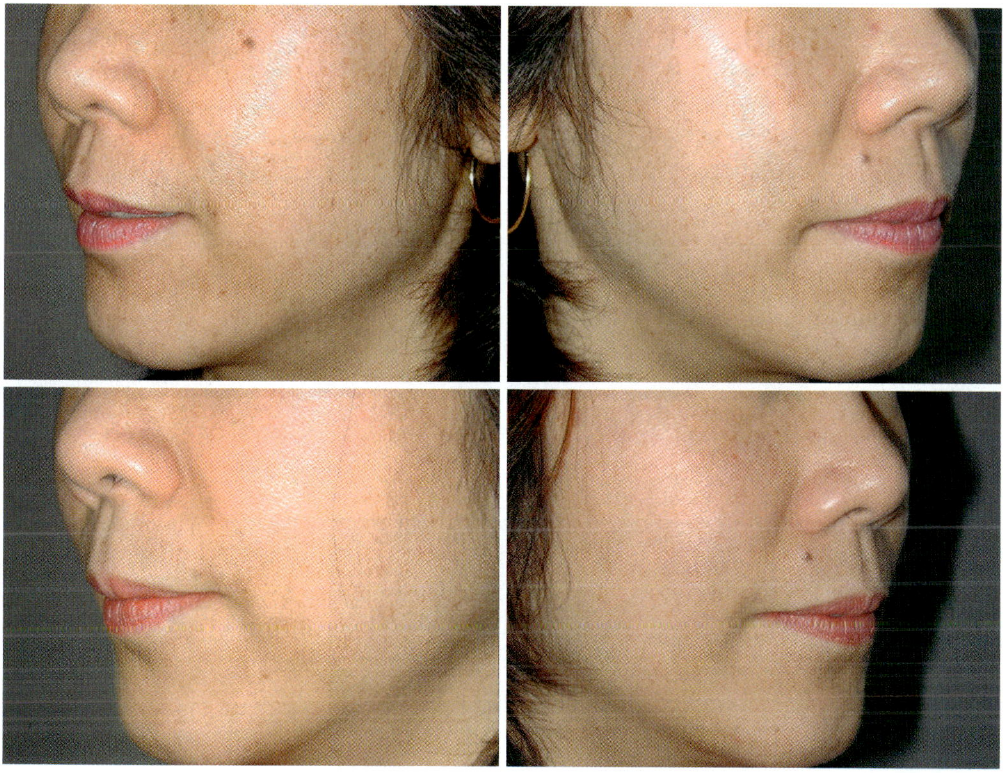

Fig. 1.26. Patient with epidermal pigmentation, before (*top*) and after (*bottom*) two treatments with a long-pulsed laser

their comparative cost advantages, recently enhanced engineering changes, and widespread popularity when used for full facial rejuvenation [74].

The broad range of wavelengths included in the intense pulsed light emission (500–1200 nm) is curtailed at the lower end (shorter wavelengths) by using of "cut off" filters. The treatment thus allows the emission of green, yellow, red, and infrared wavelengths at the same time, allowing the colored chromophores (hemoglobin and melanin) and water to be simultaneously targeted. This has the theoretical advantage of dealing with all of the common problems of photodamage at the same time. The large treatment head allows intense pulsed light treatments to be performed expeditiously (Fig. 1.27 and 1.28).

Facial rejuvenation with a variety of intense pulsed light sources is generally undertaken with a 550- to 570-nm cut off filter. Using this approach, most aspects of photodamage, such as telangiectasia, dyschromias, dilated pores, skin textural changes, and mild wrinkling can be treated [75–77]. A variety of intense pulsed light sources, made by a variety of manufacturers, are now available.

Combination Light/Laser and Radiofrequency

A novel approach to facial rejuvenation combines radiofrequency and optical energy (Aurora, Syneron Medical, Yokneam, Israel). This

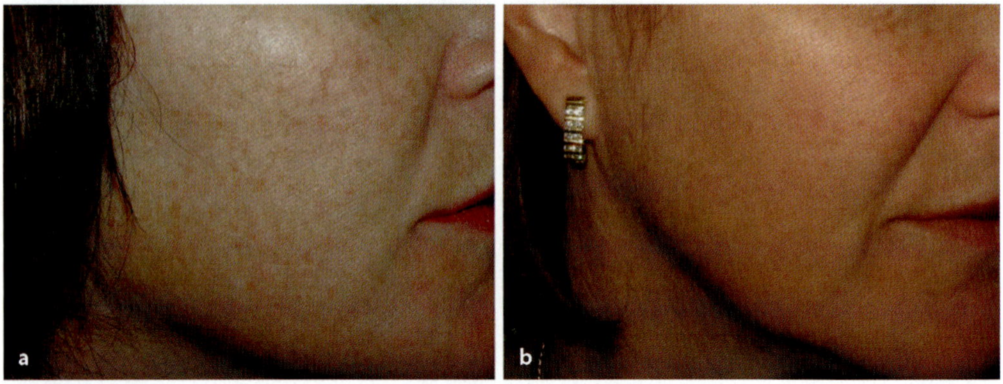

Fig. 1.27. **a** Before and **b** after intense pulsed light treatment (photographs courtesy of Dr. Philip Behhor)

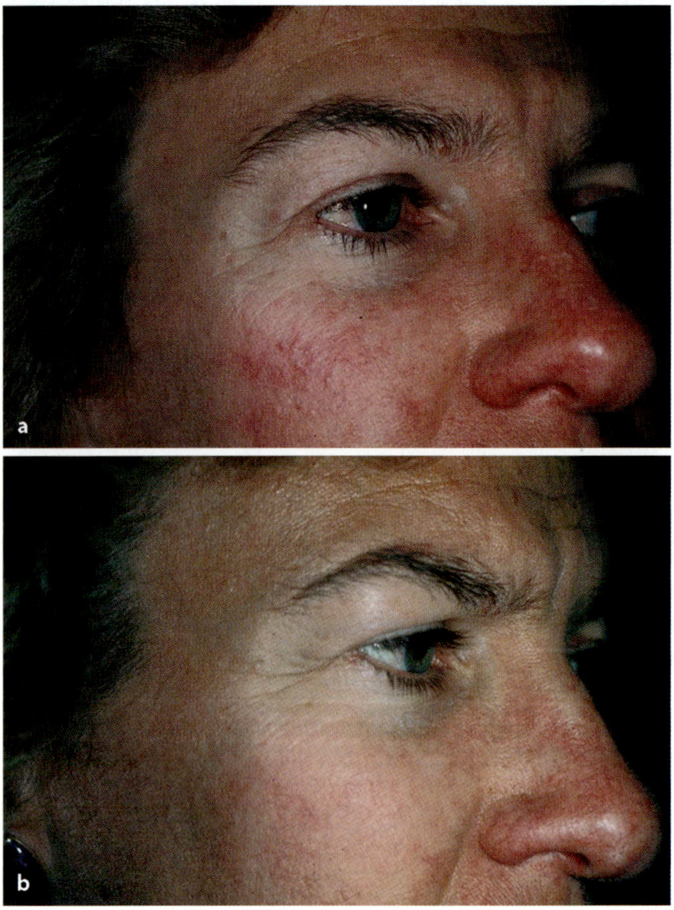

Fig. 1.28. **a** Before and **b** after intense pulsed light treatment (photographs courtesy of Dr. David Goldberg)

unique system combines an intense pulsed light, with wavelengths ranging from 580 nm to 980 nm, with a bipolar radiofrequency source delivered at a frequency of 1 MHz through a cooled handpiece. The light and radiofrequency is delivered in a synchronized pulse. The light is delivered first at low energy levels to selectively preheat vascular or pigmented lesions. Consequently, the radiofrequency current will selectively heat the preheated vessels or pigment as opposed to the surrounding tissue. The rationale underlying this technology is based on variations in conductivity in different human tissues. Improvements in conditions such as facial hyperpigmentation (78%), telangiectases (70%), and skin texture (60%) have been reported [78].

Infrared Lasers and Light Sources

As one moves from the visible to the infrared wavelengths, several changes occur in the absorption characteristics of the skin. The depth of beam penetration of the laser or light increases as colored chromophores are less specifically targeted; more transmission rather than absorption occurs. Near-infrared wavelengths, up to about 1100 nm can be absorbed by multiple available chromophores, including hemoglobin, deoxyhemoglobin, melanin, and water. With increasingly longer infrared wavelengths, water becomes the predominant target.

Lasers and light sources utilizing these wavelengths are largely attempting to remodel collagen by heating dermal water and causing some initial denaturation and eventual repair of the collagen. Although a direct heat effect on collagen has been noted, there are undoubtedly other mechanisms at play such as the role of inflammatory cytokines stimulating human skin fibroblasts to upregulate the production of extracellular matrix proteins and matrix metalloproteinases [79,80].

Infrared Lasers Targeting Hemoglobin, Melanin, and Water

The 1064-nm Nd:YAG laser

One the first attempts at nonablative resurfacing utilized the Q-switched 1064nm Nd:YAG laser for periocular or perioral rhytides (Table 1.4) [81]. At high fluences (5.5 J/cm^2), some patients appeared to improve almost as much as following ablative laser resurfacing. However, the treatment was complicated by pinpoint bleeding, petechiae, and occasional purpura. Lower fluences led to fewer postlaser concerns, but also less improvement. The 1064-nm Q-switched Nd:YAG laser has also been used with some success in the treatment of atrophic acne scarring. In one study, a three-dimensional analysis made of atrophic acne scarring showed a gradual improvement in roughness analysis from 8.9% at mid-treatment (1 month after the third treatment session), increasing to 23.3%, 31.6%, and 39.2% at 1, 3, and 6 months after the fifth treatment, respectively [82]. Clinical improvements in facial postacne scarring and facial rhytides were also seen in patients treated twice using a combined 532-/1064-nm Q-switched Nd:YAG laser.

Long-pulsed Nd:YAG lasers, in the millisecond domain, are free of the petechial and purpuric effects seen with frequency-doubled Q-switched Nd:YAG lasers. Such lasers have been used to treat deeper vascular lesions (Fig. 1.29) as well as for rejuvenation. In general, many treatments are required and the changes are often subtle [83–85]. In one study, physician-graded scores demonstrated an 11.9% decrease in coarse wrinkles, a 17.3% decrease in skin laxity, and a 20% overall improvement. In another study of 150 patients, divided into three groups, the combination of the long-pulsed 1064-nm Nd:YAG and the frequency-doubled Nd:YAG 532-nm lasers appeared to produce more improvement in the signs of photodamage than was seen with either wavelength alone.

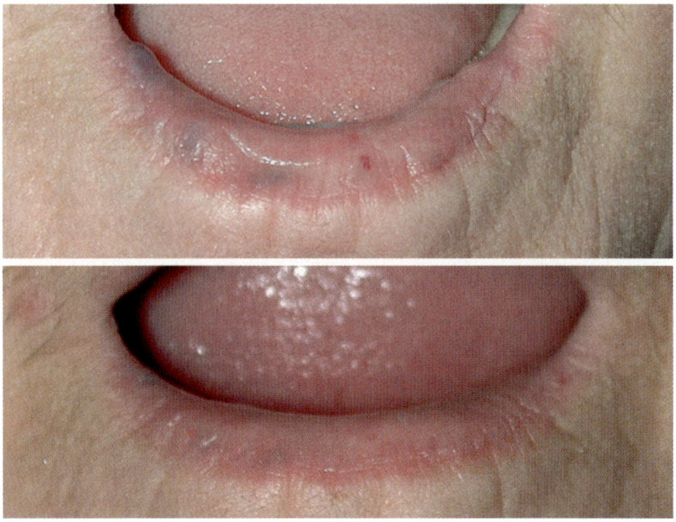

Fig. 1.29. Patient, with venous lake, before (*top*) and after (*bottom*) a single treatment with a long-pulsed 1064-nm laser

Although other wavelengths in the near-infrared range, such as 980 nm, have been used experimentally, they have shown little clinical application.

Infrared Lasers Targeting Water

A group of lasers emitting wavelengths between 1300 and 1600 nm have been used to nonselectively target the dermis by using water as the target.

The 1320-nm Nd:YAG Laser

This laser was the first of the infrared water-targeting lasers used for facial rejuvenation [86–96]. The latest model of this laser (Cool Touch 3, Cool Touch, Roseville, CA, USA) utilizes a 10-mm spot size and typical fluences of 13–20 J/cm^2 with a fixed 50-ms pulse duration. Epidermal cooling is achieved with an integrated cryogen cooling spray system. With each firing of the laser by the operator, the energy is delivered in six discreet laser pulses. The cryogen spray is delivered in three pulses. The 1320-nm wavelength has a high scattering coefficient and produces a general rise in dermal temperature inducing a wound healing response that leads to collagen denaturation and disruptions in collagen linkage. New collagen formation and collagen remodeling are seen by both histologic and clinical analysis. Early models of this laser were somewhat problematic, with a significant rate of scarring and hyperpigmentation. The later model (Cool Touch 3, Cool Touch, Roseville, CA, USA) appears to be significantly safer. Although there was early concern about short-term limited efficacy seen with this laser, longer-lasting results have now been documented.

Several studies have also shown a statistically significant, but relatively limited, subjective and objective improvement in atrophic acne scarring after three to six treatments performed at monthly intervals. However, other studies have noted less impressive results.

The 1450-nm Diode Laser

The 1450-nm infrared diode laser (Smoothbeam, Candela, Waltham, MA, USA) uses a pulse consisting of four bursts of 1450 nm infrared laser irradiation interspersed with five

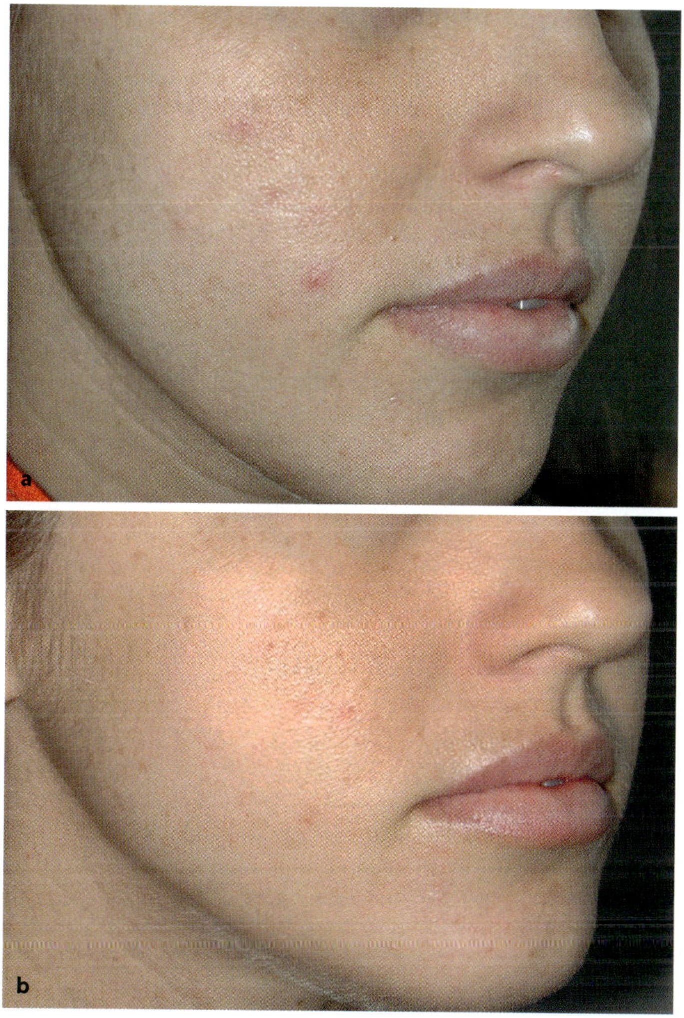

Fig. 1.30 a, b. Mild acne and acne scarring **a** before and **b** after a single treatment with the 1450-nm diode laser

bursts of cryogen spray cooling. A prelaser cooling phase is followed by a lasering phase and then followed by three more similar cooling and lasering phases (Fig. 1.30). This wavelength also primarily targets water. The cryogen spray allows for preservation of the epidermis, minimizing side effects. The 1450-nm diode infrared laser has been utilized in the treatment of acne, sebaceous hyperplasia, early rhinophyma, and periorbital rhytides [97–99].

The use of this laser for the purposes of photorejuvenation has been documented in a study of 25 women with periorbital and perioral rhytides who were treated four times at monthly intervals. Clinical and histologic analysis was undertaken both from treated and untreated control facial sites before treatment, immediately after the first treatment, and 3, 6, and 12 months after the fourth treatment [100]. An increase in collagen synthesis and deposition was noted up until 6 months after treatment. No further increase in collagen formation was evident at 12 months after the last treatment. Although there was a significant degree of hypopigmentation noted in the study, the investigators felt this was due to the laser-associated cryogen delivery, rather than from the laser itself.

The 1450-nm diode laser's effect on wrinkles has also been confirmed in other studies [101]. In one of these studies, clinical improvement occurred in 13 out of 20 patients 6 months after 2–4 treatments when the laser was used in conjunction with cryogen cooling; no improvement occurred when cryogen cooling alone was used.

A significant number of studies have also evaluated the effect of this laser on acne-induced scarring [102]. In a study comparing the 1320-nm and 1450-nm lasers for the treatment of atrophic acne scarring, a significant improvement was seen after treatment with both lasers; The 1450-nm laser appeared to produce superior results [103].

The 1540-nm Erbium:Glass Laser

The erbium:glass laser (Aramis, Quantel Medical, Clermont Ferrand, France) emits a wavelength of 1540 nm. Like the other mid-infrared lasers described above, this lasers targets dermal water through an optical fiber. In one study, 42 females were treated for perioral and periorbital rhytides; they were administered five erbium:glass laser treatments at 6-week intervals [104]. All of the subjects showed an improvement 6 months into the study and exhibited significant increases in dermal thickness. Patients were monitored until 14 months after the initial treatment and no complications were reported during that time. In another study on perioral and periorbital rhytides in 24 women, a gradual, mild to moderate improvement was noted. An increased the number of passes was delivered to the perioral region, yet the periorbital area seemed to respond better. Six months after treatment, increased dermal thickness was evident on histology. A study treating necklines and forehead rhytides of 20 female patients reported improvements in both skin tone and texture. Ultrasound evaluation showed that the neck and forehead had increased dermal thickness. One study detailed adverse reactions and lack of improvement with a 1540-nm laser on retroauricular skin. It has been suggested that since this early study utilized a different erbium glass system to that most commonly used and that the fluences were too high to allow collagen remodeling and the interval between pulses in the pulse train too short, it was not representative of the true safety and efficacy of this wavelength laser.

Fractional Photothermolysis

A laser concept termed "fractional photothermolysis" has also been developed to describe small vertical zones of full-thickness thermal damage that are produced by a mid-infrared laser [105]. This laser's effect is akin to sinking posts or drilling holes of thermal damage, with areas surrounding these posts left free of damage. This is not really a true nonablative method, but is a means of ablative resurfacing without the patient having to experience the pronounced healing phase seen after either truly ablative CO_2 or erbium laser resurfacing. This fractionated resurfacing laser approach appears to show promise in the treatment of both epidermal and dermal disease processes (Fig. 1.31). In addition, and in contrast to the effect of mid-infrared lasers, fractionated resurfacing also leads to improve-

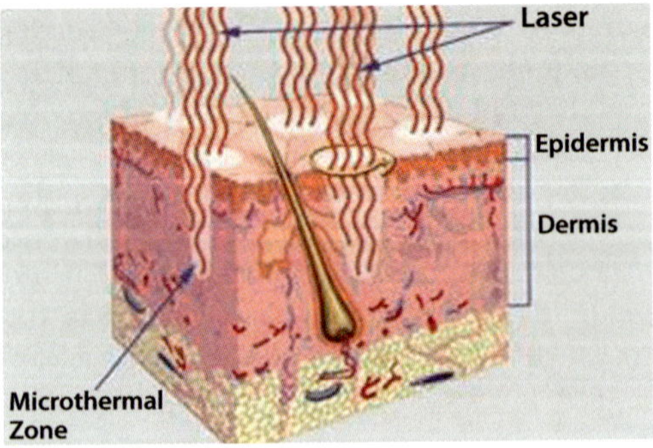

Fig. 1.31. Fractional photothermolysis (Image courtesy of Reliant Technologies)

ment in epidermal dyschromias. The major indications for fractionated treatment include melasma, acne scarring, rhytides, and other signs of photodamage (Figs. 1.32). Despite the positive results seen after treatment with this laser, it may be a relatively inefficient method of treating epidermal pigmented lesions or dyschromia when compared to treatment with intense pulsed lights or color-chromophore-seeking lasers. However, the laser is highly effective in treating such dyschromias in a patient with wrinkles or acne scarring. This laser approach may also have some advantage over other approaches for the treatment of melasma, as well as its ability to be used on nonfacial areas to treat both epidermal and dermal photoaging. In such areas, ablative resurfacing would be ill-advised. Surgical scars have also recently been successfully treated with this approach.

There are now a number of technologies that can be used for fractionated resurfacing. The most well know laser (Fraxel, Reliant, Santa Clara, CA, USA) utilizes a 1550-nm wavelength with delivered energies between 8 and 20 mJ or more, and between 125 and 250 laser-induced microthermal zones per square centimeter. Multiple passes are performed, producing between 1000 and 3000 of these microscopic zones of epidermal and dermal damage per square centimeter. Despite this, only a fraction of the available surface area of the skin is targeted. Thus, several treatment sessions (usually three to five) are required, performed approximately 2–4 weeks apart. Other fractionated laser approaches involve the use wavelengths of either 1550 nm or 2934 nm. One study has evaluated complications after 1550-nm laser fractional resurfacing. In that study, all patients undergoing fractional pho-

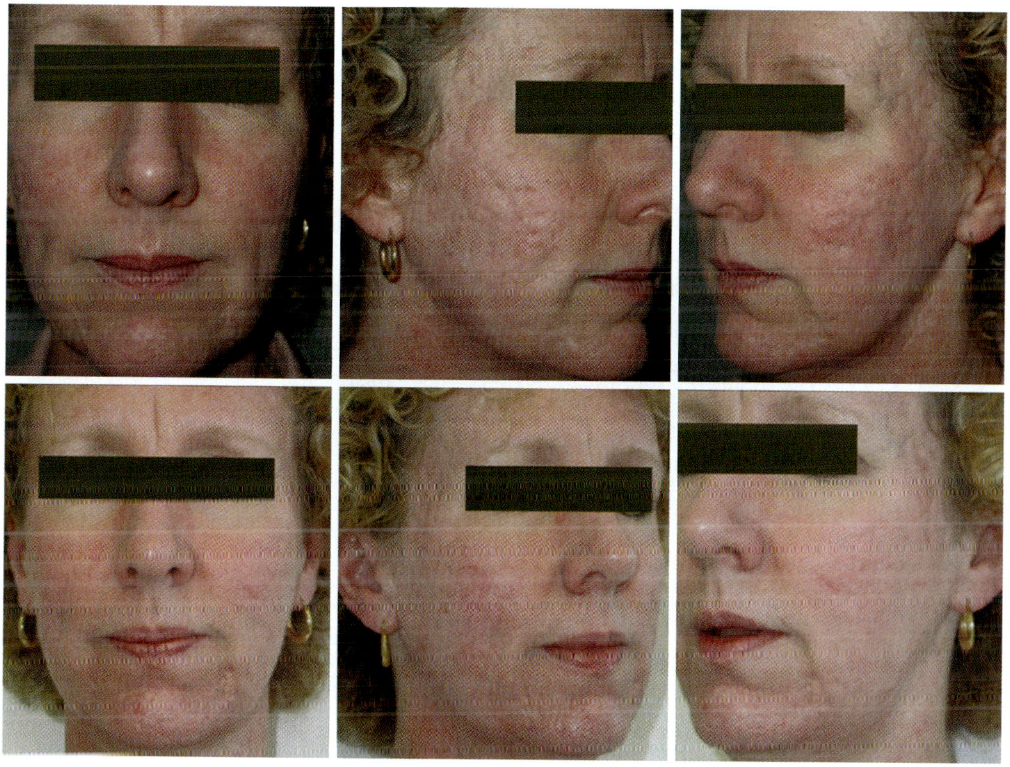

Fig. 1.32. Fractionated resurfacing, as well as fat transfer for postacne scarring. *Upper* Before treatment, *lower* after treatment. Image courtesy of Reliant Technologies

tothermolysis had transient posttreatment erythema; many had other transient reactions including facial edema (82%), dry skin (86.6%), flaking (60%), a few (one to three) small, superficial scratches (46.6%), pruritis (37%), and bronzing (26.6%). Occasional increased skin sensitivity (10%) and acneform eruption (10%) was also seen. Most patients (72%) limited their social engagements for an average of 2 days after treatment [105].

Photodynamic Therapy

Recently, PDT has become widespread in its use for the treatment of premalignant and malignant skin disease [106]. PDT will be discussed only briefly in this chapter as it is described in detail elsewhere in this book. Simplistically, this technology revolves around the use of a relevant photosensitizer and its ability to specifically accumulate in target tissues. The tissues are then irradiated at an appropriate wavelength and appropriate energy to induce an excitation product that reacts with molecular oxygen and subcellular structures to bring about cell death.

The advent of 5-aminolevulinic acid as a topical sensitizer for PDT has been largely responsible for this technology gaining popular appeal. Red light is favored for its ability to penetrate sufficiently deeply into skin to treat skin cancers and solar keratoses. However, acne and other signs of photoaging respond quite nicely to PDT treatment [107–110]. This approach, and its impact on facial rejuvenation, is described in detail in Chap. 2.

Advantages and Disadvantages of Different Technologies for Facial Rejuvenation

Ablative Lasers – Advantages

The main advantage of ablative CO_2 and erbium lasers lies in their efficacy. Throughout much of the world, they have replaced nonlaser technologies as the major tool for significant facial rejuvenation. These laser approaches still remain the gold standard by which all other ablative and nonablative technologies are compared. This applies to any analysis of wrinkles from the very fine to the very coarse,

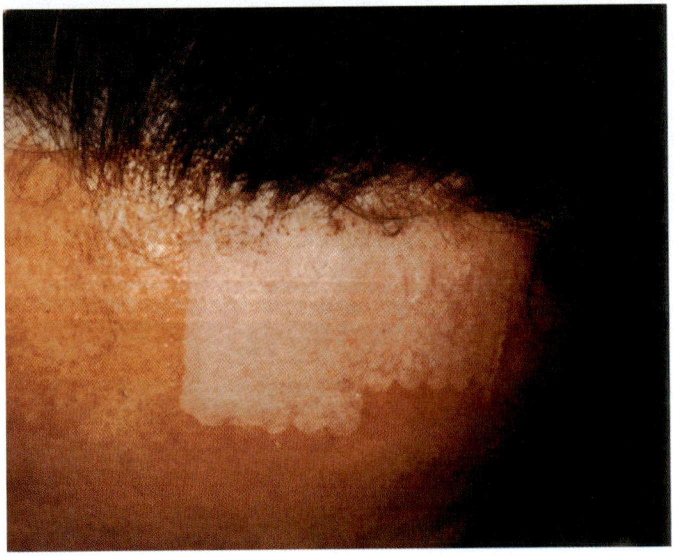

Fig. 1.33. Erbium laser showing its ablative effect on Betadine-painted skin

atrophic postacne scarring, poor skin tone, and other textural and elastotic changes.

The ability of these truly ablative lasers to treat such a wide variety of facial cosmetic issues is another of their hallmarks. They can be used to treat both epidermal and dermal photodamage in the one treatment and may be combined with other facial rejuvenation techniques described elsewhere in this book, such as botulinum toxin injections and dermal fillers (Fig. 1.33).

Another advantage of ablative CO_2 and erbium lasers lies in the physician user's ability to visualize predictable end points. One can readily determine which level in the skin one is treating by evaluating endpoints such as the loss of epidermal color and pinpoint bleeding associated with the erbium laser treatments as well as the contractile nature of the dermis most commonly associated with ablative CO_2 laser resurfacing. Other fairly reproducible end-point examples include epidermal lesion removal and wrinkle effacement. Unfortunately, the contractile nature of the laser-induced dermal interaction can lead the practitioner to overestimate the degree of long-term improvement when deep wrinkles and acne scarring are treated.

Ablative Lasers – Disadvantages

Ablative resurfacing lasers cannot provide for every aspect of facial rejuvenation. These lasers are not a substitute for techniques such as face lifting, brow lifting, or blepharoplasty, where true tissue redundancy or structural loss is a problem. Ablative laser resurfacing is also not particularly effective against expression lines or wrinkles that are dynamic in origin. Expression lines such as nasolabial lines are not well treated by lasers and should be addressed by other means such as filler materials. Muscle-induced or dynamic wrinkling is best treated with botulinum toxin injections.

Similarly, with acne scarring, ablative laser resurfacing has its limitations. It is very useful for superficial scarring but not terribly effective for deeper scars. Here, other procedures including scar subcision, filler augmentation, or small, full-thickness skin grafts may be required.

Complications such as delayed healing, scarring, hyperpigmentation and hypopigmentation can also occur. Hyperpigmentation is a temporary but disturbing complication most commonly seen in patients of olive skin type. Scarring is uncommon, but quite distressing when it does occur. Hypopigmentation is more common and is partially avoidable by decreasing the amount of energy supplied to the skin. It has been suggested by some that erbium-laser ablation may produce fewer complications than are seen after ablative CO_2 laser treatments.

Morbidity may be significant following ablative laser resurfacing, with 1–2 weeks of healing required and many further weeks of erythema after treatment being the usual case. One can also expect to see delayed, yet continuing improvement, for 3–6 months after laser resurfacing.

Maintenance of improvement after laser resurfacing is variable. Although the laser-induced effect is thought to be permanent, there is some lessening of improvement after the first 2 years. It is reasonable to assume that 50–60% of the improvement is maintained long term.

Nonablative Lasers – Advantages

The greatest advantage of nonablative lasers and light-based systems lies in their ability to improve many signs of photoaging without the prolonged healing phase associated with ablative lasers. These systems also have an enviable safety record and do not, in general, engender the degree of complications associated with more aggressive ablative laser treatments.

Colored-chromophore-seeking lights and lasers are very efficacious in removing or improving most vascular and epidermal pigmentary dyschromias (Fig. 1.34). Melasma, which has always defied ablative and nonablative laser treatments, may be improved in some, but not all patients who undergo fractional photothermolysis.

Many conditions that were formerly treated with ablative lasers can now be improved with nonablative technologies. Postacne scarring of mild to moderate degree may be treated with many of the mid-infrared lasers, as well with fractional photothermolysis. Similarly, wrinkles and skin texture are mildly improved with nonablative approaches, although for these conditions, nonablative treatments are no yet able to rival the results seen with ablative systems.

Finally, as is described elsewhere in this book, PDT to augment nonablative therapy, may in some situations augment the effect of some nonablative treatments.

Nonablative Lasers – Disadvantages

Ablative lasers usually exert their effect in a single treatment. Conversely, nonablative treatments require multiple treatments to achieve the desired effects. For some issues

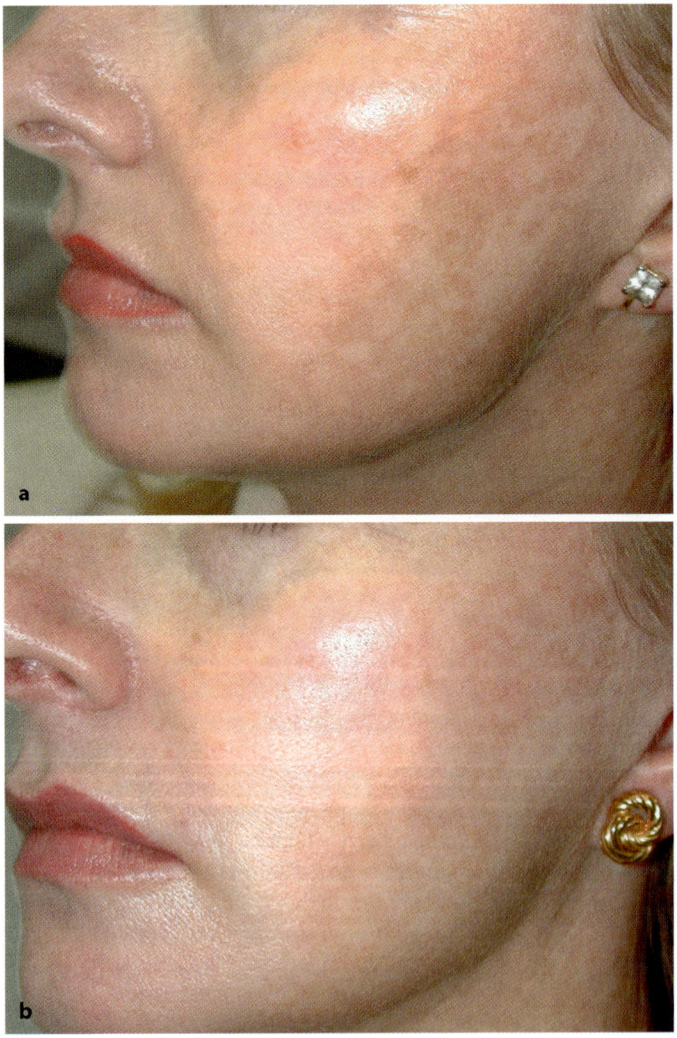

Fig. 1.34. **a** Before and **b** after visible light lasers for facial dyschromia

such as significant facial wrinkling, rhinophyma, skin laxity, and more severe signs of elastosis, nonablative lasers are not able to yet deliver satisfactory results.

Indications

Irregular Pigmentation

Among the most common pigmented lesions treated with lasers and light sources, and those often of most concern to patients, are the many epidermal lesions that are due to photoaging. In addition some epidermal pigmented lesions, such as ephelides, lentignes, seborrheic keratoses, dermatosis papulosa, and acrochordons have a hereditary predisposition.

Vascular Lesions

Vascular lesions, including telangiectasia, angiomas with venous lakes, standing erythema, and flushing disorders, are an important and accessible target for many laser and light-based technologies. Many patients who seek facial rejuvenation present with a vascular component.

Oily and Acne-Prone Skin

For those so affected, oil production and tendency toward acne and sebaceous hyperplasia is a major concern and one that recently has become a potential target for many different wavelengths. Several diode, laser, and light technologies of varying wavelengths, sometimes used with topical application of porphyrins, have been used to target both the sebaceous gland and acne-inducing bacteria (*Propionibacterium acnes*).

Skin Texture

"Skin texture" is difficult to define; skin texture abnormalities are best defined as a mixture of problems including roughness and dryness, dilated pores or wrinkling, and/or a combination of the above. Many of the available nonablative lasers and light sources may improve skin texture.

Sallow and Uneven Color

There are few colors present in the skin. The skin's appearance, from a color perspective as one ages, appears to be an interplay between red pigments (oxy- and deoxyhemoglobin), brown pigment (melanin), and scattering from changes in dermal collagen. With photodamage, uneven coloring of the skin appears because of variations in the appearance of these pigments in a scattered fashion. This, in addition to age- and ultraviolet-induced weathered collagen causes many individuals to seek facial rejuvenation. Many lasers and light-based systems can satisfactorily improve the pigmentary abnormalities. However, it is probably the reflectance off sun-damaged dermal collagen that is responsible for the sallow appearance of sun-damaged skin. Collagen improvement can be improved with both ablative and nonablative technologies.

Postacne Scarring

Postacne scarring may be atrophic or hypertrophic. Sometimes there is not true scarring, but simply pigmentary changes. Macular pigmentary changes can be brown, red, or white. Various lasers and light sources have been used treat these pigmentary changes. Atrophic scars have been dealt with by a variety of ablative, fractionated and nonablative technologies (Figs. 1.10, 1.33, and 1.35); hypertrophic scars have been treated with by vascular lasers.

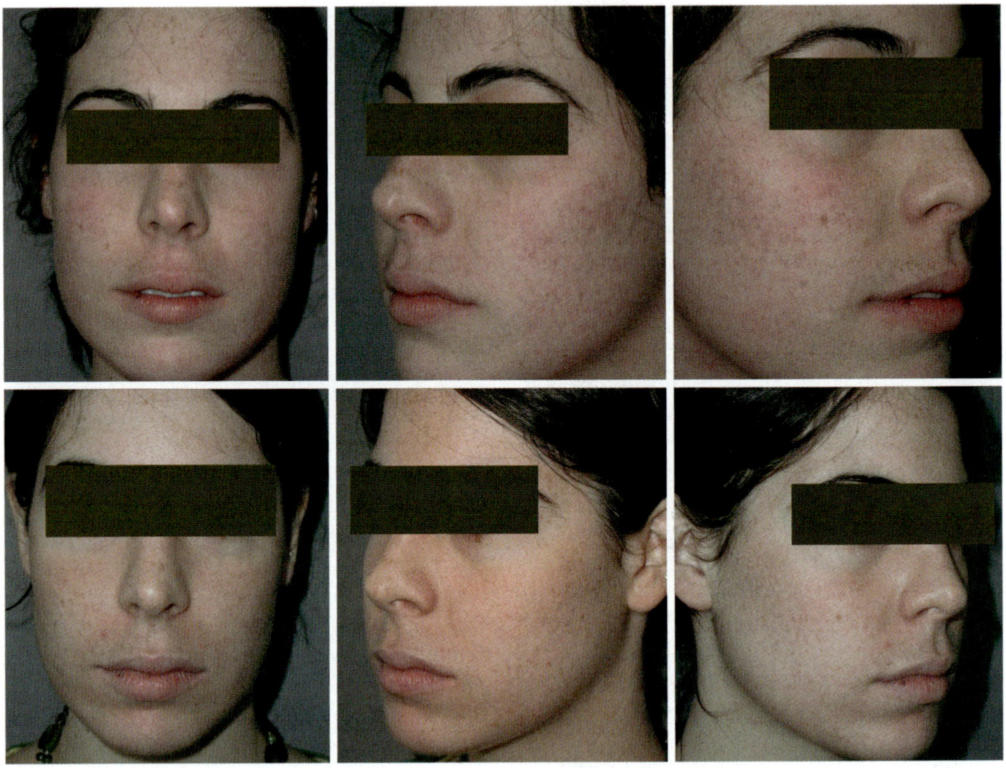

Fig. 1.35. Before (*upper*) and after (*lower*) three treatments with fractional photothermolysis

Premalignant Changes Including Actinic Keratoses

Actinic keratoses, and similar lesions, may be treated by lasers, light sources, or diode technologies, generally used with topically applied porphyrins. The usual utilized lasers include the pulsed-dye and KTP lasers. Actinic cheilitis may be targeted by either ablative lasers or PDT means.

Fine Wrinkling

Fine wrinkling may occur both with chronologic and or ultraviolet-induced aging. Fine wrinkles may be treated with ablative laser systems, but over the last decade has been increasingly targeted by nonablative technologies.

Medium Wrinkling

Medium wrinkling is more commonly seen as a manifestation of photoaging. It is best treated with ablative lasers.

Lumps and Bumps

A variety of conditions such as benign intradermal nevi, syringomas, xanthelasma, fibrous papules, and seborrheic keratoses are all conditions for which patients seek facial rejuvenation (Figs. 1.13 and 1.14).

These skin problems are well dealt with by the different lights and lasers discussed earlier in this chapter and are elaborated and weighted in their efficacy in Table 1.5.

Table 1.5. Indications for available therapies for facial rejuvenation

Treatment		Issue											
		Pigmented lesions or dyschromia	Vascular pathology	Acne and related*	Skin texture	Sallow complexion	Postacne scarring (atrophic)	Postacne scarring (hypertrophic)	Premalignant change	Mild wrinkling	Medium wrinkling	Coarse wrinkling	Skin laxity
Ablative	Carbon dioxide or combined with erbium	*	X	X	**	**	***	X	**	*	***	***	**
	Erbium laser alone	**	X	X	**	**	**	X	**	**	***	**	*
	Plasma skin resurfacing	*	X	X	**	**	**	X	?	***	**		
Non-ablative	Visible light lasers	***	***	** (***with PDT)	**	X	*	**	** (with PDT)	*	X	X	X
	IPL with or without RF	***	***	** (***with PDT)	**	*	*	X	** (with PDT)	*	X	X	X
	Infrared non-ablative	X	* (1064nm)	**	*	X	**	X	X				X
	Fractional photothermolysis	*	X	?	**	**	***	?	?	**	*	X	X
	PDT	*	X	***	**	X	X	X	***	X	X	X	X

X Not advised for this indication; ?Uncertain place in treatment at this time; *Adequate treatment; **Good treatment; ***A treatment of choice; *Acne and related (acne-prone skin, oily complexion, sebaceous hyperplasia)

Contraindications

Contraindications to skin resurfacing with ablative lasers include:

1. Koebnerising disorders such as vitiligo, warts, and mollusca.
2. Potential abnormal wound-healing states such as current or recent isotretinoin therapy or immunosuppressive therapy have been suggested contraindications. This remains controversial.
3. Decreased adnexal structures such as post-radiotherapy or burn scars.
4. Infectious diseases such as human immunodeficiency virus, hepatitis C, active herpes simplex.
5. Medical or psychological conditions likely to make the patient an anesthetic or post-operative risk.

Contraindications to nonablative technologies include:

1. Concurrent isotretinoin remains a controversial issue.
2. Current or recent tan or intention to expose to high-dosage ultraviolet radiation. This is of much greater concern in patients who seek visible laser or light source treatment.
3. Medical conditions such as epilepsy, claustrophobia, photosensitizing medications, pregnancy, or in patients psychologically unable to cope with therapy.

Informed Consent

Examples of informed consent for various lasers are given in Figs. 1.36–1.39.

Personal Approach

Glogau's or similar classifications of photodamage are useful tools in determining a personal approach (Table 1.6). However, in reality no two patients are interchangeable. However, there are some important caveats when considering lasers and light treatments for facial rejuvenation. Lasers and light-based treatments are best for surface and minor-volume facial changes. Problems of movement, marked laxity, and more marked volume change require the other therapies described in this book.

My personal approach depends both on the type of problem, the severity, and the region to be addressed. An algorithm may be established based on the patient's initial presentation. Issues of discoloration (telangiectasia, angiomas, facial redness, flushing, epidermal pigmented lesions, dyschromia) are treated with visible light lasers or intense pulsed lights. This approach leads to a patient's maximal gain with relatively little risk. If melasma is the issue and topical therapies have failed, fractionated photothermolysis may be an optimal treatment, although some practitioners

Table 1.6. Glogau categories of photodamage

Glogau category of photodamage	Photodamage skin type description
1	No keratoses, little wrinkling, no scarring, little or no requirement for make up
2	Early actinic keratoses, slight yellow skin discoloration, early wrinkling, parallel smile lines, mild scarring, small amount of make up required
3	Actinic keratoses, obvious yellow skin discoloration with telangiectasia, wrinkling present at rest, moderate acne scarring, always requires make up
4	Solar keratoses and skin cancers have occurred. Wrinkling, and cutis laxa of actinic, gravitational, and dynamic origin

Erbium or CO_2 Laser Treatment | Procedural Consent Form

A. CONDITION & PROCEDURE

The Doctor has explained that I have the following condition: *[Patient to document in patient's own words]*

....

....

The following procedure will be performed:

Laser re-texturing is a procedure involving the removal of the outer 1-2mm of the skin using laser technology.

It is useful in the treatment of wrinkling of the skin related to ageing and over-exposure to the sun, scarring or altered colour or pigmentation.

It is usually of benefit in treatment of acne scarring, however, it must be understood that the procedure will never produce totally perfect skin. It is impossible to predict those patients with acne scarring who will respond to treatment and those who will not.

Following the procedure you will experience swelling, bleeding and weeping of the skin for several days. You will need to have a dressing in place during this time to protect your skin. As a general rule 1-2 weeks is required for wound healing, at which time you may return to work. You will experience a burning feeling for 10-90 minutes after the procedure which is likened to sunburn. This is normal.

It is very important for you to notify us of any personal or family history of herpes simplex [cold sores] and/or minor skin disorders which may affect wound healing.

B. ANAESTHETIC

The procedure is usually performed under local anaesthetic. You are not required to fast prior to the procedure.

In some instances where a general anaesthetic may be required, you need to fast prior to the procedure and you should not drive yourself home following the procedure.

C. LIMITATIONS AND RISKS ASSOCIATED WITH THE PROCEDURE

They may include, but are not limited to:

(a) Wound healing: the Laser will create a superficial wound to the skin which takes several weeks to heal.

(b) Pigment changes: The treated area may heal with increased pigmentation. This often occurs more often in darker pigmented skin and following exposure to of the area to sun. You must protect yourself from the sun at all times by using a 30+ broad spectrum sunscreen and by limiting exposure for the first three months. Hyperpigmentation usually fades within three to six months. However, pigment change can be permanent. Loss of pigmentation is also possible, but extremely rare.

(c) Swelling: There will be some swelling of the skin post procedure and this will resolve within 3-7 days.

(d) Scarring: Patients who have had Roaccutane therapy have an increased risk of abnormal scarring.

(e) Eye exposure: There is risk of harmful eye exposure to laser surgery. Safeguards will be provided and it is important to keep eyes closed and wear protective eyewear during the treatment.

D. PATIENT CONSENT

I acknowledge that:

The Doctor has explained the proposed procedure. I understand the risks of the procedure, including the risks that are specific to me, and the likely outcomes.

The Doctor has explained other relevant treatment options ad their associated risks.

The Doctor has explained my prognosis and risks of not having the procedure.

I have been given a Patient Information Brochure

I was able to ask questions and raise concerns with the Doctor about the procedure, its risks and my treatment options. My questions and concerns have been discussed and answered to my satisfaction. I understand that a Doctor other than the Consultant Physician may conduct the procedure. I understand this could be a Doctor undertaking further training.

The Doctor has explained to me that if immediate life-threatening events happen during the procedure, they will be treated accordingly.

E. PATIENT PHOTOGRAPHY

I understand that photographs or video footage may be taken during my procedure. These may then be used for teaching health professionals, may be published in scientific journals and or shown for scientific reasons. I will not be identified in any photo or video. These items will remain the property of Dr. Greg Goodman.

F. PATIENT GUARANTEE

I understand that **NO** guarantee has been made that the procedure will improve my condition, and that the procedure may make my condition worse.

On the basis of the above statements, I agree to

- keep Dr. Greg Goodman and his practice informed of any details regarding my change of address, so that he may notify me of any late findings.
- I agree to cooperate with Dr. Greg Goodman in regard to my treatment after surgery until completely discharged.

I REQUEST TO HAVE THE PROCEDURE

NAME OF PATIENT:..
[PLEASE PRINT]

SIGNATURE:..Date:...........

G. PRACTITIONER STATEMENT

I have explained

- The patient's condition
- Need and type of treatment
- The procedure and the risks
- Relevant treatment options and their risks
- Likely consequences if those risks occur
- The significant risks and problems specific to this patient

I have given the patient an opportunity to

- Ask questions about any of the above matters
- Raise any other concerns

Signed:...Date:....................

Dr Greg Goodman & Associates Dermatology & Cosmetic Procedures September 2005

Fig. 1.36. Erbium and/or CO_2 laser consent form

FRAXEL™ — Procedural Consent Form

A. CONDITION & PROCEDURE

The Doctor has explained that I have the following condition: *[Patient to document in patient's own words]*

....

....

....

The following procedure will be performed: ***'Fraxel ™ Laser Treatment.*** There are risks associated with any medical procedure. Since it is impossible to state every risk or complication that may occur as a result of any treatment, the possible risks and complications listed in this informed consent may be incomplete. There may be risks or complications associated with this treatment that are unknown because Fraxel ™ Laser Treatment is a new procedure.

- I have been adequately informed of my alternative treatment options, and the risks of the proposed surgery.
- I understand that some of the areas being treated have not been cleared by the FDA (Food & Drug Administration) and give my permission for such treatment.
- I have been informed and understand that the time period for improvement [if any] is not yet known.
- I have been informed and understand that there may be a prickling sensation and some discomfort during the procedure.

B. ANAESTHETIC

The procedure is usually performed under local anaesthetic.

C. LIMITATIONS AND RISKS ASSOCIATED WITH THE PROCEDURE

They may include, but are not limited to:

(a) Mild Sunburn: you will experience a mild sunburn sensation for 1 to 2 hours after treatment.

(b) Bronzing: Your skin will have a bronze appearance for 3 to 14 days, depending on the treatment level.

(c) Flaking: Your skin will naturally and vigorously exfoliate as the reorganised skin replaces dead tissue. Use of a moisturiser will mask the appearance of flaking.

(d) Scarring: There is a small chance of skin scarring, including abnormal raised scars. Scarring is a possibility because of the disruption of the skin's surface.

(e) Bleeding: The laser treatment may cause some pinpoint bleeding which will not leave any lasting effect. In some instances bleeding may reach the upper level of the skin and may result in dark reddening of the skin. This will disappear in one to two weeks.

(f) Blistering: The laser may produce heating in the upper layers of the skin resulting in steam formation. The steam may produce a separation between the upper and middles layers of the skin resulting in a blister formation. This will subside in two to four days. Scabbing: A scab may be present after a blister forms. This will disappear during the natural healing process of the skin.

(g) Redness & Swelling: will vary depending upon your skin and the treatment. Swelling generally resolves in two to three days.

D. PATIENT CONSENT

I acknowledge that:

The Doctor has explained the proposed procedure. I understand the risks of the procedure, including the risks that are specific to me, and the likely outcomes.
The Doctor has explained my prognosis and risks of not having the procedure.

I have been given a Patient Information Brochure

I was able to ask questions and raise concerns with the Doctor about the procedure, its risks and my treatment options. My questions and concerns have been discussed and answered to my satisfaction. I understand that a Doctor other than the Consultant Physician may conduct the procedure. I understand this could be a Doctor undertaking further training.
The Doctor has explained to me that if immediate life-threatening events happen during the procedure, they will be treated accordingly.

E. PATIENT PHOTOGRAPHY

I understand that photographs or video footage may be taken during my procedure. These may then be used for teaching health professionals, may be published in scientific journals and or shown for scientific reasons. I will not be identified in any photo or video. These items will remain the property of Dr. Greg Goodman.

F. PATIENT GUARANTEE

I understand that **NO** guarantee has been made that the procedure will improve my condition, and that the procedure may make my condition worse. I understand that more than one treatment will be required.
On the basis of the above statements, I agree to:

- keep Dr. Greg Goodman and his practice informed of any details regarding my change of address, so that he may notify me of any late findings.
- I agree to cooperate with Dr. Greg Goodman in regard to my treatment after surgery until completely discharged.

I REQUEST TO HAVE THE PROCEDURE

NAME OF PATIENT:...
[PLEASE PRINT]

SIGNATURE:...**Date:**...........

G. PRACTITIONER STATEMENT

I have explained

- The patient's condition
- Need and type of treatment
- The procedure and the risks
- Relevant treatment options and their risks
- Likely consequences if those risks occur
- The significant risks and problems specific to this patient

I have given the patient an opportunity to

- Ask questions about any of the above matters
- Raise any other concerns

Signed:..**Date:**....................

Greg Goodman Dermatology & Cosmetic Procedures June 2006

Fig. 1.37. Fractionated photothermolysis (Fraxel) consent form

KTP, YAG, Vbeam® LASER, 755nm — Procedural Consent Form

A. CONDITION & PROCEDURE

The Doctor has explained that I have the following condition: *[Patient to document in patient's own words]*

....

....

....

The following procedure will be performed:

KTP, YAG,Vbeam® LASER

- Laser treatment is used to interact specifically with a target in the skin
- Birthmarks, scars and blood vessels or vascular disorders, flushing and erythema as well as pigmented lesions may be treated.
- Once the laser beam has located the target, the laser causes a localised heating that destroys the target.
- Blood vessels and red scars are usually destroyed underneath the skin and often may be treated without disrupting the top. Swelling from the newly damaged blood vessels is common and occasionally bruising may be seen.
- Brown spots are often in the top layer of the skin and their treatment will produce a scab, blister or crust.
- Laser treatment and your condition may [but not always] need more than one treatment. The degree of improvement varies between patients and conditions being treated.
- During the procedure special glasses or other protection will be worn to protect your eyes from the laser beam.
- If a healing period is required [due to scabs, blisters or crust etc] the time will vary from 1 week for facial spots, to 2-3 weeks for spots on the body. Make-up may be used if the scab is very light. Open wounds or heavy scabs will need antibiotic cream. It is important not to disturb the scab.
- A slight amount of redness around the wound may be seen and is part of normal wound healing process.
- In rare cases soreness or redness of an open wound may increase. In this event you should report this to us, as it may signify infection and antibiotics may be required.

B. ANAESTHETIC

The procedure is usually performed under local anaesthetic.

C. LIMITATIONS AND RISKS ASSOCIATED WITH THE PROCEDURE

They may include, but are not limited to:

(a) **Soreness-Redness:** In rare instances soreness and redness of an open wound may increase. In this event you should contact us as it may signify infection and antibiotics may be required.

(b) **Swelling:** This is common especially on the upper cheeks, forehead and nose. This usually subsides within a few days. Ice is applied after treatment to limit swelling, and further application at home may be helpful. Sleeping a little more upright for extensive procedures is recommended for the first two nights.

(c) **Pain:** There may be some pain during the procedure.

(d) **Pigment Loss:** In most patients with brown spots, the area loses colour temporarily. This type of reaction tends to gradually fade, returning to normal over a period of 2-4 weeks. There is a small risk of permanent pigment loss.

(e) **Hyperpigmentation**: There may be a risk of increased pigmentation as a healing reaction in olive skinned patients. If this occurs the increased pigment usually fades over a period of months and may require the use of bleaching creams. Occasionally it may last longer, but rarely is this permanent.

(f) **Scarring:** There is a very small incidence of scarring, including indented and thickened scars. Scarring is rare but may occur

(g) **Incomplete Result:** The condition being treated may not be completely or even effectively treated with one treatment and may require another session/s or the same or different modality.

D. PATIENT CONSENT

I acknowledge that:

The Doctor has explained the proposed procedure. I understand the risks of the procedure, including the risks that are specific to me, and the likely outcomes. The Doctor has explained other relevant treatment options ad their associated risks. The Doctor has explained my prognosis and risks of not having the procedure.

I have been given a Patient Information Brochure

I was able to ask questions and raise concerns with the Doctor about the procedure, its risks and my treatment options. My questions and concerns have been discussed and answered to my satisfaction. I understand that a Doctor other than the Consultant Physician may conduct the procedure. I understand this could be a Doctor undertaking further training. The Doctor has explained to me that if immediate life-threatening events happen during the procedure, they will be treated accordingly.

E. PATIENT PHOTOGRAPHY

I understand that photographs or video footage may be taken during my procedure. These may then be used for teaching health professionals, may be published in scientific journals and or shown for scientific reasons. I will not be identified in any photo or video. These items will remain the property of Dr. Greg Goodman.

F. PATIENT GUARANTEE

I understand that **NO** guarantee has been made that the procedure will improve my condition, and that the procedure may make my condition worse.

On the basis of the above statements, I agree to

- keep Dr. Greg Goodman and his practice informed of any details regarding my change of address, so that he may notify me of any late findings.
- I agree to cooperate with Dr. Greg Goodman in regard to my treatment after surgery until completely discharged.

I REQUEST TO HAVE THE PROCEDURE

NAME OF PATIENT:..

SIGNATURE:..**Date**:...........

G. PRACTITIONER STATEMENT

I have explained

- The patient's condition
- Need and type of treatment
- The procedure and the risks
- Relevant treatment options and their risks
- Likely consequences if those risks occur
- The significant risks and problems specific to this patient

I have given the patient an opportunity to

- Ask questions about any of the above matters
- Raise any other concerns

Signed:..**Date**:....................

Greg Goodman Dermatology & Cosmetic Procedures June 2006

Fig. 1.38. V Beam, potassium tritanyl phosphate (KTP), yttrium aluminum garnet (YAG), 755-nm, long-pulse consent form

SMOOTH BEAM | Procedural Consent Form

A. CONDITION & PROCEDURE

The Doctor has explained that I have the following condition:
[Patient to document in patient's own words]

....

....

....

....

The following procedure will be performed:
SMOOTHBEAM is employed to assist in the treatment of active acne lesions, acne scarring as well as fine lines and wrinkles. It does this by a combination of heating as well as cooling of the skin. A local anaesthetic cream may be applied to reduce any discomfort experienced during the treatment. During treatment a cryogen spray is applied which protects the top layer of skin [epidermis]. There may be some degree of local discomfort during the laser pulse. The Smoothbeam laser has proven to be a very safe laser with a low rate of complications.
You are required to cease using any Retin A creams prior to your Smoothbeam treatment.

B. ANAESTHETIC

The procedure is usually performed under local anaesthetic. You are not required to fast prior to the procedure.

C. LIMITATIONS AND RISKS ASSOCIATED WITH THE PROCEDURE

They may include, but are not limited to:

(a) **WOUND HEALING** The treated area will be initially pink or red. Possible papules blisters may form soon after treatment. Ice packs can be applied to reduce swelling that may occur. Make –up may be used if a scab is very light. Open wounds or heavy scabs will need an antibiotic cream. Do not disturb the scab, and you may notice a slight amount of redness around the wound – this is part of the normal healing process. If soreness and redness increase, you should report this as it may be an indication of infection.

(b) **ALLERGY** It is possible to be allergic to anaesthetic cream. If you know of any allergies you may have, please inform the doctor prior to signing t his consent.

(c) **INCOMPLETE RESULT** The condition being treated may not be effectively treated with treatment and may require further sessions of the same or different treatment modality.

(d) **HYPERPIGMENTATION** This may occur after initial healing is complete. It is more common with olive skinned patients, as well as those who expose themselves to the sun during the healing phase.

(e) **LOSS/DECREASE IN SKIN COLOUR** This is rare and is usually temporary, but on occasions could be permanent.

(f) **SWELLING** is common, especially on the upper cheeks and nose. Swelling usually subsides in a few days. Ice is applied after treatment to limit swelling, and further application at home may be helpful.

D. PATIENT CONSENT

I acknowledge that:

The Doctor has explained the proposed procedure. I understand the risks of the procedure, including the risks that are specific to me, and the likely outcomes.
The Doctor has explained other relevant treatment options ad their associated risks.
The Doctor has explained my prognosis and risks of not having the procedure.
I have been given a Patient Information Brochure
I was able to ask questions and raise concerns with the Doctor about the procedure, its risks and my treatment options. My questions and concerns have been discussed and answered to my satisfaction. I understand that a Doctor other than the Consultant Physician may conduct the procedure. I understand this could be a Doctor undertaking further training. The Doctor has explained to me that if immediate life-threatening events happen during the procedure, they will be treated accordingly.

E. PATIENT PHOTOGRAPHY

I understand that photographs or video footage may be taken during my procedure. These may then be used for teaching health professionals, may be published in scientific journals and or shown for scientific reasons. I will not be identified in any photo or video. These items will remain the property of Dr. Greg Goodman.

F. PATIENT GUARANTEE

I understand that **NO** guarantee has been made that the procedure will improve my condition, and that the procedure may make my condition worse.
On the basis of the above statements, I agree to

- keep Dr. Greg Goodman and his practice informed of any details regarding my change of address, so that he may notify me of any late findings.
- I agree to cooperate with Dr. Greg Goodman in regard to my treatment after surgery until completely discharged.

I REQUEST TO HAVE THE PROCEDURE

NAME OF PATIENT:...
[PLEASE PRINT]

SIGNATURE:...**Date:**...........

G. PRACTITIONER STATEMENT

I have explained

- The patient's condition
- Need and type of treatment
- The procedure and the risks
- Relevant treatment options and their risks
- Likely consequences if those risks occur
- The significant risks and problems specific to this patient

I have given the patient an opportunity to

- Ask questions about any of the above matters
- Raise any other concerns

Signed:...**Date:**...................

Greg Goodman Dermatology & Cosmetic Procedures June 2006

Fig. 1.39. 1450-nm Smoothbeam laser consent form

prefer Q-switched lasers or intense pulsed light sources of LED systems

1. Look for other signs of epidermal photodamage such as solar keratoses and, if present, add short-contact topical aminolevulinic acid to visible lasers, light-source, or LED treatments.
2. Look for signs of acne. If acne is predominant then consider colored light (blue, green, yellow) laser, LED, or intense pulsed light treatments with or without pretreatment with aminolevulinic acid. Mid-infrared laser treatments can also be used.
3. Look for problems of skin texture. This can usually be addressed by many of the visible light lasers and light, infrared nonablative, and ablative laser treatments.
4. Look for wrinkling. If present at rest, and mild, consider longer-wavelength cutoff filters on intense pulsed light treatments. As an alternative, consider mid-infrared (1320-, 1450-, 1540-nm) lasers. If more significant, and present at rest, consider ablation with erbium or portrait plasma skin resurfacing. If severe wrinkles are present, consider CO_2 or more aggressive erbium laser treatments. Since botulinum toxin injections have been shown to be synergistic with ablative and nonablative therapies it should probably be offered to some of these patients (see Chap. 4).
5. Look for postacne scarring. If acne scarring is mild to moderate and is saucerized in type, consider mid-infrared laser treatment. This may be undertaken with or without alternative techniques such as scar undermining (subcision). If deeper scars are present, consider fractionated, ablative, or plasma skin resurfacing (often in association with other ancillary techniques such as scar excision, punch techniques, and/or fat transfer). If hypertrophic scarring is evident then flash lamp pumped-dye laser treatments may be considered.
6. Look for unusual facial conditions that require removal. These include benign growths (seborrheic keratoses, sebaceous hyperplasia, syringomas, and fibrous papules). Such conditions require either ablative laser treatments or treatment with visible-light-based technologies, depending on their color and other characteristic presentations

Postoperative Care and Complications

Ablative Lasers

1. Guard against infection. The patient should be screened for a history of herpes simplex virus and started on appropriate antiviral treatment the day before the procedure. This should be continued throughout the postoperative period. Many practitioners add antibiotic treatment throughout the healing period; others do not. The same controversy applies to prophylactic antimonilial prophylaxis. Infection with bacteria, candida, and herpes simplex virus must be recognized and treated judiciously.
2. Moist dressings are applied to the freshly resurfaced skin throughout the reepithelialization period.
3. Psychological support. Patients who undergo ablative laser resurfacing require support during the healing phase and throughout the next several months
4. Scarring may occur if delayed wound healing occurs. This may be the result of infection, excessive treatment, or from self-inflicted trauma during the healing phase (Fig. 1.40)
5. One of the most problematic problems after ablative laser resurfacing is pigmentary alteration. This may take the form of hypo or hyperpigmentation. Hyperpigmentation is more common in olive-skinned patients and is usually temporary; hypopigmentation is more of a concern in females of Fitzpatrick skin type 1 or 2 and can be permanent (Fig. 1.41).

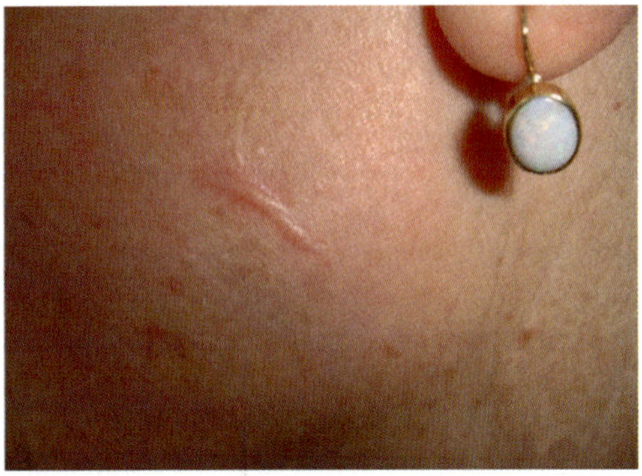

Fig. 1.40. Scar after CO_2 and erbium laser resurfacing

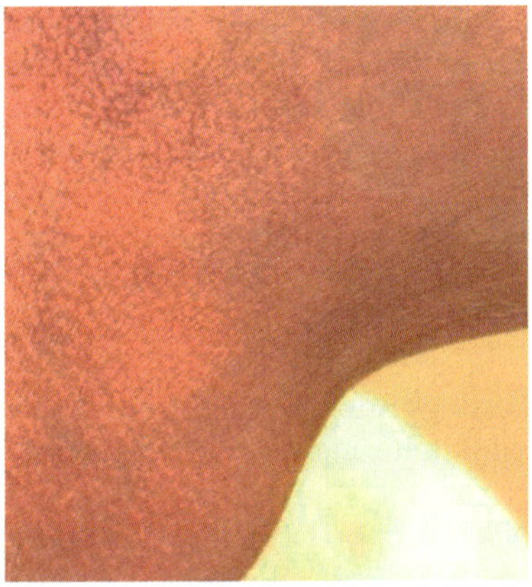

Fig. 1.41. Relative hypopigmentation due to removal of facial sun-damaged skin

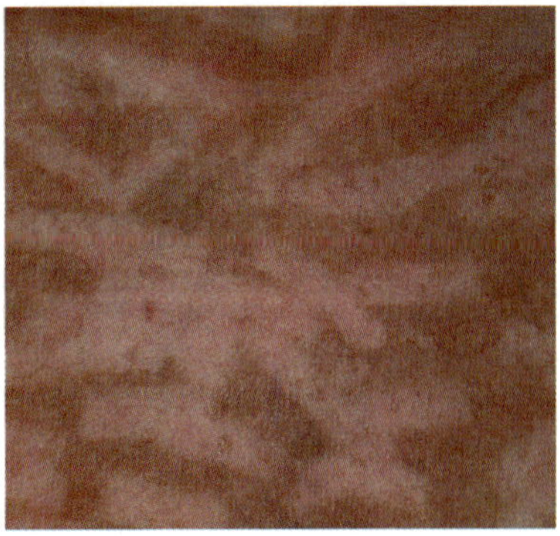

Fig. 1.42. Hypopigmentation secondary to intense pulsed light treatment on suntanned skin

Nonablative Treatments

1. Intraoperative symptoms, such as pain of treatment, are expected to some degree. This may be ameliorated by prior use of local anesthetic creams.
2. Short-term sequelae such as scabbing, crusting, blistering, and purpura may occur. Such sequelae may resolve spontaneously or may become longer-term problems.
3. Scarring and pigmentary complications or reactivation of herpes simplex virus and other infections can occur, albeit rarely considering the number of treatments performed (Fig. 1.42.)

The Future

The future of laser and light technologies is clearly dependent upon the continuing expansion of both indications and new technologies. There is likely to be continued erosion of indications for ablative treatment, with a gradual shift to nonablative therapies. Such a transition will also involve fewer required treatments and with a continuing improvement in safety profile. In addition, one can expect a continued growth of alternatives to lights and lasers such as seen with radiofrequency and plasma treatments. Innovative "intelligent" handpieces should be expected. Better anesthetic creams and better cooling devices may also lead to easier patient treatments. Fractional photothermolysis involving multiple wavelengths is likely.

Larger delivery heads, more powerful machines allowing more rapid treatment and various combinations of lights and radiofrequency may be developed. Multiplatform machines either offering many lasers within one unit, or containing lasers and lights within individual detachable handpieces are awaited. One should also expect further refinement of PDT. Finally, additional skin chromophores, such as those that occur in fat, may be found and more specifically targeted either singly or in combination with plasma, ultrasound, radiofrequency, and new light-based treatments.

References

1. Einstein A (1916) Letter to Michele Angelo Besso, November 1916
2. Anderson RR, Parrish JA (1983) Selective photothermolysis: precise microsurgery by selective absorption of pulsed radiation. Science 220:24–27
3. Asawanonda P, Anderson RR, Chang Y, et al (2001) 308-nm excimer laser for the treatment of psoriasis: a dose–response study. Arch Dermatol 137:95–96
4. Bonis B, Kemeny L, Dobozy A, et al (1997) 308 nm UVB excimer laser for psoriasis. Lancet 350:1522
5. Nistico S, Costanzo A, Saraceno R, et al (2004) Efficacy of monochromatic excimer laser radiation (308 nm) in the treatment of early stage mycosis fungoides. Br J Dermatol 151:877–879
6. Baltas E, Csoma Z, Bodai L, et al (2006) Treatment of atopic dermatitis with the xenon chloride excimer laser. J Eur Acad Dermatol Venereol 20:657–660
7. Bianchi B, Campolmi P, Mavilia L, et al (2003) Monochromatic excimer light (308 nm): an immunohistochemical study of cutaneous T cells and apoptosis-related molecules in psoriasis. J Eur Acad Dermatol Venereol 17:408–413
8. Goodman GJ, Roberts S, Bezborodoff A (2002) Studies in long-pulsed potassium tritanyl phosphate laser for the treatment of spider naevi and perialar telangiectasia. Australas J Dermatol 43:9–14
9. Marmur ES, Schmults CD, Goldberg DJ (2004) A review of laser and photodynamic therapy for the treatment of nonmelanoma skin cancer. Dermatol Surg 30:264–271
10. Dierickx CC, Anderson RR (2005) Visible light treatment of photoaging. Dermatol Ther 18:191–208
11. Weiss RA, Weiss MA, Geronemus RG, et al (2004) A novel nonthermal nonablative full panel led photomodulation device for reversal of photoaging: digital microscopic and clinical results in various skin types. J Drugs Dermatol 3:605–610
12. Fitzpatrick RE, Tope WD, Goldman MP, et al (1996) Pulsed carbon dioxide laser, trichloroacetic acid, Baker-Gordon phenol, and dermabrasion: a comparative clinical and histologic study of cutaneous resurfacing in a porcine model. Arch Dermatol 132:469–471
13. Papadavid E, Katsambas A (2003) Lasers for facial rejuvenation: a review. Int J Dermatol 42:480–487
14. Waldorf HA, Kauvar ANB, Geronemus RG (1995) Skin resurfacing of fine to deep rhytides using a char-free carbon dioxide laser in 47 patients. Dermatol Surg 21:940–946
15. Lowe NJ, Lask G, Griffin ME, et al (1995) Skin resurfacing with the Ultrapulse carbon dioxide laser. Observations on 100 patients. Dermatol Surg 21:1025–1029
16. Bernstein L, Kauvar ANB, Grossman M, et al (1998) Scar resurfacing with high-energy, short-pulsed and flashscanning carbon dioxide lasers. Dermatol Surg 24:101–107
17. Lask G, Keller G, Lowe N, et al (1995) Laser skin resurfacing with the SilkTouch flashscanner for facial rhytides. Dermatol Surg 21:1021–1024
18. Bernstein LJ, Kauvar ANB, Grossman MC, et al (1997) The short- and long-term side effects of carbon dioxide laser resurfacing. Dermatol Surg 23:519–525
19. Laws RA, Finley EM, McCollough ML, et al (1998) Alabaster skin after carbon dioxide laser resurfacing with histologic correlation. Dermatol Surg 24:633–636
20. Mulekar SV, Al Issa A, Al Eisa A, et al (2005) Genital vitiligo treated by autologous, noncultured melanocyte–keratinocyte cell transplantation. Dermatol Surg 31:1737–1739
21. Van Geel N, Ongenae K, De Mil M, et al (2001) Modified technique of autologous noncultured epidermal cell transplantation for repigmenting vitiligo: a pilot study. Dermatol Surg 27:873–876
22. Kaufmann R (2001) Role of Erbium:YAG laser in the treatment of aged skin. Clin Exp Dermatol 26:631–636
23. Kaufmann R, Hibst R (1996) Pulsed Erbium:YAG laser ablation in cutaneous surgery. Lasers Surg Med 19:324–330
24. Pozner JM, Goldberg DJ (2000) Histologic effect of a variable pulsed Er:YAG laser. Dermatol Surg 26:733–736
25. Tanzi EL, Alster TS (2003) Single-pass carbon dioxide versus multiple-pass Er:YAG laser skin resurfacing: a comparison of postoperative wound healing and side-effect rates. Dermatol Surg 29:80–84
26. Collawn SS (1999) Combination therapy: utilisation of CO_2 and Erbium:YAG lasers for skin resurfacing. Ann Plast Surg 42:21–26
27. Goldman MP, Marchell N, Fitzpatrick RE (2000) Laser skin resurfacing of the face with a combined CO_2/Er:YAG laser. Dermatol Surg 26:102–104
28. Jacob CI, Dover JS, Kaminer MS (2001) Acne scarring: a classification system and review of

treatment options. J Am Acad Dermatol 45:109–117
29. McDaniel DH, Lord J, Ash K, et al (1999) Combined CO_2/Erbium:YAG laser resurfacing of perioral rhytids and side to side comparison with carbon dioxide laser alone. Dermatol Surg 25:285–293
30. Fink B, Grammer K, Matts PJ (2006) Visible skin color distribution plays a role in the perception of age, attractiveness, and health in female faces. Evol Hum Behav 27:433–442
31. Goldberg DJ (1997) Laser treatment of pigmented lesions. Dermatol Clin 15:397–407
32. Goldman MP, Bennett MD (1987) Treatment of telangiectasia: a review. J Am Acad Dermatol 17:167–182
33. Gonzales E, Gange RW, Momtaz KT (1992) Treatment of telangiectases and other benign vascular lesions with the 577 nm pulsed dye laser. J Am Acad Dermatol 27:220–221
34. Goodman, GJ, Bekhor P, Richards S (1996) Advances in laser therapy – the importance of selective photothermolysis. Med J Aust 164:681–686
35. Hellwig S, Schonermark M, Raulin C (1995) Treatment of vascular malformations and pigment disorders of the face and neck by pulsed dye laser, Photoderm VL and Q-switched ruby laser. Laryngorhinootologie 74:635–641
36. McCoy SE (1997) Copper bromide laser treatment of facial telangiectasia: results of patients treated over five years. Lasers Surg Med 21:329–340
37. Parish LC, Witkowski JA (1991) Telangiecatasia. In: Parish LC, Lask GP (eds) Aesthetic Dermatology. McGraw Hill, New York, pp 96–100
38. Ramelet AA (1998) Telangiectases. In: Baran R, Maibach HI (eds) Textbook of Cosmetic Dermatology, 2nd edn. Martin Dunitz, London, pp 373–380
39. Thibault PK (1997) A patient's questionnaire evaluation of krypton laser treatment of facial telangiectases. A comparison with the copper vapor laser. Dermatol Surg 23:37–41
40. Chambers IR, Clark D, Bainbridge C (1990) Automation of laser treatment of port wine stains. Phys Med Biol 7:1025–1028
41. McDaniel DH, Mordon S (1990) Hexascan: a new robotized scanning laser handpiece. Cutis 45:300–305
42. Mordon SR, Rotteleur G, Buys B, et al (1989) Comparative study of the „point-by-point technique" and the „scanning technique" for laser treatment of port-wine stain. Lasers Surg Med 9:398–404
43. Rotteleur G; Mordon S; Buys B, et al (1988) Robotized scanning laser handpiece for the treatment of port wine stains and other angiodysplasias. Lasers Surg Med 8:283–287
44. Achauer BM, Vander Kam VM, Padilla JF III (1993) Clinical experience with the tunable pulsed-dye laser (585 nm) in the treatment of capillary vascular malformations. Plast Reconstr Surg 92:1233–1241
45. Garden JM, Bakus AD (1993) Clinical efficacy of the pulsed dye laser in the treatment of vascular lesions. J Dermatol Surg Oncol 19:321–326
46. Bassichis BA, Swamy R, Dayan SH (2004) Use of the KTP laser in the treatment of rosacea and solar lentigines. Facial Plast Surg 20:77–83
47. Lee MW (2003) Combination 532-nm and 1064-nm lasers for noninvasive skin rejuvenation and toning. Arch Dermatol 139:1265–1276
48. Chess C, Chess Q (1993) Cool laser optics treatment of large telangiectasia of the lower extremities. J Dermatol Surg Oncol 19:74–80
49. Dreno B, Patrice T, Litoux P, et al (1985) The benefit of chilling in argon-laser treatment of port-wine stains. Plast Reconstr Surg 75:42–45
50. Dummer R, Graf P, Greif C, et al (1998) Treatment of vascular lesions using the Versapulse variable pulse width frequency doubled neodymium:YAG laser. Dermatology 197:158–161
51. Gilchrest BA, Rosen S, Noe JM (1982) Chilling port wine stains improves the response to argon laser therapy. Plast Reconstr Surg 69:278–83
52. Nelson JS, Milner TE, Anvari B, et al (1996) Dynamic epidermal cooling in conjunction with laser induced photo thermolysis of port wine stain blood vessels. Lasers Surg Med 19:224–229
53. Waldorf HA, Alster TS, McMillan K, et al (1997) Effect of dynamic cooling on 585nm pulsed dye laser treatment of port wine stain birthmarks. Dermatol Surg 23:657–662
54. White JM, Siegfried E, Boulden M, et al (1999) Possible hazards of cryogen use with pulsed dye laser. A case report and summary. Dermatol Surg 25:250–252
55. Wang CC, Sue YM, Yang CH, et al (2006) A comparison of Q-switched alexandrite laser and intense pulsed light for the treatment of freckles and lentigines in Asian persons: a randomized, physician-blinded, split-face comparative trial. J Am Acad Dermatol 54:804–810
56. Huang YL, Liao YL, Lee SH, et al (2002) Intense pulsed light for the treatment of facial freckles in Asian skin. Dermatol Surg 28:1007–1012
57. Moody BR, McCarthy JE, Hruza GJ (2003) Collagen remodeling after 585-nm pulsed dye laser irradiation: an ultrasonographic analysis. Dermatol Surg 29:997–999
58. Dang Y, Ren Q, Hoecker S, et al (2005) Biophysical, histological and biochemical changes

after non-ablative treatments with the 595 and 1320 nm lasers: a comparative study. Photodermatol Photoimmunol Photomed 21:204–209
59. Dang Y, Ren Q, Li W, et al (2006) Comparison of biophysical properties of skin measured by using non-invasive techniques in the KM mice following 595 nm pulsed dye, 1064 nm Q-Switched Nd:YAG and 1320 nm Nd:YAG laser non-ablative rejuvenation. Skin Res Technol 12:119–125
60. Omi T, Kawana S, Sato S, et al (2003) Ultrastructural changes elicited by a nonablative wrinkle reduction laser. Lasers Surg Med 32:46–49
61. Zelickson B, Kist D (2000) Effect of pulsed dye laser and intense pulse light source in dermal extracellular matrix remodeling. Lasers Surg Med S12: 68
62. Hsu TS, Zelickson B, Dover JS, et al (2005) Multicenter study of the safety and efficacy of a 585-nm pulsed-dye laser for the nonablative treatment of facial rhytides. Dermatol Surg 31:1–9
63. Bjerring P, Clement M, Heickendorff L, et al (2000) Selective non-ablative wrinkle reduction by laser. J Cutan Laser Ther 2:9–15
64. Patel N, Clement M (2002) Selective nonablative treatment of acne scarring with 585 nm flashlamp pulsed dye laser. Dermatol Surg 28:942–945
65. Rostan E, Bowes LE, Iyer S, et al (2001) A double-blind, side-by-side comparison study of low fluence long pulse dye laser to coolant treatment for wrinkling of the cheeks. J Cosmet Laser Ther 3:129–136
66. Goldberg DJ, Sarradet D, Hussain M, et al (2004) Clinical, histologic, and ultrastructural changes after nonablative treatment with a 595-nm flashlamp-pumped pulsed dye laser: comparison of varying settings. Dermatol Surg 30:979–982
67. Trelles MA, Allones I, Levy JL, et al (2004) Combined nonablative skin rejuvenation with the 595- and 1450-nm lasers. Dermatol Surg 30:1292–1298
68. Kono T, Manstein D, Chan HH, et al (2006) Q-switched ruby versus long-pulsed dye laser delivered with compression for treatment of facial lentigines in Asians. Lasers Surg Med 38:94–97
69. Bitter PH (2000) Noninvasive rejuvenation of photodamaged skin using serial, full-face intense pulsed light treatments. Dermatol Surg 26:835–842
70. Kligman DE, Zhen Y (2004) Intense pulsed light treatment of photoaged facial skin. Dermatol Surg 30:1085–1090
71. Raulin C, Weiss RA, Schonermark MP (1997) Treatment of essential telangiectasias with an intense pulsed light source (PhotoDerm VL). Dermatol Surg 23:941–945
72. Sadick NS, Weiss R, Kilmer S, et al (2004) Photorejuvenation with intense pulsed light: results of a multi-center study. J Drugs Dermatol 3:41–49
73. Schroeter CA, Neumann HA (1998) An intense light source. The photoderm VL-flashlamp as a new treatment possibility for vascular skin lesions. Dermatol Surg 24:43–48
74. Ross EV (2006) Laser versus intense pulsed light: competing technologies in dermatology. Lasers Surg Med 38:261–272
75. Weiss RA, Weiss MA, Beasley KL (2002) Rejuvenation of photoaged skin: 5 years results with intense pulsed light of the face, neck, and chest. Dermatol Surg 28:1115–1119
76. Weiss RA, Weiss MA (2006) Devices for nonablative photorejuvenation. In: Goldman MP (ed) Cutaneous and Cosmetic Laser Surgery. Mosby Elsevier, Philadelphia, pp 249–262
77. Bjerring P, Christiansen K, Troilius A, et al (2004) Facial photo rejuvenation using two different intense pulsed light (IPL) wavelength bands. Lasers Surg Med 34:120–126
78. Bitter P (2002) Report of a new technique for enhanced non-invasive skin rejuvenation using a dual mode, pulsed light and radio-frequency energy source: selective radio-thermolysis. J Cosm Dermatol 1:142–145
79. Cutroneo KR (2003) How is Type I procollagen synthesis regulated at the gene level during tissue fibrosis. J Cell Biochem 90:1–5
80. Kondo S (2000) The roles of cytokines in photoaging. J Dermatol Sci 23:S30–36
81. Goldberg DJ, Whitworth J (1997) Laser skin resurfacing with the Q-switched Nd:YAG laser. Dermatol Surg 23:903–906
82. Friedman PM, Jih MH, Skover GR, et al (2004) Treatment of atrophic facial acne scars with the 1064-nm Q-switched Nd:YAG laser: six-month follow-up study. Arch Dermatol 140:1337–1341
83. Dayan S, Damrose JF, Bhattacharyya TK, et al (2003) Histological evaluations following 1,064-nm Nd:YAG laser resurfacing. Lasers Surg Med 33:126–131
84. Dayan SH, Vartanian AJ, Menaker G, et al (2003) Nonablative laser resurfacing using the long-pulse (1064-nm) Nd:YAG laser. Arch Facial Plast Surg 5:310–315
85. Muccini JA Jr, O'Donnell FE Jr, Fuller T, et al (1998) Laser treatment of solar elastosis with epithelial preservation. Lasers Surg Med 23:121–127
86. Anvari B, Milner TE, Tanenbaum BS, et al (1995) Selective cooling of biological tissues: application for thermally mediated therapeutic procedures. Phys Med Biol 40:241–252

87. Goldberg DJ (1999) Non-ablative subsurface remodeling: clinical and histologic evaluation of a 1320-nm Nd:YAG laser. J Cut Las Ther 1:153–57
88. Kelly KM, Nelson JS, Lask GP, et al (1999) Cryogen spray cooling in combination with nonablative treatment of facial rhytides. Arch Dermatol 135:691–694
89. Lask G, Lee PK, Seyfzadeh M, et al (1997) Nonablative laser treatment of facial rhytids. SPIE Proc 2970:338–349
90. Nelson JS, Miller TE, Dave D, et al (1997) Clinical study of non-ablative laser treatment of facial rhytides. Lasers Surg Med 95:32–33
91. Bhatia AC, Dover JS, Arndt KA, et al (2006) Patient satisfaction and reported long-term therapeutic efficacy associated with 1,320 nm Nd:YAG laser treatment of acne scarring and photoaging. Dermatol Surg 32:346–352
92. Fatemi A, Weiss MA, Weiss RA (2002) Short-term histologic effects of nonablative resurfacing: results with a dynamically cooled millisecond-domain 1320 nm Nd:YAG laser. Dermatol Surg 28:172–176
93. Menaker GM, Wrone DA, Williams RM, et al (1999) Treatment of facial rhytides with a nonablative laser: a clinical and histologic study. Dermatol Surg 25:440–444
94. Goldberg DJ (2000) Full-face nonablative dermal remodelling with a 1320 nm Nd:YAG laser. Dermatol Surg 26:915–918
95. Rogachefsky AS, Hussain M, Goldberg DJ (2003) Atrophic and a mixed pattern of acne scars improved with a 1320-nm Nd:YAG laser. Dermatol Surg 29:904–908
96. Chan HH, Lam LK, Wong DS, et al (2004) Use of 1,320 nm Nd:YAG laser for wrinkle reduction and the treatment of atrophic acne scarring in Asians. Lasers Surg Med 34:98–103
97. Apikian MA, Goodman GJ, Roberts S (2007) Management of mild to moderate rhinophyma with a 1450-nm diode laser: report of five patients. Dermatol Surg (in press)
98. No D, McClaren M, Chotzen V, et al (2004) Sebaceous hyperplasia treated with a 1450-nm diode laser. Dermatol Surg 30:382–384
99. Paithankar DY, Ross EV, Saleh BA, et al (2002) Acne treatment with a 1450-nm wavelength laser and cryogen spray cooling. Lasers Surg Med 31:206–214
100. Tanzi EL, Williams CM, Alster TS (2003) Treatment of facial rhytides with a nonablative 1450 nm diode laser: a controlled clinical and histologic study. Dermatol Surg 29:124–128
101. Hardaway CA, Ross EV (2002) Nonablative laser skin remodeling. Dermatol Clin 20:97–111
102. Chua SH, Ang P, Khoo LS, et al (2004) Nonablative 1450-nm diode laser in the treatment of facial atrophic acne scars in type IV to V Asian skin: a prospective clinical study. Dermatol Surg 30:1287–1291
103. Tanzi EL, Alster TS (2004) Comparison of a 1450-nm diode laser and a 1320-nm Nd:YAG laser in the treatment of atrophic facial scars: a prospective clinical and histologic study. Dermatol Surg 30:152–157
104. Dahan S, Lagarde JM, Turlier V, et al (2004) Treatment of neck lines and forehead rhytids with a nonablative 1540-nm Er:glass laser: a controlled clinical study combined with the measurement of the thickness and the mechanical properties of the skin. Dermatol Surg 30:872–879
105. Fisher GH, Geronemus RG (2005) Short-term side effects of fractional photothermolysis. Dermatol Surg 31:1245–1249
106. Gupta AK, Ryder JE (2003) Photodynamic therapy and topical aminolevulinic acid: an overview. Am J Clin Dermatol 4:699–708
107. Piacquadio DJ, Chen DM, Farber HF, et al (2004) Photodynamic therapy with aminolevulinic acid topical solution and visible blue light in the treatment of multiple actinic keratoses of the face and scalp: investigator-blinded, phase 3, multicenter trials. Arch Dermatol 140:41–46
108. Goldman M, Atkin D (2003) ALA/PDT in the treatment of actinic keratosis: spot versus confluent therapy. J Cosmet Laser Ther 5:107–110
109. Taub AF (2004) Photodynamic therapy in dermatology: history and horizons. J Drugs Dermatol 3:S8–25
110. Ruiz-Rodriguez R, Sanz-Sanchez T, Cordoba S (2002) Photodynamic photorejuvenation. Dermatol Surg 28:742–744

Chapter 2

Photodynamic Photorejuvenation

2

Michael Gold

Core Messages

- Photodynamic photorejuvenation involves the use of a topical photosensitizer and a light source.
- A 20% solution of 5-aminolevulinic acid and a 20% methyl ester cream of 5-aminolevulinic acid are the two most commonly used topical photosensitizers.
- A variety of visible lasers and non-laser light sources can be used to activate the topical photosensitizer.
- Many aspects of photodamage can be treated with photodynamic photorejuvenation.

History

The field of aesthetic and cosmetic laser surgery has been enhanced by some of the outstanding contributions made by many who paved the way into aesthetic medicine before it was in vogue. Clinicians and researchers such as Kligman et al., who pioneered the early work with topical tretinoin [1] and showed its beneficial effects on the skin surface [2], and Voorhees et al. [3], who were the first to describe the effects of tretinoin on wrinkles and rhytides of the face have made significant early contributions. These studies were followed by those of Van Scott and Yu [4], who described the effects of alpha hydroxy acids and their usefulness in improving skin texture and tone.

Not to be outdone, groups of dermatologists forged ahead in the cosmetic aesthetic surgical arena, led by pioneering works in dermabrasion and chemical peeling of the skin. Physicians such as Kromeyer [5], Burks [6], Harmon and Yarborough [7], and Roenigk [8] taught us that through the use of diamond fraises or wire brushes, skin rejuvenation was possible. Physicians could produce outstanding cosmetic results when the devices were used properly and by skilled clinicians. Others, such as Brody and Hailey [9], Monheit [10], Coleman and Futrell [11], and Rubin [12], among others, laid the foundation for the use of superficial and medium-depth chemical peeling to cause a controlled wound to the skin, with the resultant healing leading to an enhanced cosmetic effect.

Lasers soon entered into the cosmetic foray, and through the early work of Goldman and Rockwell [13], and Anderson and Parish [14], and others, the term selective photothermolysis became commonplace in many dermatologic and aesthetic practices, allowing the clinician to treat an enormous array of cosmetic and aesthetic concerns. In the early 1990s, Goldman et al. [15] described the use of what is now simply known as the IPL, or the intense pulsed light device, for the treatment of vascular lesions of the skin. This broadband wave light source provided physicians with the opportunity to selectively target a variety of concerns within photodamaged skin, allowing a new era of rejuvenation treatments to begin. Research quickly spread with the use of IPLs, including its expanded use into the world of permanent hair removal and pigmented lesion removal. Subsequent work by Goldberg and Cutler [16] and Zelickson et al. (personal communication) showed that, with several IPL treatments, collagen formation was achieved. Elastin studies demonstrated normalization of dermal structures, thus improving the skin's texture. By adding all of the benefits achieved with IPL, the era of "photorejuvenation" was created. Photorejuvenation, no more than an early laser company marketing tool, quickly became one of the most commonly performed cosmetic and aesthetic laser or "light-based" treatments. The reason for this phenomenon was really quite simple: IPL therapy led to a global improvement in patients' extensive photodamage. Vascular damage, manifest by telangectasias (pigmented changes, manifest by mottled hyperpigmentation and lentiginous lesions) and collagen changes, as seen in histologic analysis, were all improved.

Photorejuvenation, as a named procedure for aesthetic and cosmetic laser surgeons, took hold when Bitter, in 2000, published the first clinical manuscript on the topic of photorejuvenation [17]. In Bitter's study, more than 90% of the patients studied (n=49) had a greater than 75% improvement in rosacea symptoms (facial erythema and flushing), 84% had an improvement in their fine wrinkles, 78% had significant changes in their facial pigment, and 49% noted an improvement in their pore size. Each patient in that study received five full-face IPL treatments at a 1-month intervals. This is still the standard of care performed today. Others also noted improvements in photodamage (i.e., photorejuvenation with the IPLs), including several studies by Goldberg, Weiss, and Sadick [18–21]. In the studies by Goldberg [18, 19], one-third of the individuals (n=30) noted substantial improvements with their IPL treatments, while one-half of the subjects noted some improvement with the IPL. Weiss et al. [20], in a retrospective analysis of his IPL treated patients, found, that at 5 years, patients still maintained improvement in their skin texture (83%), telangectasias (82%), and dyschromia (79%). Furthermore, in work reported by Sadick [21], more than 90% of treated patients had improvement in their wrinkle appearance. Other important investigations included clinical studies by Negishi et al. [22], showing the effectiveness of IPL photorejuvenation treatments in the Asian population, and by Hernandez-Perez [23] showing improvement in patients of Hispanic ethnicity.

IPL photorejuvenation has become a mainstay in the aesthetic and cosmetic arena; it improves both vascular and pigmented concerns, and improves the collagen and elastic tissue changes associated with photodamaged skin. The procedure has become predictable and, in the right hands, with the proper training and guidance, is very safe and effective, with consistent results and minimum downtime. The fact that these treatments result in minimum downtime for patients is very significant and is one of the main reasons for its popularity today. As a result, the use of IPL has increased tremendously over the past several years, with now almost every laser company producing an IPL to compliment their laser portfolio. IPLs on the market today are better than ever, with squared-off pulses and efficient cooling systems being common features of today's devices. The various IPLs currently available are shown in Table 2.1.

IPL photorejuvenation is safe, effective, predictable, and is a minimum-downtime procedure. The success of IPL treatments has led to the obvious question. Is it possible to improve on the use of this procedure? A variety of clinical investigators have been pondering these questions for the past several years. Many believe this can be done through the use of photodynamic therapy (PDT) to enhance the photorejuvenation process.

PDT, in its simplest form, is a procedure that requires a photosensitizer, light, and oxygen. The most common photosensitizer available for use with PDT is 20% 5-aminolevulinic acid (ALA). Once applied to the skin, ALA is transformed into protoporphyrin IX (PpIX), the active ingredient required for a PDT reaction to occur. Previous work has shown that PpIX is absorbed into actinically damaged skin cells and into the pilosebaceous units of the skin. Upon exposure to a light source of a

Table 2.1. Intense pulsed light sources. IPL Intense pulsed light, FPL fluorescent pulsed light

Manufacturer	Brand Name
Adept Medical Concepts	SpectraPulse McCue Ultra Variable Pulsed Light™
American Medical Bio Care	Omnilight FPL Novalight FPL
Candela	Ellipse FPL
Cutera	CoolGlide Xeo Xeo SA Genesis Plus
Cynosure	Cynergy PL Cynergy III PhotoSilk Plus
DermaMed USA	Quadra Q4 Platinum Series
Laserscope	Solis
Lumenis	IPL Quantum SR VascuLight Elite Lumenis One
McCue	Ultra VPL
MedSurge Advances	Prolite II
Novalis	Clareon SR Solarus SR
Palomar	StarLux System MediLux System EsteLux System
Radiancy	SkinStation S P R
Sciton	Profile-MP Profile-S BBL
Syneron	Aurora SR Galaxy

proper wavelength, singlet oxygen is formed and a PDT reaction will occur, causing destruction of the cells in which PpIX has accumulated. The absorption curve for PpIX is shown in Fig. 2.1. Research with ALA-PDT initially focused on its use on actinic keratoses (AKs) and, in the United States, with blue light. Blue light was chosen because it coincides with the largest absorption band of PpIX, known as the Soret Band. But this wavelength is not the only wavelength that will activate ALA, and other lasers and light sources, as will be described below, also play key roles in the concept of "photodynamic photorejuvenation" [24].

Two ALA photosensitizing products are currently on the worldwide market, but only one at present, is on the market in the USA. Levulan Kerastick is a 20% ALA solution and is manufactured by Dusa Pharmaceuticals (Wilmington, MA, USA). Metvix, as the product is known in Europe and Australia, and Metvixia, as the product will be known in the USA, is the 20% methyl ester cream form of ALA, also readily identified as MAL. It is manufactured by PhotoCure ASA, Norway and is marketed by Galderma (Ft. Worth, TX, USA). Each one will be further described below.

In the USA, ALA, in the form of Levulan, has been approved by the Food and Drug Administration (FDA) for the treatment of nonhyperkeratotic AKs of the face and scalp, utilizing a 14- to 18-h drug incubation followed by exposure to blue light for 16 min 40 s [24]. Pivotal FDA trials have confirmed the effectiveness and safety of the product. In phase II clinical trials, 39 patients with extensive AKs of the face and scalp were subjected to 16 min 40 s of blue light after a 14- to 18-h ALA drug incubation. Pain associated with the light treatment was common, as was posttreatment erythema and edema, which eventually led to a crust formation, lasting up to 1 week. At the first evaluation point, 8 weeks following the ALA-PDT treatment, 66% of the individually treated AKs had cleared. Those AKs not cleared received a second treatment and at 16 weeks had an improved clinical efficacy of 85% [25]. A larger phase III clinical trial was subsequently undertaken in which 243 individuals participated. Individualized AKs were again treated with the ALA incubated for 14–18 h, then exposed to 16 min 40 s of blue light.

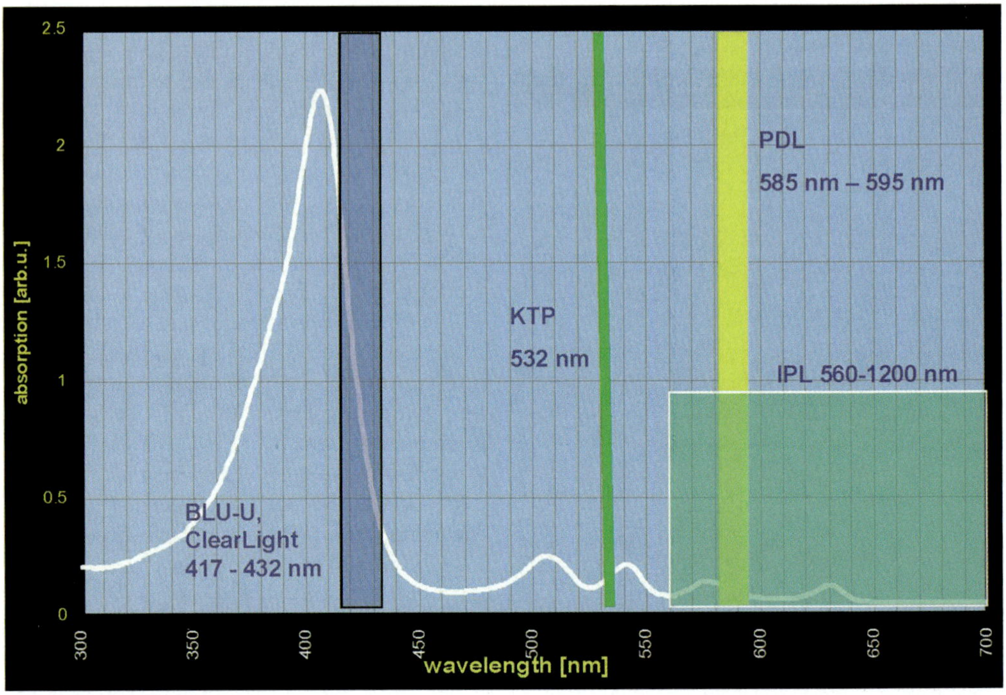

Fig. 2.1. Protoporphyrin IX (*PpIX*) absorption in vivo. *BLU-U* Blue light source, *KTP* potassium tritanyl phosphate, *PDL* pulsed-dye laser, *IPL* intense pulsed light

Study results showed that there was a greater than 70% complete clearance of the individual AKs at 12 weeks. Those AKs not cleared were once again treated and at the end of 24 weeks, the authors concluded that 88% of the individuals in the clinical trial had a greater than or equal to 75% clearance of their AKs as compared to 20% in the placebo group. An example of an AK treated during this trial is shown in Fig. 2.2. Posttreatment downtime, sometimes referred to as the "PDT effect," and pain associated with the light therapy were evident in the majority of individuals participating in this clinical trial. A secondary endpoint of this trial was that 94% of the individuals in the clinical trial rated their cosmetic appearance as either excellent or good [26]. The noted cosmetic improvement has stimulated further, more exciting clinical research.

Armenakas-Armenakas and Geronemus [27] reported on the use of a long-pulsed-dye laser (PDL) in the treatment of AKs of the face and scalp. These investigators noted that a short drug incubation with ALA was as successful as long drug incubation in the treatment of individual AKs.

In 2002, this author published his first experiences with ALA-PDT and a blue light source and noted that besides resolution of the treated AKs, some response was also being seen in contiguous areas, resulting in a "rejuvenation" effect, as shown in Fig. 2.3 [28]. A PDT effect was also quite evident in this series of patients. In order to address the PDT effect and to make the treatment easier and more acceptable to use amongst laser and aesthetic/cosmetic physicians, studies soon began focusing on shorter drug incubation times and full-face treatments, so that both clinical and subclinical AKs would be treated as a result of this therapy. In one of the most important studies evaluating ALA-PDT and this new treatment paradigm of full-face therapy, Touma et al. [29]

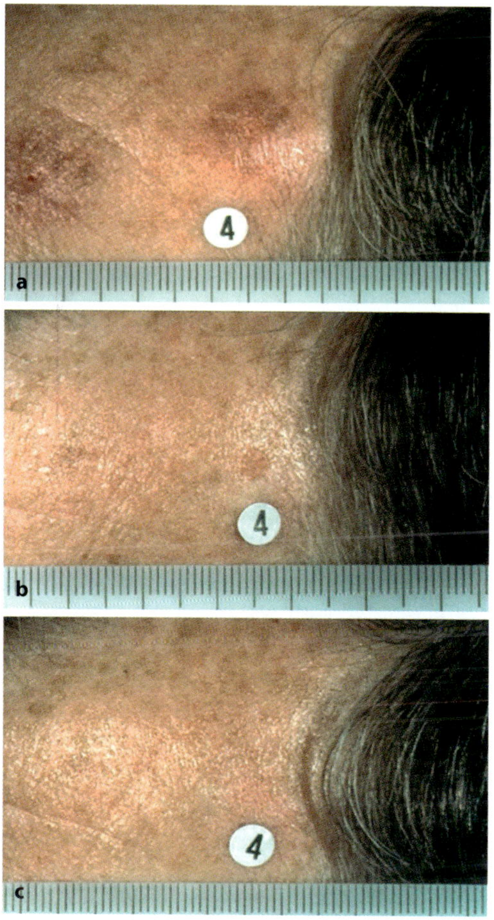

Fig. 2.2 a–c. Clinical example from a Levulan phase III trial. Photos courtesy of Dusa Pharmaceuticals, Wilmington, MA, USA

presented evidence that a 1-h drug incubation time was as efficacious as 14–18 h in improving the parameters of photodamage (i.e., photorejuvenation). Patients noted improvements in facial skin sallowness, fine wrinkling, and mottled hyperpigmentation. This study utilized a blue light source as the ALA activator.

Another important clinical trial was that of Ruiz-Rodriquez et al. [30], who also looked at a shorter drug incubation time (3 h). Their patients received IPL therapy, the first real report of "Photodynamic photorejuvenation." This was the first reported clinical trial that

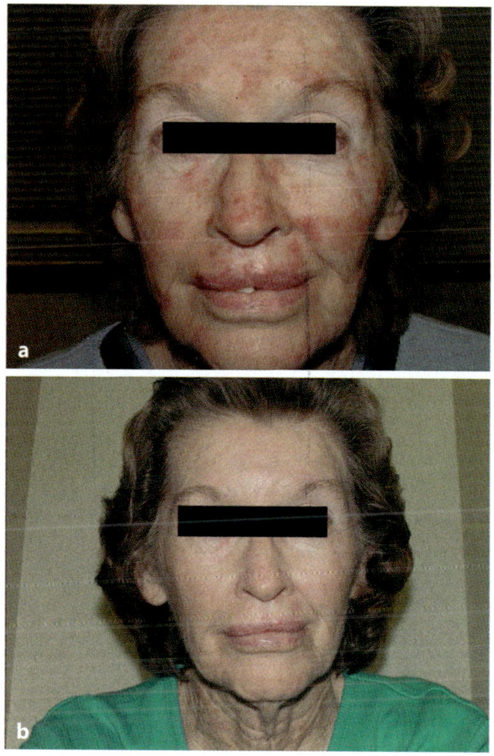

Fig. 2.3 a, b. Actinic keratoses (Aks) treated with 5-aminolevulinic (ALA)-photodynamic therapy (PDT) and blue light (**a**) resulting in a "rejuvenation" effect (**b**).

looked at photorejuvenation parameters with a medical device other than a blue light source. They treated 17 patients with an IPL device and showed that after 2 IPL sessions, the cosmetic appearance was excellent as a result of the therapy.

Other important clinical trials with a variety of lasers and light sources soon followed [31–34]. These are shown in Table 2.2. The results of these clinical trials showed clearly that the use of full-face ALA application and exposure to a variety of lasers and light sources is useful in the treatment of photodamaged skin (i.e., photorejuvenation). The studies also pointed out that by using ALA-PDT, "typical" photorejuvenation treatment protocols could be modified. One or two therapies with ALA-PDT could be equivalent, if not superior, to

Table 2.2. Light sources. *PDL* Pulsed dye laser, *AK* actinic keratoses, *ALA* 5-aminolevulinic acid, *PDT* photodynamic therapy

Authors	Light source	Drug incubation (number of patients)	Significant results	Other significant notes
Gold et al. [31]	Blue light	30–60 minutes (10 patients)	83% AKs responded; 90% crow's feet, 100% skin roughness, hyperpigmentation 90%, facial erythema 70%	
Goldman et al. [32]	Blue light	1 hour (32 patients)	90% AKs responded; improvement in skin texture 72%, pigment change 59%	62.5% preferred ALA-PDT over cryotherapy
Avram et al. [33]	IPL	1 hour (17 patients)	69% AKs responded; telangiectasia 55%, pigment change 48%, skin texture 25%	One treatment with ALA-PDT/IPL compatible to five IPL alone treatments (?)
Alexiades-Armenakas et al. [34]	PDL	2–3 hours (19 patients)	Actinic cheilitis – 68% clearance at 12 months	

the routine five or six IPL photorejuvenation treatments usually performed.

In order to verify the results seen in the aforementioned "open" clinical trials, split-face trials were subsequently performed. To date, five of these trials have been published in the peer-reviewed literature. The first of these split-face trials, by Alster et al. [35], compared ALA with an IPL on one side of the face compared to IPL alone on the other side of the face in ten individuals. They found that the side of the face receiving ALA-IPL showed a greater improvement in photorejuvenation when compared to the side treated with IPL alone. Key [36] looked at subjects utilizing a PDL with ALA on one half of the face; results were similar to those of Alster's group. The photorejuvenation parameters improved more on the ALA-PDL-treated side than on the side treated with PDL alone. Goldberg's group [37] looked at a split-face ALA-IPL versus an IPL-alone protocol and performed biopsy sampling on individuals to examine at the production of type I collagen production. They found that there was a greater increase in type I collagen production in those patients receiving ALA-IPL than in those receiving IPL alone.

Dover et al. [38] looked at an ALA-IPL split face protocol where patients received three split-face ALA-IPL treatments at 3-week intervals followed by two additional IPL full-face treatments. All patients were evaluated at 4 weeks following the final IPL treatment. They found improvements in the global score for photoaging (80% versus 50%), mottled hyperpigmentation (95% versus 65%), and in fine lines (55% versus 20%). Interestingly, in their group of 29 individuals there was no statistical change in tactile skin roughness or sallowness over baseline levels.

Gold et al. [39] recently reported their split-face analysis utilizing ALA-IPL on one half of the face and only IPL on the other half. The protocol included three split-face treatments performed at 4-week intervals, with follow-up at 1 and 3 months following the final treatment. Of the 13 individuals studied, they found greater improvements in

Table 2.3. Split-face study

Authors	Light source	Drug incubation (number of patients)	Significant results	Other significant notes
Alster et al. [35]	IPL	1 hour (10 patients)	ALA-IPL side higher clinical scores for photorejuvenation	
Key [36]	PDL	1 hour	ALA-PDL more significant than PDL alone for photorejuvenation	
Marmur et al. [37]	IPL	1 hour (7 patients)	Ultrastructural analysis: increase in type I collagen – more so when pretreated with ALA	
Dover et al. [38]	IPL	1 hour (20 patients)	Improvement in global photoaging scale for ALA-IPL side (80–50%), hyperpigmentation (95–65%), fine lines (55–20%)	Three split-face treatments, then two full-face IPLs
Gold et al. [39]	IPL	1 hour (13 patients)	Improvements on ALA-IPL side versus IPL alone: AKs (78–54%), crow's feet (55–20%), skin roughness (55–30%), hyperpigmentation (60–37%), facial erythema (85–54%)	

the ALA-IPL side versus the IPL side in the following parameters: AKs (78% versus 53.6%), crows feet (55% versus 28.5%), tactile skin roughness (55% versus 29.5%), mottled hyperpigmentation (60.3% versus 37.2%), and in erythema (84.6% versus 53.8%).

These split-face clinical trials confirmed the earlier "open" clinical trials showing the effectiveness of ALA-PDT in the treatment of photorejuvenation. They are summarized in Table 2.3. Subsequent clinical evaluations will further define the protocols for each type of device on the market to be used, including the various blue lights, IPLs, and PDLs.

The second photosensitizer, Metvix, or MAL, has European Union (EU) clearance for the treatment of nonhyperkeratotic AKs of the face and scalp, and basal cell carcinomas (BCCs) that are not amenable to conventional surgery. In the USA, at the time of this writing, FDA approval is for the treatment of nonhyperkeratotic AKs of the face and scalp [24]. A further description of MAL will follow. MAL is best utilized with a red light source at 630 nm. Clinical trials supporting its effectiveness in the treatment of AKs are numerous, well designed, and all show convincing results [40–48]. These studies are summarized in Table 2.4. Clinical trials for photorejuvenation with MAL are in their infancy at the time of the writing, with several skilled European investigators studying MAL for photorejuvenation with red light sources as well as with a variety of other lasers and light sources.

Currently Available Technology

At this time, as noted earlier, there are two photosensitizers currently available for use. One is Levulan Kerastick, shown in Fig. 2.4. The Levulan Kerastick is a 20% weight/volume ALA solution with 48% alcohol. It was

Table 2.4. Methyl aminolaevulinate (MAL) AK trials. CR Complete response

STUDY	No. of Patients	No of lesions treated with MAL PDT (PP)	Dosage regimen	Results (lesion CR) at 3 months
Phase II study Braathen [40]	110	384 MAL PDT	Dose and regime-finding study	Metvix 160 mg/g for 3 hours optimal (compared: 1 and 3 hours, 80 and 160 mg/g) Second Metvix PDT increased CR from 67% to 89% (lesions were prepared) Efficacy is better with lesion preparation than without
1x Metvix PDT vs. double freeze-thaw cryotherapy Szeimies et al. [41]	202	367 MAL PDT	1 x MAL PDT session For lesions on face & scalp = 93% of lesions vs double cycle cryotherapy	Complete lesion response at 3 months: 1 x Metvix session (69%) as effective as double freeze-thaw cryotherapy (75%) 96% patients had excellent or good cosmetic outcome vs 81% with cryotherapy 74% patients preferred Metvix PDT to previous other therapies
European double-blind, placebo-controlled trial Bjerring et al. [42]	39		1 x MAL PDT session vs placebo	Complete lesion response at 3 months: 1x Metvix session (76%) > placebo (18%)
2 x Metvix PDT vs single cryotherapy, placebo controlled Freeman et al. [43]	200	295 MAL PDT	2 x MAL PDT sessions 7 days apart vs. single cycle cryotherapy	Complete lesion response at 3 months: 2x Metvix sessions (91%) > cryotherapy (68%) > placebo (30%) 84% of patients had an excellent cosmetic outcome with Metvix PDT vs cryotherapy (51%) 98% had excellent or good cosmesis with Metvix! 85% of patients rated Metvix better (61%) or equal 14%) to previous treatments

Table 2.4. *Continued*

STUDY	No. of Patients	No of lesions treated with MAL PDT (PP)	Dosage regimen	Results (lesion CR) at 3 months
US double-blind, 2x Metvix PDT vs placebo-controlled trial Pariser et al. [44]	80	260 MAL PDT	2 x MAL PDT sessions 7 days apart vs. placebo	Complete lesion response at 3 months: 2 x Metvix sessions (89%) > placebo (38%) 97% of patients had excellent or good cosmetic outcome with Metvix PDT. 73% of patients preferred Metvix PDT to other previous therapies
Single Metvix PDT vs. dual Metvix PDT Tarstedt et al. [45]	211	400 MAL PDT	1 x MAL PDT session, retreat only non complete responding lesions at 3 months (19%) Regime I vs 2 x MAL PDT 7 days apart Regime II	At 3 months: For thin lesions, complete lesion response similar with 1 x Metvix (93%) and 2 x Metvix (89%) For thicker lesions, CR better with 2 x Metvix (84%) than 1 x Metvix (70%), which improved after repeat treatment at 3 months (88%) Regime I is not inferior to regime II Overall: Regime I: 92% (81% after first session); Regime II: 87% For thin lesions: Regime I 97%; Regime II 89% For thicker lesions: Regime I: 88%; Regime II: 84%

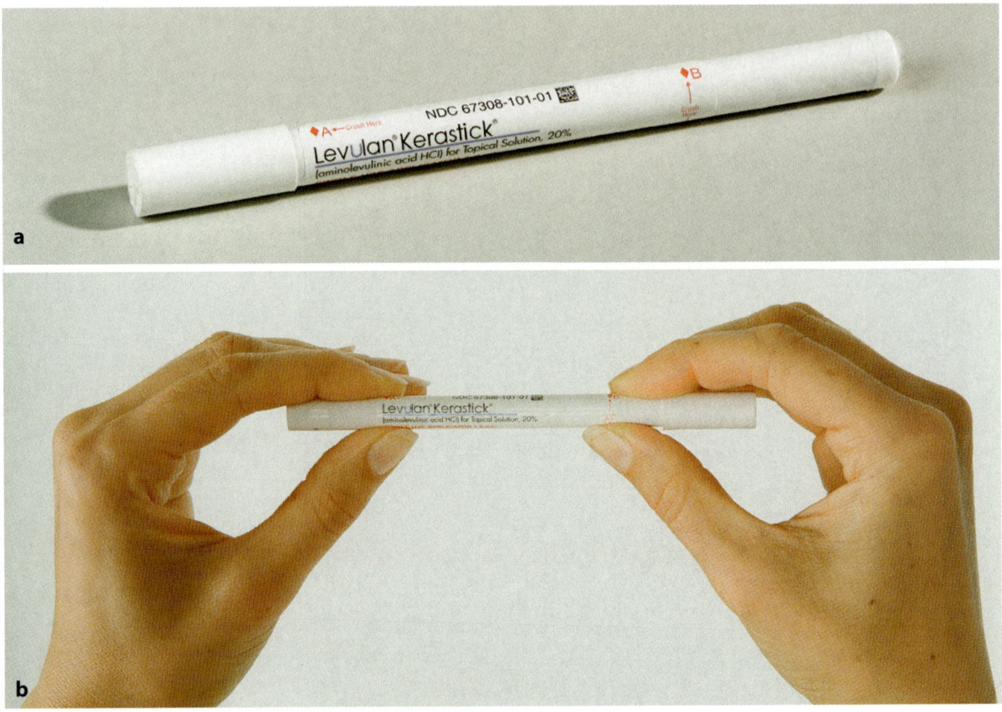

Fig. 2.4 a, b. Levulan Kerastick (Dusa Pharmaceuticals, Wilmington, MA, USA)

developed to have a roll-on special dermatologic applicator at one of the ends to allow easy and accurate application of the medicine to the area(s) being treated. This applicator tip is applied to a flexible glass tubing that contains two glass vials. One of the vials contains the ALA in a powder form; the other contains the alcohol. Light manual pressure upon the glass vials in the Kerastick will break the vials, allowing for mixture of the two by gentle rotation in a back-and-forth direction. Three minutes of mixing is recommended prior to the application of the 20% ALA [24].

The recommended light source for ALA is a blue light source, for which there are currently three popular brands: the Blu-U (Dusa Pharmaceuticals, Wilmington, MA, USA); the ClearLight (CureLight, Yokneam, Israel), and the IClear (CureLight, Yokneam, Israel). These are shown in Figs. 2.5–2.7.

As noted, a variety of IPLs and PDLs, as well as the potassium tritanyl phosphate (KTP) lasers can also activate ALA. The IPLs have already been listed (Table 2.1) and examples are shown in Figs. 2.8 and 2.9. A variety of PDLs are also on the market, one of which is shown in Fig. 2.10. Finally, some LED sources can also be highly effective in activating ALA (see Chapter 3).

Metvix, or Metvixia, is the methyl ester of ALA. The recommended treatment protocols for the proper use of MAL includes the gentle scraping or curettage of the affected area/lesion prior to the application of the MAL cream. This area is then occluded for upwards of 3 h under before being subjected to the recommended red light source [24].

Advantages

The advantages of utilizing ALA-PDT or MAL-PDT in the treatment of photorejuvena-

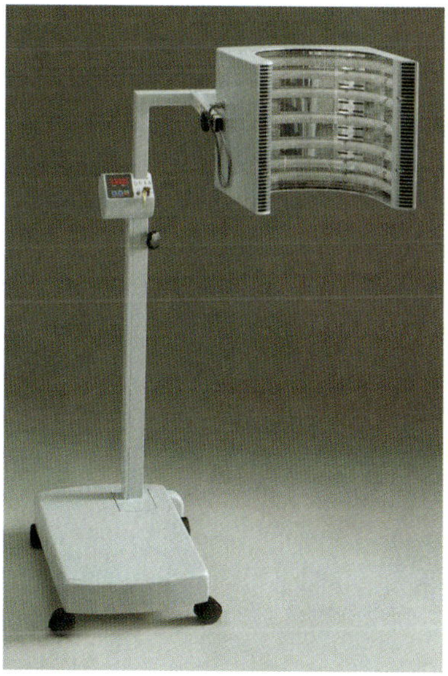

Fig. 2.5. BluU (Dusa Pharmaceuticals, Wilmington, MA, USA)

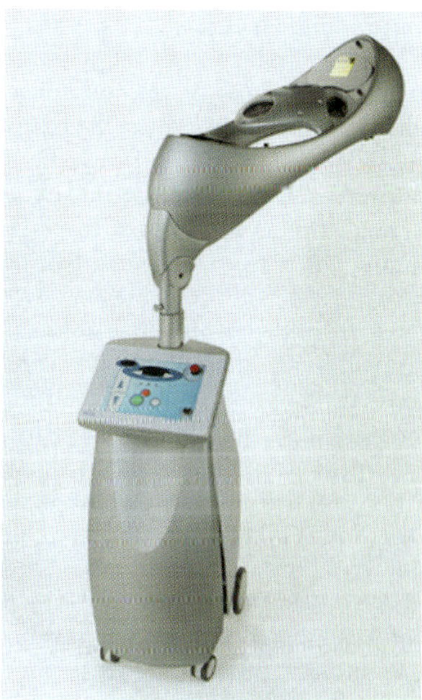

Fig. 2.6. ClearLight (CureLight, Yokneam, Israel)

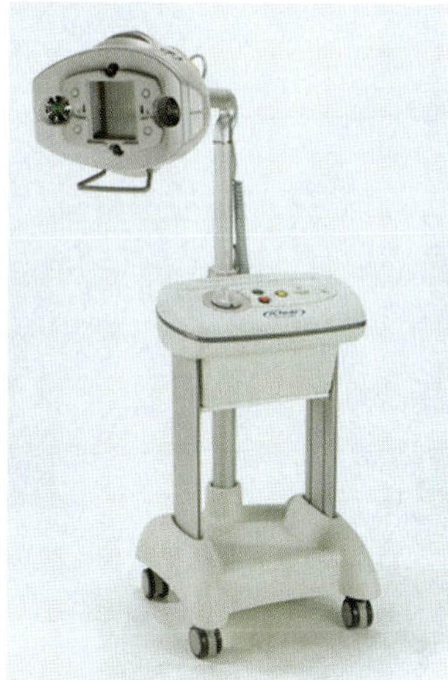

Fig. 2.7. IClear (CureLight, Yokneam, Israel)

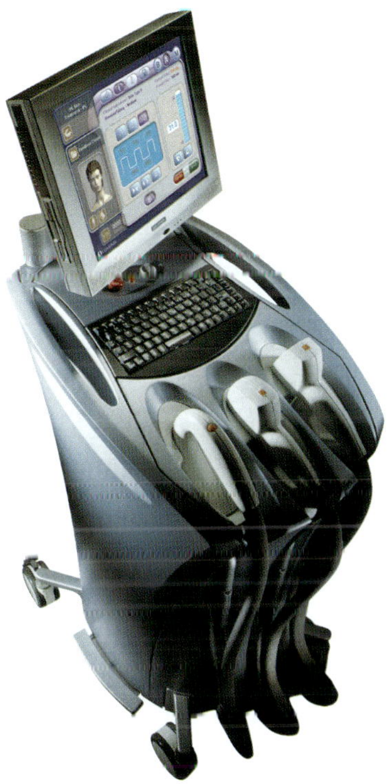

Fig. 2.8. Lumenis One (Lumeni, Santa Clara, CA, USA)

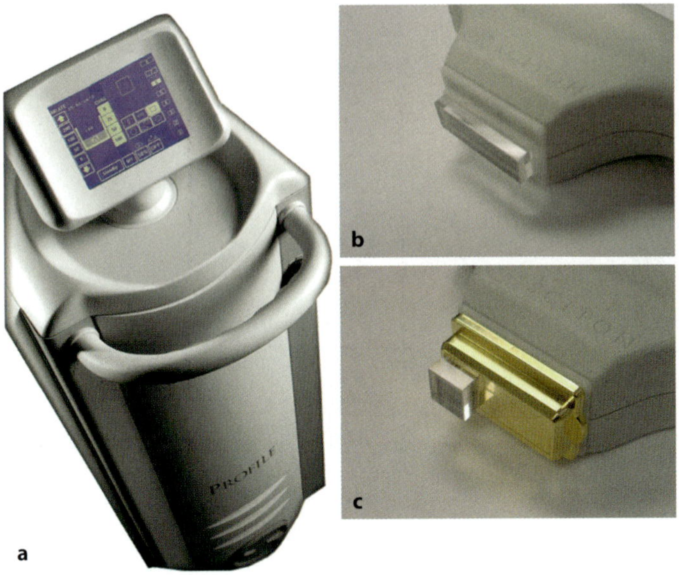

Fig. 2.9. Sciton BBL (Sciton, Palo Alto, CA, USA)

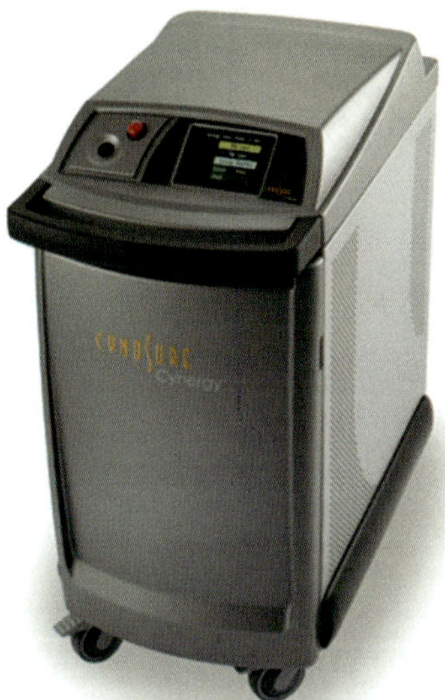

Fig. 2.10. Cynergy (Cynosure Lasers, Chelmsford, MA, USA)

tion have been elucidated earlier in this text. The use of ALA has been studied more for the treatment of photorejuvenation and associated Aks, while MAL has been studied more extensively for nonhyperkeratotic AKs as well as for nonmelanoma skin cancers.

It has been shown conclusively that ALA, with either blue light sources or IPLs, or lasers such as PDL or KTP lasers, can be used successfully to treat all of the associated signs of photodamage. What seems evident from the clinical trials presented is that with ALA-PDT and any of the presented lasers or light sources, one can treat the signs of photodamage faster than without the use ALA. In the clinical trials, most investigators used anywhere from one to three ALA sessions to achieve the results presented; this is in contrast to plain IPL treatments, which routinely need five to six sessions.

Also evident from the clinical trials is that although conventional therapies have centered predominantly upon the use of the IPL, photorejuvenation can be effected by other protocols. Clinical trials with ALA have shown that not only IPLs, but also blue light sources, PDLs, and KTP lasers are effective in the treatment of photodamage and associated AKs. They too can activate ALA.

The use of MAL has not been fully evaluated in the treatment of photodamage/photorejuvenation. Once investigators utilizing MAL can modify their current protocols so that downtime is minimized and the potential for adverse events lessened, perhaps MAL too will play a role in photorejuvenation.

One final advantage for the use of both ALA and MAL in the treatment of photorejuvenation is that each of these agents is potentially useful as a chemopreventative agent. This treatment may be useful as a prevention for the development of further AKs and nonmelanoma skin cancers. Several studies, first on animal models [49,50], and in patients with basal cell nevus syndrome [51,52], as well as in immunocompromized patients suggest that both ALA and MAL [53] can prevent the development of new AKs and basal cell carcinomas following PDT. Further clinical research will define the roles of chemoprevention with ALA and MAL (Fig. 2.11).

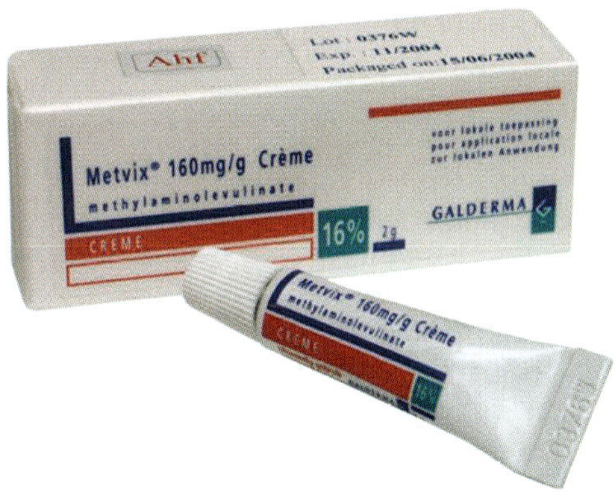

Fig. 2.11. Medvix MAL cream

Disadvantages

There are several potential disadvantages to the use of both ALA and MAL in the process of photorejuvenation. Clinicians are working toward minimizing these disadvantages. The major disadvantage of ALA and MAL for PDT is the potential development of photosensitivity as a result of the therapy. The "PDT effect" has been described as pain and discomfort during and following the treatment. This has been shown to last up to 1 week following the therapy [24]. In the initial reports with ALA, as shown in both phase II and III clinical FDA trials, many of the subjects reported pain during the procedure. This pain, although seen on occasion with some of the newer protocols, is directly attributable to the long, 14- to 18-h drug incubation time followed by exposure to the blue light source. With short contact, full-face ALA therapy, usually from 30 min to 1 h, and with the use of the newer light sources, even with the use of blue light sources, most patients do not complain of a great deal of discomfort. If patients are still concerned about the potential pain experienced during the therapy, one may use hand-held fans or other cooling devices during the treatments. One common cooling device is the SmartCool (Cynosure, Westford, MA, USA) as shown in Fig. 2.11.

Following ALA-PDT treatment, especially when spot AK treatment is performed, it was not uncommon to see the treated lesions become erythematous and edematous, crust, and require upwards of up to 1 week for healing to occur. This is seen in Fig. 2.2. With the new protocols being used by most clinicians today, this adverse event is rarely seen.

MAL-PDT does cause pain during treatment. Patients with lesions amenable to MAL-PDT treatment generally have the lesions "prepped" with a gentle curettage prior to application of MAL. Once the MAL is applied, the areas are usually occluded for upwards of 3 h before application of the red light. Most reports of MAL therapy report pain as a result of the red light therapy, perhaps as a result of the curettage, occlusion of MAL, and the red light itself, which penetrates deeper into the skin than any of the other lasers or light sources described previously. The "PDT effect" is commonly seen with MAL treatments [24]. This is something that will need to be addressed when MAL becomes more common place in photorejuvenation therapy, so that downtime can be eliminated.

The most serious of the disadvantages associated with the use of ALA-PDT or MAL-PDT is the potential for phototoxicity [24].

Both of these sensitizers can result in phototoxicity; an example of which is shown in Fig. 2.12. Phototoxicity can be minimized by removing any residual ALA or MAL from the skin following the PDT treatment, ensuring that the patient remains out of the sun for the first 24–48 h following their PDT session, and assuring the proper use of sunscreen immediately following the PDT treatment.

Other adverse events directly related to ALA-PDT or MAL-PDT treatment are distinctly rare. Of course whenever a laser is used for any reason, potential adverse reactions are possible, such as burning, blistering, hyperpigmentation, hypopigmentation, and scarring. These procedures and these devices should only be performed under the auspices of a physician who is well versed in lasers, light sources, PDT, and wound healing.

Indications

The indications for the use of ALA-PDT and MAL-PDT have been reviewed previously in this chapter. The FDA and EU approvals have also been described. In the USA, the primary indications for the use of ALA-PDT are photorejuvenation and any associated AKs, acne vulgaris, sebaceous gland hyperplasia, and hidradenitis suppurativa. These are all off-label indications for use of ALA-PDT in the USA, as noted by the FDA approvals. In Europe, the primary indication for MAL-PDT is for the treatment of nonmelanoma skin cancers and Bowen's Disease, or squamous cell carcinoma in situ. The use of MAL-PDT in the treatment of acne vulgaris and photorejuvenation were still in their infancy at the time of this writing.

Contraindications

There are no specific contraindications to the use of ALA or MAL. ALA-PDT can be used successfully on patients of all skin types (I–VI). When ALA-PDT is used on darker skin types, a blue light source should be used rather than a lasers or an IPL system.

Informed Consent

A copy of the patient consent form used for photodynamic treatment is given in Fig. 2.13.

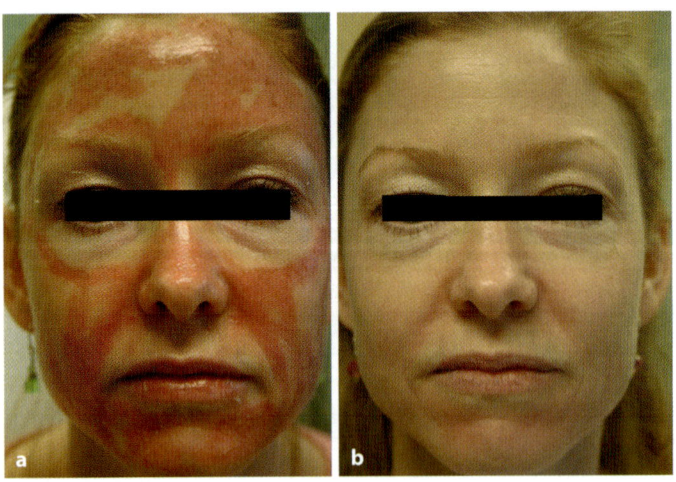

Fig. 2.12 a, b. Phototoxicity – case report. Patient with phototoxic reaction 2 days after PDT for AKs utilizing topical ALA and a blue light source (**a**) and 25 days of twice daily cream application showing complete skin restoration with no evidence of AK lesions (**b**). Permission to reproduce figures was obtained from the Journal of Drugs in Dermatol September 2006, Gold, MH, in press

Levulan (Aminolevulinic acid 20%) is a naturally occurring photosensitizing compound which has been approved by the FDA and Health and Welfare Canada to treat pre-cancerous skin lesions called actinic keratosis. Levulan is applied to the skin and subsequently "activated" by specific wavelengths of light. This process of activating Levulan with light is termed Photodynamic Therapy. The purpose of activating the Levulan is to improve the appearance and reduce acne rosacea, acne vulgaris, and sebaceous hyperplasia, decrease oiliness of the skin, and improve texture and smoothness by minimizing pore size. Any pre-cancerous lesions are also simultaneously treated. The improvement of these skin conditions (other than actinic keratosis) is considered an "off-label" use of Levulan.

I understand that Levulan will be applied to my skin for 30–120 minutes. Subsequently, the area will be treated with a specific wavelength of light to activate the Levulan. Following my treatment, I must wash off any Levulan on my skin. I understand that I should avoid direct sunlight for 24 hours following the treatment due to photosensitivity. I understand that I am not pregnant.

Anticipated side effects of Levulan treatment include discomfort, burning, swelling, blistering, scarring, redness and possible skin peeling, especially in any areas of sun damaged skin and pre-cancers of the skin, as well as lightening or darkening of skin tone and spots, and possible hair removal. The peeling may last many days, and the redness for several weeks if I have an exuberant response to treatment.

I consent to the taking of photographs of my face before each treatment session. I understand that I may require several treatment sessions spaced 1-6 weeks apart to achieve optimal results. I understand that I am responsible for payment of this procedure, as it is not covered by health insurance.

I understand that medicine is not an exact science, and that there can be no guarantees of my results. I am aware that while some individuals have fabulous results, it is possible that these treatments will not work for me. I understand that alternative treatments include topical medications, oral medications, cryosurgery, excisional surgery, and doing nothing.

I have read the above information and understand it. My questions have been answered satisfactorily by the doctor and his staff. I accept the risks and complications of the procedure. By signing this consent form I agree to have one or more Levulan treatments.

____

Signature

____

Name

________________________ ________________________

Date Witness

Fig. 2.13. Patient consent for photodynamic treatment

Personal Approach

At the time of this writing there were no standards that specifically state the ideal approach to the utilization of ALA-PDT in the USA. Several investigators have commented on their favorite approaches and each clinician will develop their own guidelines and procedures that will optimize the use of PDT in their office. A recent United States Consensus Paper does outline steps that one may follow when beginning to use PDT in the clinical setting [54]. The following describes how ALA-PDT is utilized in my clinic, with antidotes from other authors included where appropriate.

Initially, a thorough review with the patient is required that documents the risks and benefits of the procedure. Signed, written consent to undergo the procedure will verify that one has reviewed the necessary information and potential sequelae with a patient. At the time of this writing, the use of ALA-PDT for photorejuvenation off-label according to the FDA; this should also be explained to your patient.

Since the majority of PDT treatments are performed on the face, the face will be used as the example for the procedure. If a patient has a history of herpes simplex, it is prudent to have started the appropriate antiviral medication at least 2–3 days prior to undertaking the procedure. The face must be thoroughly cleansed with a mild cleanser. A degreasing procedure is performed next to enhance the skin's absorption of ALA. There are two major ways to degrease the skin, microdermabrasion and an acetone scrub. I prefer to use an acetone scrub as it is a less expensive additive procedure than microdermabrasion, but there is growing evidence that the use of microdermabrasion does enhance the penetration of ALA. If a microdermabrasion is to be done, there are options here as well, including standard microdermabrasion with crystals, crystalless microdermabrasion, and paddle-enhanced microdermabrasion. We utilize crystalless microdermabrasion systems or the paddle method when we choose to use microdermabrasion in our patient population. Examples of these are shown in Figs. 2.14 and 2.15.

Next, the Levulan Kerastick (a 20% weight/volume ALA solution with 48% alcohol) is broken and mixed, as has been previously explained in this chapter. It has a special roll-on dermatologic applicator at one of the ends to allow easy and accurate application of the medicine to the area(s) being treated. This applicator tip is applied to a flexible glass tubing that contains two glass vials. One of the vials contains the ALA in a powder form; the other contains the ethanol. Light manual pressure upon the glass vials in the Kerastick will break the vials, allowing the two contents to be mixed by gentle rotation in a back-and-forth direction. Three minutes of mixing is recommended prior to the application of the 20% ALA [24]

Once the Kerastick is prepared, it will be "painted" in a uniform manner over the forehead, cheeks, chin, and nose area. If there are AKs present, a second "coat" of medicine is routinely applied. The drug is then allowed to incubate on the skin. For all practical indications, drug incubation is 1 h for photorejuvenation and AKs. For each successive treatment, drug incubation will be increased by approximately 15–30 min.

The patient is now ready for their light or laser administration. If an IPL light source is going to be used, it is recommended that the skin be once again cleansed prior to the use of

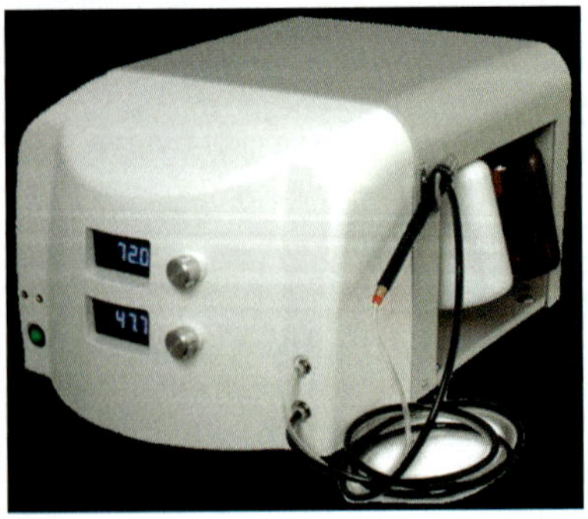

Fig. 2.14. Silkpeel (eMed, Westlake Village, California, USA)

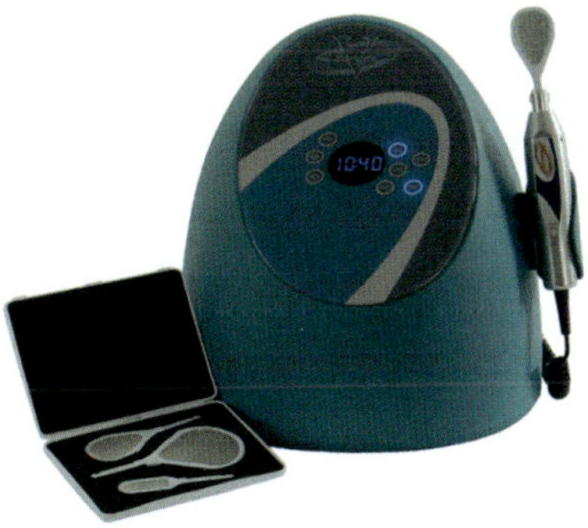

Fig. 2.15. Vibraderm (Vibraderm, Grand Prairie, Texas, USA)

the light source. One will find that the coupling medium, or gel, often used with an IPL will not remain on the skin surface after the application of the ALA without prior cleansing. If a blue light source or PDL is to be used, most would still recommend the skin to be cleansed once again, although it is not mandatory. All of our treatments are carried out with the aid of air cooling, which the patient holds and uses as needed.

Postoperative Care and Complications

After the therapy is completed, there are several very important steps to be performed before discharging the patient. First, any remaining ALA needs to be thoroughly removed from the skin. Many clinicians find that if they perform an IPL or PDL treatment followed by a short, 5-min blue light "quenching," all excess ALA will be removed. This may also serve to give an additional benefit to the patient, although clinical trials with regard to this concept have not been performed at the time of this writing. Next, we employ the use of ice onto the treated areas, which helps with any patient discomfort or skin burning. During this time we begin our discussions of proper skin care and sun protection, which are crucial for the patient to follow to avoid the only real adverse effect of the procedure, phototoxicity. Phototoxicity can be minimized by following several very simple rules. The patient must remain out of the sun for the first 24–48 h following the procedure. Sunscreen use, with a minimum sun protection factor of 30, is required, and in our office it is applied prior to the patient leaving our office. There are many new creams and lotions that are being evaluated to help reduce any erythema that may be associated with treatment with lasers and light sources without the use of ALA; these are also being investigated for their potentials with ALA. These include Neocutis Bio-restorative Skin Cream [55], Biafine [56], and Avene Gel D'eau [57], studies of which have recently been presented.

As noted, phototoxicity is the only major concern that may be seen following an ALA-PDT procedure. By following the simple rules outlined above, this is routinely minimized in our clinical setting. Our patients may note some desquamation of the skin after several days, but proper use of moisturizers or "spray" waters will minimize this effect.

Patients ideally should have a thorough understanding of "how many" treatments with ALA-PDT they will require for a given effect. Unfortunately, this remains an elusive question at this time. Because all patients are different, it is not possible to give a precise answer to the question.

Complications, which are rare, have been described elsewhere in this chapter.

Results and Photographs

Clinical results are shown in Figs. 2.16–2.20.

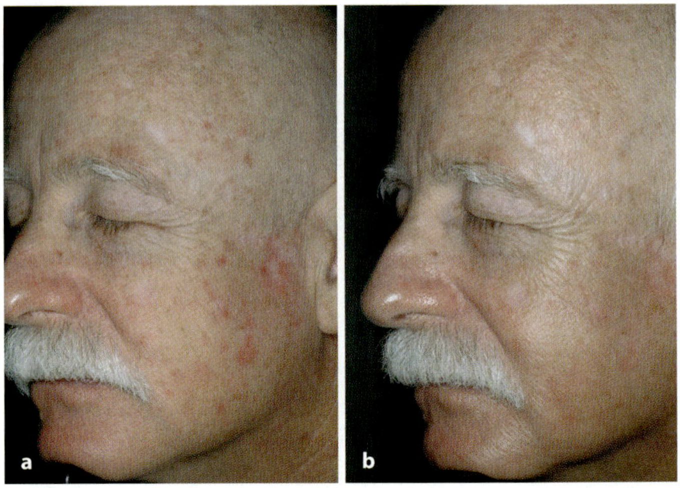

Fig. 2.16 a, b. Before treatment (**a**); After one treatment with acetone scrub, 30-min Levulan incubation and Lumenis IPL at 30 J/cm^2 (**b**). Photographs courtesy of Dore Gilbert, M.D, Newport Beach, California, USA

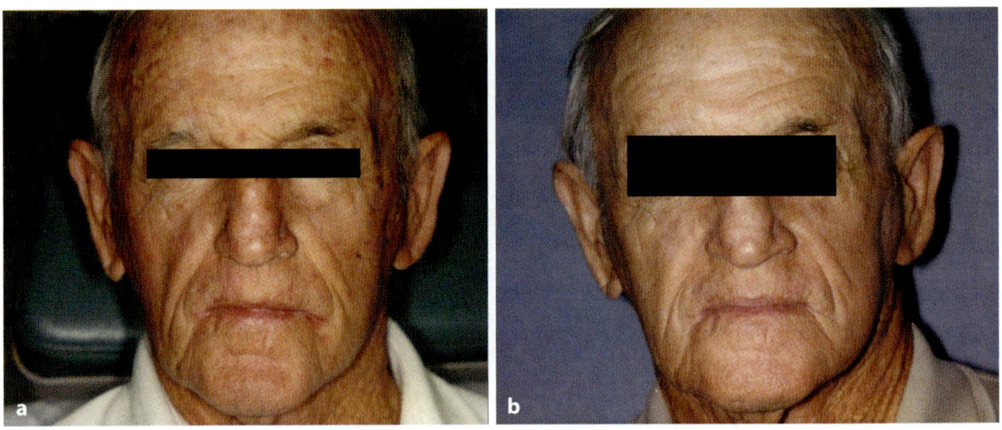

Fig. 2.17 a, b. Before treatment (**a**); After ALA-PDT treatment (**b**). Clinical photographs courtesy of Mark S. Nestor, M.D, Aventura, FL, USA

The Future

The future for ALA-PDT and MAL-PDT looks very exciting. Further clinical trials will continue to define protocols and parameters for the use of ALA-PDT for photorejuvenation. Research with MAL-PDT will also determine its future roll in the treatment of photodamaged skin.

The role of both ALA-PDT and MAL-PDT in chemoprevention is perhaps the most exciting and most important of the future potential uses for PDT. Researchers are actively studying this issue and they are encouraged to continue this very exciting and important work.

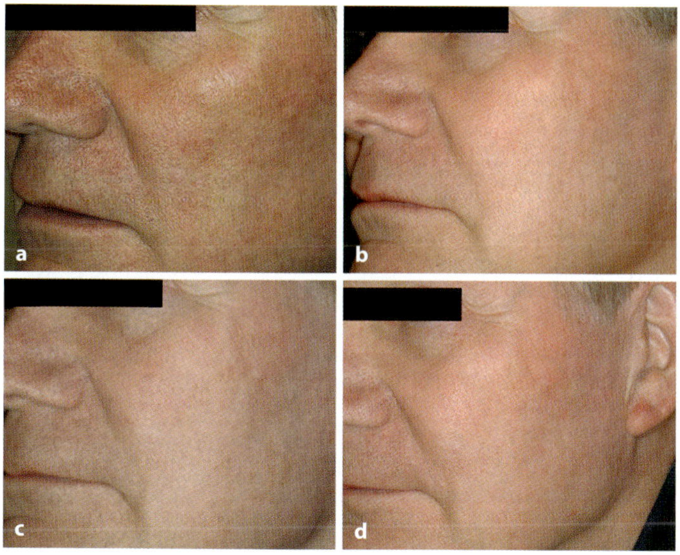

Fig. 2.18 a–d. Before treatment consisting of acetone scrub, 60-min Levulan incubation and Lumenis IPL at 30 J/cm^2 (**a**); 1 year after treatment (**b**); 2 years after treatment (**c**); 3 years after treatment (**d**). Photographs courtesy of Martin Braun, M.D, Vancouver, Canada

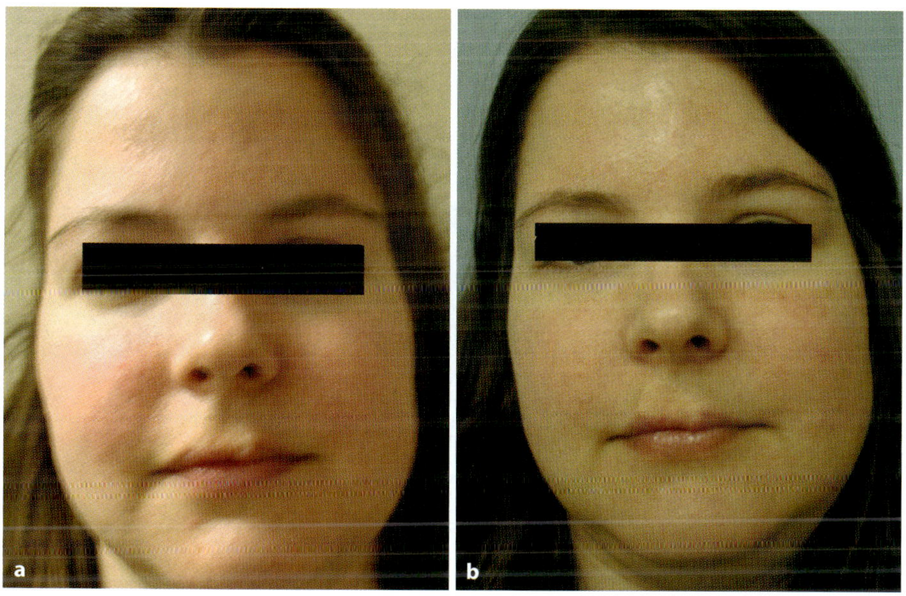

Fig. 2.19 a, b. Patient with rosacea before treatment (**a**); After four ALA-IPL and IPL only alternating treatments with Levulan and Lumenis One (**b**). All four treatments consisted of 60 min of Levulan incubation.

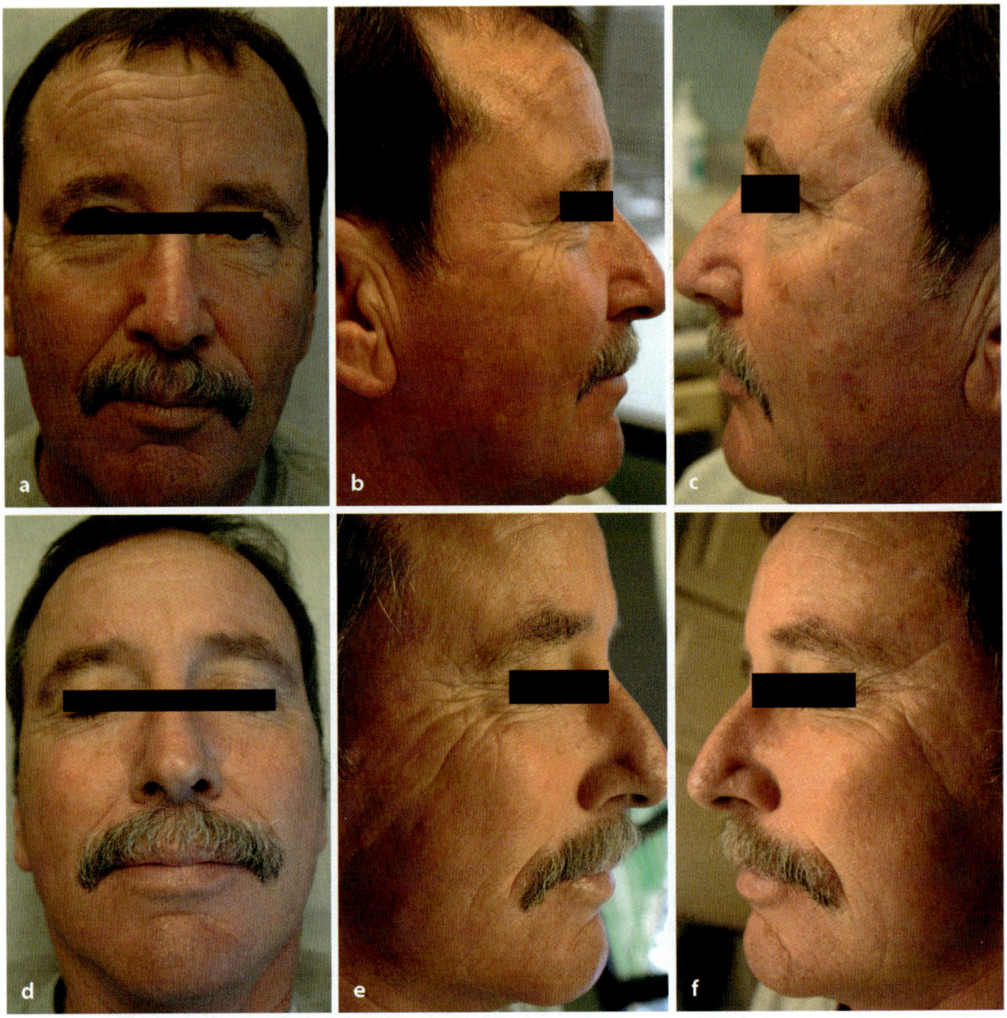

Fig. 2.20 a–f. Patient before treatment (**a–c**); after three ALA-IPL treatments with Levulan and Lumenis One (d–f). The first treatment comprised a 30-min Levulan incubation; the second and third treatments comprised 45-min Levulan incubations.

References

1. Kligman A, Fulton JE Jr, Plewig G (1969) Topical vitamin A acid in acne vulgaris. Arch Dermatol 99:469–476
2. Kligman AM, Grove GL, Hirose R, et al (1986) Topical tretinoin for photoaged skin J Am Acad Dermatol 15:836–859
3. Talwar HS, Griffiths CE, Fisher GJ, et al (1995) Reduced type I and type III procollagens in photodamaged adult human skin. J Invest Dermatol 105:285–290
4. Van Scott EJ, Yu RJ (1984) Hyperkeratinization, corneocyte cohesion and alpha hydroxy acids. J Am Acad Dermatol 11:867–879
5. Kromeyer E (1930) Cosmetic Treatment of Skin Complaints. Oxford University Press, New York

6. Burks JW (1956) Wire Brush Surgery. Charles C. Thomas, Springfield
7. Harmon CB, Yarborough JM (1996) Scar revision by dermabrasion. In: Roenigk NH, Roenigk RK (eds) Dermatology Surgery, 2nd edn. Marcel Decker, New York, pp 911–921
8. Roenigk HH (1996) Dermabrasion. In: Roenigk NH, Roenigk RK (eds) Dermatology Surgery, 2nd edn. Marcel Decker, New York, pp 1089–102
9. Brody JH, Hailey CW (1986) Medium depth chemical peeling of the skin: a variation of superficial chemosurgery. J Dermatol Surg Oncol 12:1268–1275
10. Monheit G (1989) The Jessner's + TCA peel: a medium depth chemical peel. J Dermatol Surg Oncol 15:945–950
11. Coleman WP, Futrell JM (1994) The glycolic acid + trichloroacetic acid peel. J Dermatol Surg Oncol 20:76–80
12. Rubin MG (1995) The efficacy of a topical lidocaine/prilocaine anesthetic gel in 35% trichloroacetic acid peels. Dermatol Surg 21:223–225
13. Goldman L, Rockwell R (1968) Laser systems and their applications in medicine and biology. Adv Biomed Eng Med Phys 1:317–382
14. Anderson RR, Parish JA (1983) Selective photothermolysis: precise microsurgery by selective absorption of pulsed radiation. Science 220:524–527
15. Goldman M, Eckhouse S (1996) Photothermal sclerosis of leg veins. Dermatol Surg 22:323–330
16. Goldberg DJ, Cutler KB (2000) Non-ablative Treatment of rhytids with intense pulsed light. Lasers Surg Med 26:196–200
17. Bitter PH (2000) Noninvasive rejuvenation of photodamaged skin using serial, full-face intense pulsed light treatments. Dermatol Surg 26:835–842
18. Goldberg DJ, Cutler KB (2000) Nonablative treatment of rhytids with intense pulsed light. Lasers Surg Med 26:196–200
19. Goldberg DJ, Samady JA (2001) Intense pulsed light and Nd:YAG laser non-ablative treatment of facial rhytids. Lasers Surg Med 28:141–144
20. Weiss RA, Weiss MA, Beasley KL (2002) Rejuvenation of photoaged skin: 5 years results with intense pulsed light of the face, neck and chest. Dermatol Surg 28:115–119
21. Sadick NS (2003) Update on non-ablative light therapy for rejuvenation: a review. Lasers Surg Med 32:120–128
22. Negishi K, Tezuka Y, Kushikata N, et al (2001) Photorejuvenation for Asian skin by intense pulsed light. Dermatol Surg 27:627–631; discussion 632
23. Hernandez-Perez E (2002) Gross and microscopic findings in patients submitted to nonablative full-face resurfacing using intense pulsed light: a preliminary study. Dermatol Surg 28:651–655
24. Gold MH, Goldman MP (2004) 5-Aminolevulinic acid photodynamic therapy: where we have been and where we are going.. Dermatol Surg 30:1077–1084
25. Jeffes EW, McCullough JL, Weinstein GD, et al (2001) Photodynamic therapy of actinic keratoses with topical aminolevulinic acid hydrochloride and fluorescent blue light. J Am Acad Dermatol 45:96–104
26. Jeffes EW (2002) Levulan: the first approved topical photosensitizer for the treatment of actinic keratosis. J Dermatolog Treat 13:S19–23
27. Alexiades-Armenakas MR, Geronemus RG (2003) Laser-mediated photodynamic therapy of actinic keratoses. Arch Dermatol 139:1313–1320
28. Gold MH (2002) The evolving role of aminolevulinic acid hydrochloride with photodynamic therapy in photoaging. Cutis 69:8 13
29. Touma D, Yaar M, Whitehead S, et al (2004) A trial of short incubation, broad-area photodynamic therapy for facial actinic keratoses and diffuse photodamage. Arch Dermatol 140:33–40
30. Ruiz-Rodriguez R, Sanz-Sanchez T, Cordoba S (2002) Photodynamic photorejuvenation. Dermatol Surg 28:742–744
31. Gold MH, Bradshaw VL, Boring MM, et al (2004) Treatment of sebaceous gland hyperplasia by photodynamic therapy with 5-aminolevulinic acid and a blue light source or intense pulsed light source. J Drugs Dermatol 3:S6–9
32. Goldman MP, Atkin D, Kincad S (2002) PDT/ALA in the treatment of actinic damage: real world experience. J Lasers Surg Med 14:24
33. Avram DK, Goldman MP (2004) Effectiveness and safety of ALA-IPL in treating actinic keratoses and photodamage. J Drugs Dermatol 3: S36–39
34. Alexiades-Armenakas MR, Geronemus RG (2004) Laser-mediated photodynamic therapy of actinic cheilitis. J Drugs Dermatol 3:548–551
35. Alster TS, Tanzi EL, Welch EC (2005) Photorejuvenation of facial skin with topical 20% 5-aminolevulinic acid and intense pulsed light treatment: a split-face comparison study. J Drugs Dermatol 4:35–38
36. Key DJ (2005) Aminolevulinic acid-pulsed dye laser photodynamic therapy for the treatment of photoaging. Cosm Derm 18:31–36
37. Marmur ES, Phelps R, Goldberg DJ (2005) Ultrastructural Changes Seen After ALA-IPL photorejuvenation: a pilot study. J Cosmet Laser Ther 7:21–24

38. Dover JS, Bhatia AC, Stewart B, et al (2005) Topical 5-aminolevulinic acid combined with intense pulsed light in the treatment of photoaging. Arch Dermatol 141:1247–1252
39. Gold MH, Bradshaw VL, Boring MM, et al (2006) Split-face comparison of photodynamic therapy with 5-aminolevulinic acid and intense pulsed light versus intense pulsed light alone for photodamage. Dermatol Surg 32:795–801; discussion 801–803
40. Braathen LR, Szeimies RM, Basset-Seguin N, et al (2006) Guidelines on the use of photodynamic therapy for nonmelanoma skin cancer: an international consensus. J Am Acad Dermatol 56:125–143
41. Szeimies RM, Karrer S, Radakovic-Fijan S, et al (2002) Photodynamic therapy using topical methyl 5-aminolevulinate compared with cryotherapy for actinic keratosis: a prospective, randomized study. J Am Acad Dermatol 47:258–262
42. Bjerring P, Funk J, Poed-Petersen J, et al (2001) Randomized double blind study comparing photodynamic therapy (PDT) with Metvix to PDT with placebo cream in actinic keratosis. Abstract accepted at the 29th Nordic Congress of Dermatology and Venereology, 7–10 June, Gothenborg, Sweden, 2001
43. Freeman M, Vinciullo C, Francis D, et al (2003) A comparison of photodynamic therapy using topical methyl aminolevulinate (Metvix) with single cycle cryotherapy in patients with actinic keratosis: a prospective, randomized study. J Dermatolog Treat 14:99–106
44. Pariser DM, Lowe NJ, Stewart DM, et al (2003) Photodynamic therapy with topical methyl aminolevulinate (Metvix) is effective and safe in the treatment of actinic keratosis: results of a prospective randomized trial. J Am Acad Dermatol 48:227–232
45. Tarstedt M, Rosdahl I, Berne B, et al (2005) A randomized multicenter study to compare two treatment regimens of topical methyl aminolevulinate (Metvix)-PDT in actinic keratosis of the face and scalp. Acta Derm Venereol 85:424–428
46. Morton C, Campbell S, Gupta G, et al (2006) Intraindividual, right-left comparison of topical methyl aminolaevulinate-photodynamic therapy and cryotherapy in subjects with actinic keratoses: a multicentre, randomized controlled study. Br J Dermatol 155:1029–1036
47. Bissonnette R, Bergeron A, Liu Y (2004) Large surface photodynamic therapy with aminolevulinic acid: treatment of actinic keratoses and beyond. J Drugs Dermatol 3:S26–31
48. Caty V, Liu Y, Viau G, et al (2006) Multiple large surface photodynamic therapy sessions with topical methylaminolaevulinate in PTCH heterozygous mice. Br J Dermatol 154:740–742
49. Itkin A, Gilchrest BA (2004) Aminolevulinic acid and blue light photodynamic therapy for treatment of multiple basal cell carcinomas in two patients with nevoid basal cell carcinoma syndrome. Dermatol Surg 30:1054–1061
50. Chapas AM, Gilchrest BA (2006) Broad area photodynamic therapy for treatment of multiple basal cell carcinomas in a patient with nevoid basal cell carcinoma syndrome. J Drugs Dermatol 5:3–5
51. Wulf HC, Pavel S, Stender I, et al (2006) Topical photodynamic therapy for prevention of new skin lesions in renal transplant recipients. Acta Derm Venereol 86:25–28
52. Gold MH, Nestor MS, Kauvar AN, et al (2006) The use of photodynamic therapy in dermatology: results of a consensus conference. J Drugs Dermatol 5:140–154
53. Gold MH, Biron JA (2006) A novel skin cream containing a mixture of human growth factors and cytokines for the treatment of adverse events associated with photodynamic therapy. J. Drugs Dermatol 5:796–798
54. Gold MH (2006) A single center, split face, double–blind, randomized clinical trial of the effects of an emulsion containing trolamine verses a petrolatum ointment post erbium micro laser peel for seven days. Poster presentation at the 2006 Summer American Academy of Dermatology meeting, 26–30 July, San Diego, CA, USA
55. Gold MH, Ribet V, Gral N, et al (2006) Calming efficacy and tolerance of Avene spring water gel after cepilatory laser treatment combined to healing cream in adults. Poster presentation at the 2006 Summer American Academy of Dermatology meeting, 26–30 July, San Diego, CA, USA
56. Gold MH (2006) Single-center, split-face, double-blind, randomized clinical trial of the efficacy of a Trolamine-containing topical emulsion and a topical petrolatum-based product in reducing redness and peeling after treatment with a micro-laser peel. Poster presentation at the American of Academy Dermatology Summer meeting 2006, 26–30 July, San Diego, CA, USA
57. Ribet V, Gral N, Gold MH, et al (2006) Calming efficacy and tolerance of Avene Spring Water Gel after depilatory laser treatment combined to healing cream in adults. Poster presentation at the American of Academy Dermatology Annual meeting 2006, 26–30 July, San Francisco, CA, USA

Chapter 3

LED Low-Level Light Therapy

3

Robert A. Weiss

Core Messages

- Light-emitting diode (LED) treatments, unlike lasers and light sources, do not produce any thermal impact on skin.
- LED treatments photomodulate human cells.
- LED technology, much like lasers and light sources, can produce energy of varying wavelengths.
- Various LED wavelengths appear to have varying effects on human skin

History

Photorejuvenation is the process whereby light energy sources are utilized to reverse or repair the process of sun-induced aging or environmental damage to the skin. Nonablative photorejuvenation refers to the controlled use of thermal energy to accomplish this without disturbance of the overlying epidermis. Nonablative modalities include intense pulsed light (IPL), pulsed-dye laser (PDL), 532-nm green light (potassium tritanyl phosphate, KTP laser) and various infrared wavelengths including 1064 nm, 1320 nm, 1450 nm, and 1540 nm [1]. All of these devices involve thermal injury either by heating the dermis to stimulate fibroblast proliferation or by heating blood vessels for photocoagulation [2,3]. Light-emitting diode (LED) photomodulation is the newest category of nonthermal light treatment designed to regulate the activity of cells rather than to invoke thermal wound-healing mechanisms [4]. This incurs far less risk than other light modalities when treating patients.

The use of LED and low energy light therapy (LILT) for stimulating cell growth has been investigated in plants [5] and in wound healing for oral mucositis [6]. The notion that cell activity can be up- or downregulated by low-energy light has been entertained in the past, but consistent or impressive results have been lacking [6,7]. Wavelengths previously examined include a 670-nm LED array [6], a 660-nm array [8], and higher infrared wavelengths [9]. Fluence in these studies was variable, with energy as high as 4 J/cm^2 required for results [6].

To investigate LED light for modulating skin properties, a model of fibroblast culture has been used in addition to clinical testing. Particular packets of energy with specific wavelengths, combined with using a very specific propriety pulse-sequencing "code," has been found to upregulate collagen I synthesis in fibroblast culture using reverse transcriptase-polymerase chain reaction to measure collagen I [10]. The upregulation of fibroblast collagen synthesis correlates with the clinical observation of increased dermal collagen on treated human skin biopsy samples [11]. In both the fibroblast and clinical model, collagen synthesis is accompanied by a reduction of matrix metalloproteinases (MMPs), in particular MMP-1, or collagenase being greatly reduced with exposure to 590-nm low-energy light (Fig. 3.1). The model of using very low energy, narrow-band light with specific pulse-code sequences and durations is termed LED photomodulation [10].

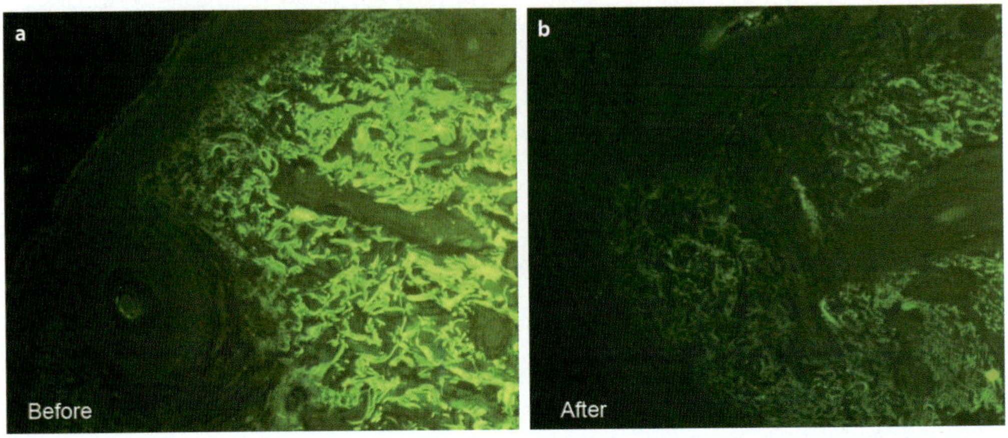

Fig. 3.1. **a** Immunostaining for matrix metalloproteinases (MMP) of human skin before yellow 590 nm light-emitting diode (LED) treatments. **b** MMP immunostaining of human skin after yellow LED treatments; note reduced staining

Currently Available Technologies

Photorejuvenation

LED photomodulation can be used both alone and in combination with a variety of common nonablative rejuvenation procedures in an office setting. Several anti-inflammatory and wound-healing applications are also emerging. Treatments can be delivered using the Gentlewaves yellow light, 590-nm LED photomodulation unit (LightBioScience, Virginia Beach, VA, USA) with a full-face panel device. With this LED technology, energy density is set at 0.15 J/cm^2. One hundred pulses are delivered with a pulse duration of 250 ms and an off interval of 100 ms. Treatment time is less than 1 min. We have treated more than 1000 patients over the last 2 years. Of these treatments, 30% were LED photomodulation alone and 70% were photomodulation concomitant with a thermal-based photorejuvenation procedure. Using specific pulsing sequence parameters, which are the basis for the "code" of LED photomodulation, a multicenter clinical trial was conducted with 90 patients receiving a series of 8 LED treatments over 4 weeks [11–14]. This study showed very favorable results, with over 90% of patients improving by at least one Fitzpatrick photoaging category and 65% of the patients demonstrating a global improvement in facial texture, fine lines, background erythema, and pigmentation. Results peaked at 4–6 months following completion of a series of eight treatments [14]. Another study using the same 590-nm LED array demonstrated similar results confirmed by digital microscopy (Fig. 3.2) [15].

Goldberg and his group have shown that other wavelengths of LED light, using red and infrared wavelengths, may be effective for improvement in skin texture [16]. With this approach, each treatment is given in a continuous mode with a treatment time of 20 min using 633 nm and 830 nm as an LED array (Omnilux, Phototherapeutics, Lake Forest, CA, USA).

In their report of 36 patients receiving 9 treatments over a 5-week period, these investigators not only evaluated improvements in skin textural changes, but also undertook biopsy sampling to determine the ultrastructural posttreatment changes in collagen fibers. They noted a statistically significant improvement in wrinkles, as evaluated by profilometric analysis. The majority of subjects reported improvements in softness, smoothness, and firmness at the end of treatment. Finally, electron microscopic analysis

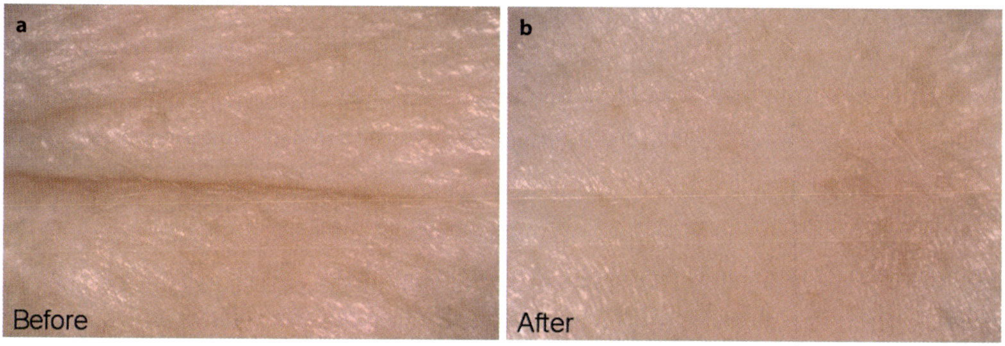

Fig. 3.2. **a** Digital microscopy before yellow LED treatments. **b** Improvement in digital microscopic changes in skin after a series of yellow LED treatments

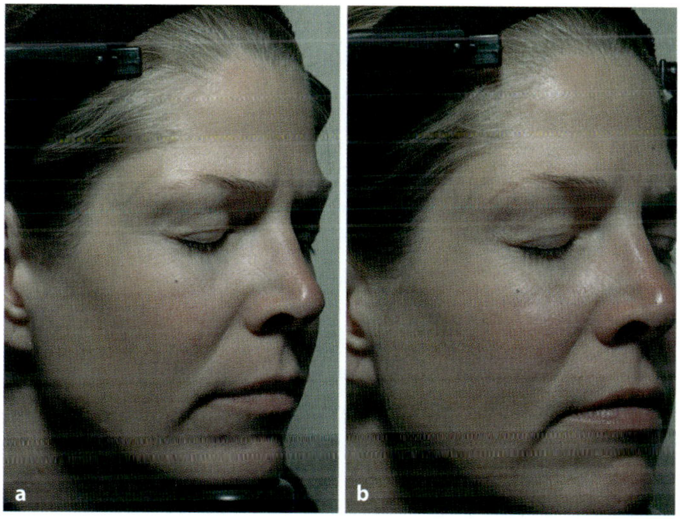

Fig. 3.3. **a** Before a series of red/infrared LED treatments. **b** Improvement in skin quality after a series of red/infrared LED treatments (photographs courtesy of David J. Goldberg, MD)

showed evidence of LED-treatment-induced thicker collagen fibers (Figs. 3.3 and 3.4)

When LED photomodulation is given alone with the yellow 590-nm pulsing array, patients with mild to moderately severe photo aging receive eight treatments over a 4-week period. Alternatively, patients may receive LED photomodulation immediately following a nonablative treatment such as IPL, PDL, KTP, or infrared lasers including 1064 nm, 1320 nm or 1450 nm. We find that using LED photomodulation in combination with other modalities results in more effective clinical results as well as faster resolution of erythema. It is believed that the faster resolution of erythema is a result of the anti-inflammatory effects of LED photomodulation. Some patients may receive a series of yellow LED photomodulation treatments for atopic eczema or to reduce bruising and/or second-degree burns. It is unknown whether other LED wavelengths including red or blue are effective for anti-inflammatory effects.

LED treatments may also improve facial acne [17]. In one study, 24 subjects with Fitzpatrick skin types II–V, with mild to severe symmetric facial acne vulgaris, were treated over 8 sessions, with alternating 415-nm blue

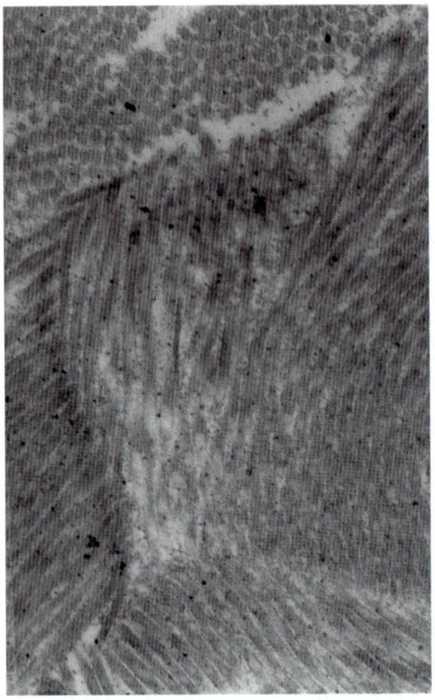

Fig. 3.4. Ultrastructural evidence of type I collagen formation after a series of red/infrared LED treatments (photograph courtesy of David J. Goldberg, MD)

light (20 min/session, 48 J/cm^2) and 633-nm red light (20 min/session, 96 J/cm^2) from an LED-based therapy system. Patients also received a mild microdermabrasion before each session. Acne was assessed at baseline and weeks 2, 4, 8, and 12.

Twenty-two patients completed the trial. A mean reduction in lesion count was observed at all follow-up points. At the 4-week follow-up, the mean lesion count reduction was significant at 46% (p=0.001). At the 12-week follow-up, the mean lesion count reduction was also significant at 81% (p=0.001). Patient and physician assessments were similar. Severe acne showed a marginally better response than mild acne. Side effects were minimal and transitory. Comedones did not respond as well as inflammatory lesions.

The investigators of this study concluded that a combination of blue and red LED therapy appears to have excellent potential in the treatment of mild to severe acne [17].

Photodynamic Therapy

Red light (630 nm) has been used for many years in combination with a sensitizer (levulinic acid) for photodynamic therapy (PDT) [18]. When exposed to light of the proper wavelength, the sensitizer produces an activated oxygen species, singlet oxygen, which oxidizes the plasma membrane of targeted cells. Due to a lower metabolic rate, there is less sensitizer in the adjacent normal tissue, hence a lesser reaction. One of the absorption peaks of the metabolic product of levulinic acid, protoporphyrin, absorbs strongly at 630 nm red. A red LED panel emitting at 630 nm (Omnilux PDT, Phototherapeutics, Lake Forest, CA, USA) has been used for this purpose [18]. We have also used the full-panel 590 nm LED array for facilitating PDT. This therapy is delivered by application of levulinic acid (Levulan DUSA, Wilmington, MA, USA) for 45 min and exposure to continuous (nonpulsed) 590 nm LED for 15 min for a cumulative dose of over 70 J/cm^2. This approach is further described in Chap. 2 of this textbook.

Mechanism of Action

The primary means for photomodulated upregulation of cell activity by LED is the activation of energy-switching mechanisms in mitochondria, the energy source for cellular activity. Cytochrome molecules are believed to be responsible for the light absorption in mitochondria. Cytochromes are synthesized from protoporphyrin IX and absorb wavelengths of light from 562 nm to 600 nm. It is believed that LED light absorption causes conformational changes in antenna molecules within the mitochondrial membrane. Proton translocation initiates a pump, which ultimately leads to energy for conversion of ADP to ATP. This essentially recharges the "cell battery" and provides more energy for cellular activity.

Others have confirmed that mitochondrial ATP availability can influence cellular growth and reproduction, with lack of mitochondrial ATP associated with oxidative stress [19]. Cellular aging may be associated with decreased mitochondrial DNA activity [20]. Previous work has also demonstrated rapid ATP production within mitochondria of cultured fibroblasts exposed to 590 nm yellow LED light only with the proper pulsing sequence [4,21]. New ATP production occurs rapidly after LED photomodulation, triggering subsequent metabolic activity of fibroblasts [13]. There also appear to be receptor-like mechanisms that result in modulation of the expression of gene activity producing up- or down-regulation of gene activity as well as wide-ranging cell signaling pathway actions. The choice of photomodulation parameters plays a vital role in determining the overall pattern of gene up/downregulation. In our experience, use of LED yellow light without the proper pulsing sequence leads to minimal or no results on mitochondrial ATP production. Others have found that LED without pulsing produces clinical results, although no cellular activity in fibroblast cultures have been reported [16].

LED arrays are useful for collagen stimulation and textural smoothing. Wound healing studies show slightly accelerated wound resolution. Initial experience and observations confirm that combinations of thermal nonablative photorejuvenation and nonthermal LED photomodulation have a synergistic effect. LED photomodulation is delivered immediately subsequent to the thermal-based treatment for its anti-inflammatory effects, which may reduce the thermally induced erythema of nonablative treatments.

Blue light therapy (415 nm) is effective at activating coproporphyrin III and protoporphyrin IX, subsequently destroying the *Propionibacterium acnes* bacteria. There is a marked correlation between the reduction in numbers of *P. acnes* bacteria and clinical improvement in patients with acne [11]. Red light (633 nm) is less effective at activating coproporphyrin III than blue light, but is a potent activator of protoporphyrin IX, also found in *P. acnes* bacteria [7]. Since red light penetrates deeper into tissue than blue, it is possible that red light actively destroys any *P. acnes* bacteria residing in the lower regions of the sebaceous gland. Furthermore red light has noted anti-inflammatory properties. Young et al. demonstrating that red light influences the production of anti-inflammatory cytokines from macrophages while at the same time increasing the synthesis of fibroblast growth factor from photoactivated macrophage-like cells [12].

The effect of visible red light on the local vasculature is also well recognized. The red light will bring more oxygen and nutrients into the area, further helping to reduce inflammation and enhance the wound repair process

Lam et al. [22] demonstrated that in vitro irradiation of fibroblasts with a 633-nm-wavelength LED light increased procollagen synthesis fourfold from baseline while exhibiting no effect on the activity of the collagen-regulating proteolytic enzymes collagenase and gelatinase. Irradiation with this red light increased fibroblastic growth factor synthesis from photoactivated macrophages and accelerated mast cell degeneration [23].

Light at a wavelength of 830 nm (near infrared) is absorbed in the cellular membrane rather than in cellular organelles, which remain the target when using light in the visible spectrum. Irradiation at 830 nm leads to accelerated fibroblast–myofibroblast transformation and mast-cell degranulation. In addition, chemotaxis and phagocytic activity of leucocytes and macrophages is enhanced through cellular stimulation by this wavelength [24,25].

Advantages

Patients who receive pure Gentlewaves LED photomodulation alone without concomitant treatment report that they observe a softening of skin texture, and reduction of roughness and fine lines that ranges from significant to

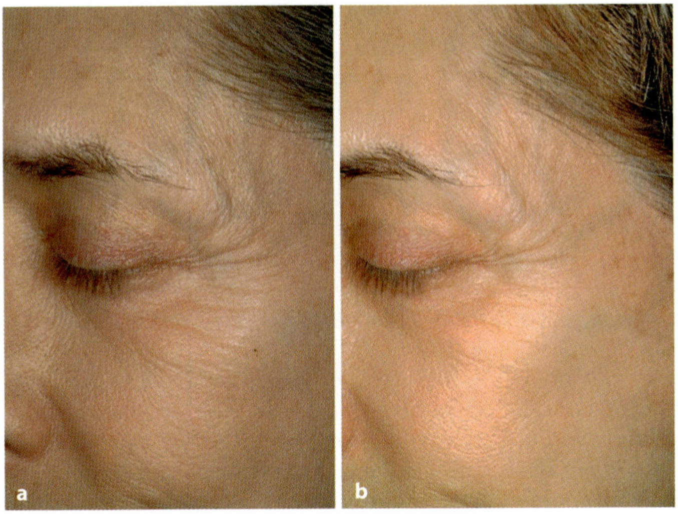

Fig. 3.5. **a** Before a series of yellow LED treatments. **b** Reduction in roughness and fine lines after a series of yellow LED treatments

sometimes subtle changes (Fig. 3.5). The USA FDA recently cleared LED devices to be used in the reduction of periocular wrinkles. Gentlewaves was the initial device approved; Omnilux followed. Studies have borne out that textural changes with reduction in fine lines can be observed on photoaged skin.

Consent

LED treatments present very little risk. Nevertheless, a similar consent to that used for laser treatments is commonly provided to patients (see Chap. 1)

Personal Approach

Our clinical experience over the last 2 years in a busy cosmetic dermatologic surgery practice indicates that these effects of LED photomodulation on skin texture and fine lines, although subtle, are observed on a much larger number of patients than reported in the original clinical studies.

Patients having a thermal photorejuvenation laser or light- source treatment with no LED photomodulation versus with LED treatment report noticeable reduction in posttreatment erythema and an overall impression of increased efficacy with an accompanying LED treatment [26,27]. Anecdotal treatment of atopic eczema in patients withdrawn from all topical medications has led to rapid resolution within three to four treatments.

Future

Pilot studies for atopic eczema indicate that there is the potential to further utilize the specific anti-inflammatory properties of LED photomodulation. Preliminary data from DNA microarray analyses of the entire human genome of certain skin cell lines after LED photomodulation and also after ultraviolet injury and subsequent LED therapy are currently being analyzed and support a versatile role for LED photomodulation in enhancing cellular energy production as well as diverse effects on gene expression. LED photomodulation may even negate some of the negative aspects of ultraviolet exposure [22]. Many clinical and basic science research pathways await further exploration for this exciting new nonthermal, low-risk technology.

References

1. Weiss RA, McDaniel DH, Geronemus RG (2003) Review of nonablative photorejuvenation: reversal of the aging effects of the sun and environmental damage using laser and light sources. Semin Cutan Med Surg 22:93–106
2. Weiss RA, Goldman MP, Weiss MA (2000) Treatment of poikiloderma of Civatte with an intense pulsed light source. Dermatol Surg 26:823–827
3. Fatemi A, Weiss MA, Weiss RA (2002) Short-term histologic effects of nonablative resurfacing: results with a dynamically cooled millisecond-domain 1320 nm Nd:YAG Laser. Dermatol Surg 28:172–176
4. McDaniel DH, Weiss RA, Geronemus R, Ginn L, Newman J (2002) Light–tissue interactions I: photothermolysis vs photomodulation laboratory findings. Lasers Surg Med 14:25
5. Whelan HT, Smits RL Jr, Buchman EV, Whelan NT, Turner SG, Margolis DA, et al (2001) Effect of NASA light-emitting diode irradiation on wound healing. J Clin Laser Med Surg 19:305–314
6. Whelan HT, Connelly JF, Hodgson BD, Barbeau L, Post AC, Bullard G, et al (2002) NASA light-emitting diodes for the prevention of oral mucositis in pediatric bone marrow transplant patients. J Clin Laser Med Surg 20:319–324
7. Whelan HT, Buchmann EV, Dhokalia A, Kane MP, Whelan NT, Wong-Riley MT, et al (2003) Effect of NASA light-emitting diode irradiation on molecular changes for wound healing in diabetic mice. J Clin Laser Med Surg 21:67–74
8. Walker MD, Rumpf S, Baxter GD, Hirst DG, Lowe AS (2000) Effect of low-intensity laser irradiation (660 nm) on a radiation-impaired wound-healing model in murine skin. Lasers Surg Med 26:41–47
9. Lowe AS, Walker MD, O'Byrne M, Baxter GD, Hirst DG (19998) Effect of low intensity monochromatic light therapy (890 nm) on a radiation-impaired, wound-healing model in murine skin. Lasers Surg Med 23:291–298
10. McDaniel DH, Weiss RA, Geronemus R, Ginn L, Newman J (2002) Light–tissue interactions II: photothermolysis vs photomodulation clinical applications. Lasers Surg Med 14:25
11. Weiss RA, McDaniel DH, Geronemus R, Weiss MA (2005) Clinical trial of a novel non-thermal LED array for reversal of photoaging: clinical, histologic, and surface profilometric results. Lasers Surg Med 36:85–91
12. McDaniel DH, Newman J, Geronemus R, Weiss RA, Weiss MA (2003) Non-ablative non-thermal LED photomodulation – a multicenter clinical photoaging trial. Lasers Surg Med 15:22
13. Geronemus R, Weiss RA, Weiss MA, McDaniel DH, Newman J (2003) Non-ablative LED photomodulation – light activated fibroblast stimulation clinical trial. Lasers Surg Med 25:22
14. Weiss RA, McDaniel DH, Geronemus R, Weiss MA, Newman J (2004) Non-ablative, non-thermal light emitting diode (LED) phototherapy of photoaged skin. Lasers Surg Med 16:31
15. Weiss RA, Weiss MA, Geronemus RG, McDaniel DH (2004) A novel non-thermal non-ablative full panel led photomodulation device for reversal of photoaging: digital microscopic and clinical results in various skin types. J Drugs Dermatol 3:605–610
16. Goldberg DJ, Amin S, Russell BA, Phelps R, Kellett N, Reilly LA (2006) Combined 633-nm and 830-nm LED treatment of photoaging skin. J Drugs Dermatol 5:748–753
17. Goldberg DJ, Russell BA (2006) Combination blue (415 nm) and red (633 nm) LED phototherapy in the treatment of mild to severe acne vulgaris. J Cosmet Laser Ther 8:71–75
18. Tarstedt M, Rosdahl I, Berne B, Svanberg K, Wennberg AM (2005) A randomized multicenter study to compare two treatment regimens of topical methyl aminolevulinate (Metvix)-PDT in actinic keratosis of the face and scalp. Acta Derm Venereol 85:424–428
19. Chen HM, Yu CH, Tu PC, Yeh CY, Tsai T, Chiang CP (2005) Successful treatment of oral verrucous hyperplasia and oral leukoplakia with topical 5-aminolevulinic acid-mediated photodynamic therapy. Lasers Surg Med 37:114–122
20. Zhang X, Wu XQ, Lu S, Guo YL, Ma X (2006) Deficit of mitochondria-derived ATP during oxidative stress impairs mouse MII oocyte spindles. Cell Res 16:841–845
21. Sorensen M, Sanz A, Gomez J, Pamplona R, Portero-Otin M, Gredilla R, et al (2006) Effects of fasting on oxidative stress in rat liver mitochondria. Free Radic Res 40:339–347
22. Lam TS, Abergel RP, Meeker CA, Castel JC, Dwyer RM, Uitto J (1986) Laser stimulation of collagen synthesis in human skin fibroblast cultures. Lasers Life Sci 1:61–77
23. Young S, Bolton P, Dyson M, Harvey W, Diamantopoulos C (1989) Macrophage responsiveness to light therapy. Lasers Surg Med 9:497–505
24. Osanai T, Shiroto C, Mikami Y (1990) Measurement of Ga ALA diode laser action on phagocytic activity of human neutrophils as a possible therapeutic dosimetry determinant. Laser Ther 2:123–134
25. Dima VF, Suzuko K, Liu Q (1997) Effects of GaALAs diode laser on serum opsonic activity assessed by neutrophil-associated chemiluminescence. Laser Ther 9:153–158

26. Weiss RA, Weiss MA, McDaniel DH, Newman J, Geronemus R (2003) Comparison of non-ablative fibroblast photoactivation with and without application of topical cosmeceutical agents. Lasers Surg Med 15:23

27. Weiss RA, McDaniel DH, Geronemus RG, Weiss MA, Beasley KL, Munavalli GM, et al (2005) Clinical experience with light-emitting diode (LED) photomodulation. Dermatol Surg 31:1199–1205

Chapter 4

Botulinum Toxins

Joel L. Cohen and Kenneth Beer

4

Core Messages

- Botulinum toxin injections have revolutionized the field of nonfacial rejuvenation.
- In the USA, Botox® is the only approved botulinum toxin A used for facial rejuvenation.
- Other botulinum toxins available elsewhere in the world are currently being evaluated for use in the USA.
- Botulinum toxin A is an ideal primary agent or adjunctive agent for facial rejuvenation.

Introduction

In the 15 years since Jean and Alastair Carruthers reported the use of botulinum toxins (BTXs) for cosmetic indication, this procedure has become the most popular cosmetic procedure in the United States [1,2]. At a time when use of this neurotoxin was limited to treatments for strabismus, torticollis, and other dystonias, the Carruthers' recognized the potential for aesthetic areas of treatment.

Since those initial reports, core aesthetic physicians have explored new indications for BTX injections – both alone as well as in conjunction with fillers, lasers, and light sources. The utility of BTX injections has not only expanded into a myriad of cosmetic usages, but also into a wide range of therapeutic areas. Newer applications of the toxin have led to a better understanding of the anatomic intricacies of the face as it relates to minimally invasive aesthetic surgery. Aesthetic areas once considered difficult to treat with BTX, such as the perioral area, are now routinely being injected and improved. In addition, brow sculpting and facial asymmetries are now just some of the other aesthetic areas being addressed with injections of BTX.

Over time, injectors have learned many important lessons, such as tailoring dosing regimens. Whereas physicians once injected enough material to eliminate movement in a given area, many now choose to leave some residual movement to preserve a more youthful look without having the appearance of a "deer in the headlights" (with the forehead being the best example of physicians decreasing dosages over the past few years). Injections of BTX may also be used to postpone more invasive procedures (such as surgical repair of mild blepharochalasis) and to enhance the results of more invasive surgical procedures such as laser resurfacing of the periocular area, browlifts, and facelifts in general [3,4]. Noncosmetic applications are also expanding beyond strabismus and dystonias and now include the treatment of migraines, hyperhidrosis, postherpetic neuralgia, anal fissures, and even tennis elbow [5–8]. Psychological benefits have also been attributed to BTX type A (BTX-A) injections, and it is believed that this mechanism of action relies upon the ability of BTX-A to improve a patient's facial affect and to help convey a more positive and relaxed emotion [9].

As the therapeutic and cosmetic uses have expanded, so, naturally, have the reports of potential complications. Instances such as the loss of expression after injection and diffusion of toxin into unintended muscles have resulted in patients who have detrimental cosmetic outcomes rather than enhancements. Injections by various types of nonaesthetic physicians, and especially nonphysicians have also resulted in an increase in the number of bad outcomes from this product [10]. Experienced injectors now strive to obtain a relaxed "natural" look for their patients rather than total paralysis. In addition, core aesthetic physicians have the training and know-how to offer their patients a range of combination therapies previously unimaginable.

With the number of people being treated with BTX-A exceeding 3 million people per year and increasing [2], it behooves all physicians injecting this product to have a complete understanding of its strengths, potential complications, relevant anatomy, and complementary treatments that can be used to achieve optimal outcomes.

The goal of this section is to provide a thorough understanding of BTX-A physiology and relevant facial anatomy. How to best use this product for an ever-expanding variety of cosmetic procedures will also be a primary focus. Becoming a proficient injector requires not only mastery of the technical aspects of injections, but also an understanding of the potential pitfalls associated with various injections. A realistic understanding of what may and may not be accomplished with this modality is also presented.

The Product

BTX has seven subtypes (A–G). Of these, two are clinically relevant at the present time (types A and B). Differences between the two type A products (Botox® and Reloxin) are important to understand, particularly their respective dosing regimens. Differences between type A products and the type B product (Myobloc) are more profound, involving mechanisms of action as well as dosing and migration characteristics.

The Anatomy

It is impossible to have precise placement of BTX without a solid understanding of the underlying structures where you intend to place it. For this to occur, the relevant anatomy of each area injected must be thoroughly appreciated. In addition to an understanding of anatomy as it appears in a textbook, functional variations that occur from patient to patient must also be appreciated so that individualized treatments are tailored for best patient outcomes.

The Patient

It is imperative that the physician impart to the patient a realistic understanding of what can be accomplished in his or her face. Before injecting any product, it is essential to carefully assess the patient's face. Special attention to preexisting asymmetries as well as existing rhytides and scars should be documented in the patient record and, whenever possible, photographs should be taken (especially for first-time patients). For every cosmetic procedure undertaken, a careful discussion of the proposed plan including its limitations, risks, and need for recurring treatments should occur prior to the treatment.

Pretreatment Consultations

When treating patients with BTX, it is essential to minimize the risk of patient dissatisfaction. Each patient should be made aware of the duration of correction, the potential side effects, and the fact that uses for areas other than the glabella constitute an "off-label" indication for BTX-A in the United States at the present time. Consent should be in the form of an oral discussion as well as a written document signed and dated, preferably in several places (on each page or in areas indicating salient issues). All patients should be made aware that the typical duration of BTX-A is often 3–4 months for most aesthetic indications (the perioral area tends to be a bit shorter). And again, all preexisting conditions, such as asymmetries and scars should be discussed, documented, and preferably photographed prior to treatment.

Indications by Area

Glabella

At the present time, the glabella is the only United States Food and Drug Administration (FDA)-approved site for the cosmetic injection of Botox®. It also represents the most common site of aesthetic BTX-A treatment. Patients and aesthetic physicians frequently begin their experiences with BTX-A with injections in this area as they are technically the most easily accomplished and are well tolerated from the patient's perspective. Treatment of the glabellar complex frequently results in a high degree of patient satisfaction, and quite often their desire to return for additional treatments in this and other areas.

When injecting the glabella (and brow), it is important to avoid potential BTX-A diffusion (through the orbital septum) to the levator palpebrae superioris muscle of the upper lid. If static rhytides (etched-in lines at rest) are present in addition to the dynamic ones (lines that form with muscular contraction), it is best to show and document to the patient the lines that are imprinted in the skin and not expected to significantly improve after BTX-A This may be accomplished by stretching the skin and showing the creases that may be present following treatment with BTX. This demonstration is also an opportunity to discuss the adjunctive use of fillers such as Cosmoderm or hyaluronic acid products that can be used to soften these imprinted lines. The synergistic usage of fillers and BTX-A has been well documented, and in many patients their concomitant use can not only result in a better correction, but also a more durable response than with an injectable aesthetic product used alone [11].

Several patients who have had excellent results from glabellar injections may have less effective treatments over time. This is typically the result of recruitment of adjacent musculature from the midbrow area, leading to some muscular movement at the lateral glabellar complex. Specifically, this is caused by medial pull of orbicularis oculi fibers toward the tail of the corrugator muscle. The potential for this eventuality should be discussed with patients and may be demonstrated by using a mirror to show the inactivity of the corrugator complex and the "push" from the midbrow area that is causing the medial brow to move. Failure to discuss and/or treat this component may lead patients to believe that BTX-A did not effectively address their concerns. Prior to injecting the glabellar area, it is also important to evaluate the length, direction, and bulk of the corrugators as well as the prominence of the procerus and nasalis muscles as they relate to the proposed treatments, so that the individualized dosing and injection pattern can be most accurately decided upon for each unique patient.

Forehead

Many patients seek treatment of prominent or evolving horizontal forehead lines through injection of the frontalis muscle. When considering treatment of this area, it is important not to look at the frontalis in isolation since it is anatomically intertwined with the eyebrow and eyelid below. For this reason, redundant upper eyelid skin in patients should be noted prior to forehead BTX-A injections. In particular, this should be discussed with patients who desire correction of every last line of their foreheads, especially patients concerned about the most inferior forehead rhytides just above the lateral brow. Patients with blepharochalasis typically have imprinted lines in their foreheads above the lateral brow due to their frontalis trying to compensate for their bow-lid redundancy by hoisting the lateral upper lids cephalad. Treatment of this area in such patients and in those with dermatochalasis is very likely to accentuate their brow ptosis by relaxing these inferior frontalis fibers being relied upon to compensate for brow-lid redundancy [12].

Patients seeking treatment in the forehead and brow should also be helped to understand the gender differences between male and female brow shape and position. Whereas males tend to have horizontally oriented brows, females tend to have brows that are arched. Each of these shapes may be maintained or achieved through well-considered injection sites. To achieve an arched feminine brow, BTX-A injections should spare the lateral elevators (lateral frontalis) but treat the lateral brow depressors (lateral aspect of the orbicularis oculi). In general, the lower 2–3 cm of the frontalis elevates and shapes the brow, and this area should be avoided in most women. This will avoid brow heaviness in patients who rely upon the frontalis to pull the brow and lids upward while at the same time preserving some brow expression.

Mid and Lower Face

Treatment of the mid and lower face is best reserved for experienced injectors and patients who have already enjoyed the benefits of successful BTX-A in the upper face. The lower face requires more advanced knowledge of anatomy and technique, and is less forgiving. Misadventures in the lower face may result in significant facial asymmetry and speech impediments. Thus, before embarking upon a treatment session involving the lower face, one should have a thorough discussion with each patient as to what the likely and potential effects of such treatments are upon the position of the mouth, contour of the lips, and ability to animate the perioral area. A detailed discussion of other treatments such as soft-tissue augmentation alone or in combination with BTX-A should also occur at this time.

Lips

Injections of BTX-A into and/or around the lips has several caveats unique to this site [13]. Treatment of this area does have risks including decreasing the ability to purse the lips, create a seal around a spoon, drink from a straw, whistle, or enunciate some words (especially with "p, b, j, or g). Occasionally, patients can complain of difficulty applying lipstick as well. Treatments in this area should therefore be avoided in those patients who rely upon their lips for either their vocation or avocation. This may include those who are avid scuba divers or are broadcast journalists, public speakers, or play wind instruments.

Patients considering BTX-A treatments of the lips need to understand what the procedure can accomplish for them. In the right patient, injections of the lip can soften the vertical muscular columns that appear when a patient speaks or chews. Treatment of these columns can in some patients also lead to the appearance of fuller lips. This latter effect is accomplished by diminishing the hollowing appearance of the vertical muscular bands, offering a "pseudoaugmentation." However, treatment of this area will not completely prevent and will certainly not obliterate etched-in vertical lip lines. Patients with deep perioral rhytides would be best treated with fillers and/or resurfacing lasers. To be very clear, patients with prominent muscular vertical columns who do not yet have significant etched-in cutaneous lines are the specific types of patients who may benefit most from BTX-A alone or in combination with fillers.

For patients who are candidates, be sure to communicate to them that the musculature of this area and the small dosages used its treatment translate into shorter duration of effect than in other areas. Since each area is treated with only a few units, treatments usually have an average duration of about 6–8 weeks.

Unfortunately, any discussion of the therapeutic or cosmetic uses of BTX-A is clouded by concerns about infections with its derivational agent *Clostridium botulinum*. This bacterium is an anaerobic, spore-forming organism that, under the proper conditions, can germinate and create a deadly toxin.

Beginning in the 1920s and through the 1930s, investigators including Herman Sommer and Justinius Kerner began exploration of the therapeutic potential of BTX. Kerner suggested potential therapeutic uses of toxin to block abnormal motor movements (such as chorea) and speculated on its use in disorders with hypersecretion [14,15].

Type A toxin was isolated in 1946 by Edward Shantz for the United States Army, which briefly considered its use as a warfare agent. It was also Shantz who, more than 30 years later in 1979, prepared the first batch of what would later be called "Botox®." This initial batch served as the source of all BTX-A used clinically in humans in the United States until 1997, when the FDA approved the BTX-A source used by Allergan (Irvine, CA, USA).

A study published in 1973 demonstrated that injections of BTX-A could weaken extraocular muscles in monkeys. This led the way to its use in humans in 1977. Two years later, the FDA granted limited approval to use BTX-A for strabismus; in 1985, this approval was expanded to include blepharospasm. Allergan acquired the BTX-A source in 1989 from Oculinum, then owned by early proponent ophthalmologist Alan Scott. It was during this period that the FDA approved the use of BTX-A for strabismus, blepharospasm, and hemifacial spasm. Despite FDA limitations, BTX-A was tried for nystagmus, torticollis, spasmodic dystonia, and many other diseases related to muscle dysfunction.

In 1987, Canadian ophthalmologist Jean Carruthers recognized the cosmetic potential of BTX-A. While treating patients for benign essential blepharospasm, Dr. Carruthers noted that several patients treated for blepharospasm had significant improvement of dynamic rhytides in the glabellar region. Following this observation, Drs. Alastair and Jean Carruthers began more systematic studies of BTX-A for cosmetic indications. In 1991, the Carruthers reported their initial findings of cosmetic treatment with BTX-A at North American Dermatology and Ophthalmology meetings. Their first publication on this topic was in 1992, demonstrating the safe and effective treatment of dynamic rhytides in the glabella with BTX-A [1]. In 1993, Blitzer and colleagues described the use of BTX for rhytides of the forehead [16]. Over the next decade, reports ensued of the efficacy of BTX-A in the many cosmetic areas reviewed in this chapter. Finally in 2003, BTX-A (Botox®) was approved for the treatment of glabellar rhytides. BTX-A continues to be investigated and there are reports of efficacy in a wide range of medical and aesthetic areas including the treatment of hyperhidrosis, headaches, and depression.

Currently Available BTXs

Currently in the United States, the only FDA-approved brand of BTX-A is Botox®. Other brands are available elsewhere in the world, some of which are currently being evaluated in the United States. This chapter will focus on Botox®, with the recognition that the described core principles apply to all BTX-As.

The integrity of the BTX-A product as well as its proper handling and reconstitution are essential aspects of any treatment. As was amply demonstrated during a botulism poisoning from the use of imported raw BTX (South Florida in 2004), the use of nonapproved toxins or BTXs that are extemporaneously compounded may have significant deleterious consequences.

Botox® (Allergan, CA, USA), is manufactured and distributed in a lyophilized form. The powder is subsequently reconstituted using saline. Although the manufacturer recommends reconstitution with preservative-free saline, substitution with preserved saline may afford a more comfortable injection without altering its efficacy [17]. Once reconstituted, the manufacturer suggests that BTX-A be refrigerated at 2–8°C. Other additives have been mixed during the reconstitution of Botox®. A single case report exists of adding hyaluronidase to Botox® in an effort to facilitate its spread and decrease the overall dosage required in the treatment of axillary hyperhidrosis [18].

Dilution of the Toxin for Cosmetic Purposes

Various experienced injectors have different techniques for reconstituting the Botox® brand of BTX. For every 100-unit bottle, most injectors will dilute with between 1 and 4 ml of saline. Larger volumes of diluent result in a more dilute solution that is potentially more likely to diffuse. This type of diffusion may be desirable for certain areas (for instance the forehead or orbicularis oris), where diffuse or sphincter-like muscles require broad areas of treatment [19]. More concentrated solutions (from 1 to 2.5 ml per bottle) may be more suited to injections of discrete muscles that are smaller and easily identified or isolated (for instance the corrugators).

Several studies have demonstrated that efficacy is based upon the total number of units used [20,21], making overall dosage more important than the dilution of the product [22]. At the present time, there is no uniformly accepted dilution for Botox® and no consistently reliable method (short of electromyogram devices) to identify the exact location of the muscles targeted. Therefore, it is necessary to understand the principles of BTX diffusion before embarking upon patient treatments with this product.

Needles

As with the wide variation of reconstitution techniques that exist among experienced injectors, there is a range of needles used by those same physicians. Some injectors espouse the use of a 32-gauge needle with the belief that the smaller size results in more comfortable injections and is less likely to inadvertently traumatize a small vessel in the area. Others use 30-gauge needles because they believe that these needles are sharper than the 32-gauge needles. A third contingent advocates the Becton-Dickinson integrated syringe-needle combination because the 31-gauge needles with this device have a short hub, so potentially there is less loss of product in the needle itself. Suffice it to say, whatever needle one chooses, it is imperative to change it frequently so that it does not become dulled following injections into the skin. Additional caveats include avoiding the same needle being used to penetrate the rubber stopper and then inject the patient, as this will most certainly be a dull needle being inserted into the patient's skin.

Advantages of BTX Injections

By now, it is widely known that the approved BTX-A formulation (Botox®) is safe and effective for many cosmetic and therapeutic indications. Over the span of more than 15 years, Botox® has offered outstanding clinical outcomes for facial rhytides, with minimal recovery time and no permanent side effects.

The ease and cost-effectiveness of aesthetic treatments with BTXs have spurred several million people per year to undergo these treatments. More than 3.3 million people per year undergo treatment and some report the boost in self-esteem that can accompany an improved appearance [9]. It can also improve the lives of those with facial asymmetries (such as Bell's Palsy), or an unintentional sad affect (frown or downturned smile) [23].

Disadvantages of BTX Injections

One disadvantage of BTX-A is the relatively short duration of its clinical effect compared to other common aesthetic procedures such as fillers and lasers. Although recurring treatments with BTX-A may result in an increased duration of overall efficacy, generally injections need to be repeated every 3–4 months.

Other potential BTX-A complications are often related to poor technique or inappropriate patient selection – or a combination thereof. Frequent complications may include bruising, swelling, and transient headache [24]. Ptosis of the eyelid occurs in usually less than 1% of patients (even much less so, in the opinion of the authors, with the more experienced injectors) and generally resolves within 2–3 weeks [25]. Occasionally, patients may observe more effect on one side than the other, causing an asymmetric or unbalanced appearance. This may be corrected with additional "enhancement" injections (a term we prefer over "touch-up"). Strabismus is a temporary side effect that has been infrequently reported. Although rare, some patients may develop resistance to treatment with BTX. These are usually patients treated with large amounts of toxin for medical rather than cosmetic indications (such as cervical dystonia, where average dosages used are over 300 units of Botox®), and was far more common prior to 1997 when the protein load in Botox® was 80% higher [25]. Rashes can also occur following injections with toxins, but they are infrequent and transient [24].

Indications

At the present time, the treatment of glabellar lines remains the only FDA-approved cosmetic indication for Botox®. However, as is common with most drugs, its off-label uses in other areas are diverse and they continue to expand. For medical dermatological indications, it is used for the treatment of focal hyperhidrosis, but is FDA-approved only for the axillary form of this entity.

Injections of BTX benefit some patients with headaches, spasticity, dystonia, torticollis, hemifacial spasm, blepharospasm, Meige syndrome, spastic dysphonia, Frey's syndrome, writer's cramp, or tremors. It has also been reported to be safe and effective in the treatment of bladder dysfunction [26].

Contraindications

Contraindications to treatment with BTX-A include patients who are pregnant, breastfeeding or have neuromuscular diseases, such as myasthenia gravis, Eaton-Lambert syndrome, or amyotrophic lateral sclerosis (Lou Gehrig's Disease). Patients allergic to albumin or who are known to be allergic to any ingredient in the BTX-A formulation should also avoid treatment.

Informed Consent

Appropriate management of patient expectations is of paramount importance in all cosmetic procedures. The use of written informed consent is recommended for most cosmetic procedures. Typically, the consent should state that the cosmetic use of BTX (Botox®) in any area other than the glabella currently constitutes an "off-label" indication in the United States. Patients should also be aware of their pretreatment appearance, and the use of pretreatment photography to provide documentation is certainly recommended. The use of photographs mitigate the risk that patients will blame the treatment itself for lines that "magically" appear following the injections (this typically occurs when the lines that were a patient's primary source of concern disappear after treatment and their attention shifts to another line or area). The consent process should also indicate the fact that subsequent treatments incur additional costs (this avoids the discussion with patients who occasionally think that the treatment was promised to have an efficacy of at least 3–4 months). Injections of BTX-A are intended to treat hyperdynamic lines, *not lines at rest*, and this distinction should be part of the consent process as well.

A proper informed consent should be specific for the areas of treatment. It should mention complications including headache, flu-like symptoms, bruising, eyelid drooping, anaphylaxis, smile asymmetry, speech enunciation changes, or even very rare cases of dysphagia [24,25].

During the patient consultation, it is helpful to explain the dose–response curve for BTX-A. As an extension of this, it is also helpful to explain that the number of units used by the treating physician are believed to be the correct dose for relaxing the target musculature, but that each person is different and that he or she may require more or less than the average patient. Because each person has different anatomy, it is possible that a particular individual may require more or less units than recommended averages published in consensus papers [27]. In the event that more is required, a waiting period of approximately 14 days is recommended – as it is most helpful to wait sufficient time for the onset of maximal action of the product. It is imperative to study the anatomy of the patient being treated, and it may be helpful to demonstrate the muscles involved in a particular rhytide using a mirror. Having muscular diagrams available and/or drawing the normal anatomy (with muscle fiber orientation) for patients allows them to observe the function of the various muscles.

Personal Approach

The patient treatment approach described in this section emphasizes the importance of not only a thorough understanding of the physiology of BTX-A, but also a mastering of the underlying anatomy of the areas being treated.

Prevention and Management of Patient Discomfort

To minimize the risks of swelling and bruising, patients can be advised (if medically feasible) to discontinue aspirin, vitamin E, and nonsteroidal anti-inflammatory drugs at least 1 week prior to treatment. However, there is to date no clinical trial comparing the incidence of bruising and swelling in patients that have and have not discontinued these products. To help minimize the discomfort associated with any injection, it may be helpful to pretreat a small minority of needle-phobic patients with topical anesthetic products, such as lidocaine. Pre- and posttreatment application of ice to the injection sites may decrease the incidence of bruising and swelling through some degree of vasodilation in the treatment area. In addition, many patients find that the application of ice makes the procedure more comfortable.

Prior to applying topical anesthetics, it is important to identify patients with potential allergies to components contained therein. This is especially true for topical anesthetic products as many contain ester derivatives, which contain a sulfur moiety analog. Prior to any facial injection, it is important to thoroughly cleanse the area of makeup, lipstick, or any foreign substance containing dyes. It is recommended that alcohol be used to clean the sites, and also that this chemical is allowed to thoroughly evaporate prior to the injection of BTXs (as there is a theoretic risk of alcohol inactivating the toxin).

Approaches to Specific Areas

Glabella

Please refer to Figs. 4.1 and 4.2.

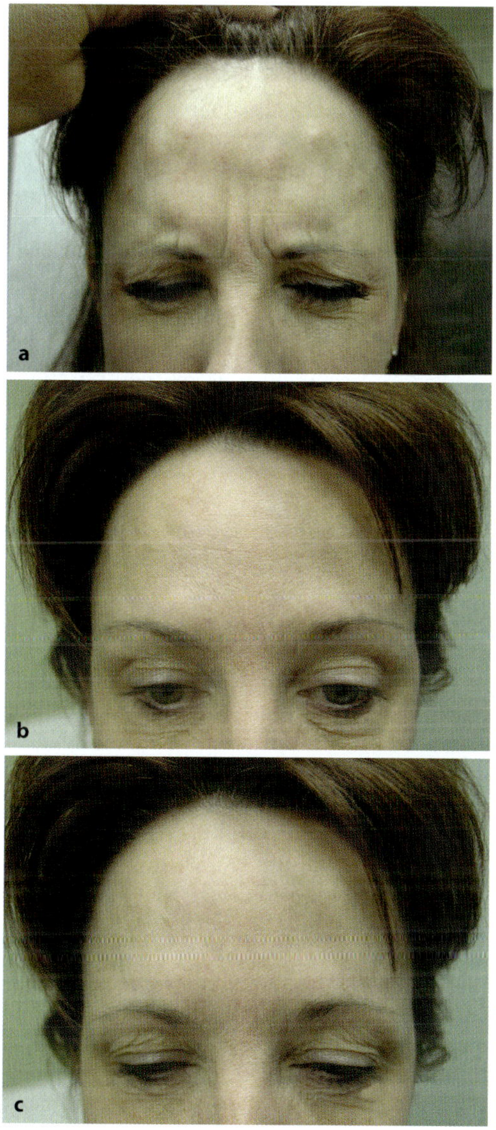

Fig 4.1 **a** Glabellar folds, pretreatment, with maximum frown. **b** Glabellar folds, posttreatment, at rest. **c** Glabellar folds, posttreatment, with maximum frown

Glabellar Anatomy

The glabella remains the most frequently injected cosmetic site for BTX-A. At the present time, it remains the only site that is FDA-approved for cosmetic Botox® injections. Its

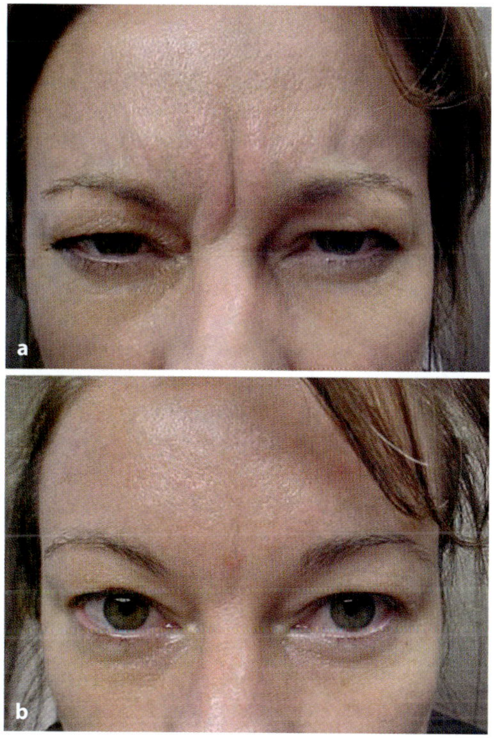

Fig. 4.2. **a** Glabella , pretreatment. **b** Glabella, posttreatment

anatomy is best understood not only by picturing the individual muscles independently, but also through understanding that the glabella area functions as a complex of interrelated muscles that work in the intertwined manner belied by their anatomy.

Relevant brow anatomy is considered in two distinct aspects: the medial brow and lateral brow. Medial brow anatomy includes the depressor supercilii, procerus, corrugator supercilii, and frontalis. Lateral brow anatomy includes the lateral portion of the orbicularis oculi and the frontalis muscles, and it will be considered in the periorbital section below.

The depressor supercilii originates on the nasal bridge and inserts into the skin of the midbrow area. It draws the middle and medial portions of the brow inferiorly and medially. The corrugators also draw the mid and medial brow in these directions. These corrugator muscles originate on the nasal bone and insert into the skin of the brow above the pupil. Due to variations in anatomy, the insertion point into the brow may be more lateral in some people than in others. This variation is occasionally responsible for movement of the brow even after the glabella treatment has been properly dosed. In addition to these two muscles, the third muscle that forms the medial brow complex is the procerus. Unlike the other two muscles, which tend to form vertical lines by drawing the skin medially, the procerus forms horizontal lines by drawing the skin inferiorly. The procerus muscle originates on the nasal bridge and inserts into the skin of the midglabella directly above it. As these muscles contract, they form etched-in lines perpendicular to the direction of their action. Treatment of the glabellar area with BTX typically addresses the muscles in concert. Opposing these brow depressor muscles is the frontalis, which is a brow elevator. The frontalis may be a solitary wispy sheet that invests the entire forehead, or it may be two muscles (in a "V-shape") separated by a thin fascial component in the mid forehead

As the corrugator and depressor supercillii muscles function as medial brow depressor, BTX-A treatment of them results in a medial brow lift that is cosmetically desirable. This effect is distinct from reduction of the "scowl" lines associated with activity of these muscles. Due to the proximity of the frontalis muscle, treatment of the glabella may result in diffusion to some of its central inferior fibers. This may result in some degree of relaxation of lower and medial aspects of the frontalis muscle. If significant diffusion to the frontalis occurs, the medial brow lift may be offset due to the brow elevation function of the frontalis being weakened. This weakening of the inferomedial frontalis fibers can result in a compensatory hyperactivity of the superior and lateral frontalis fibers. This provides increased muscular tone, and sometimes a lateral brow lift as a result. Thus, this compensatory lateral frontalis activity may be the most important mechanism in producing the brow lift that follows glabellar injections of BTX.

Injection Techniques for the Glabella

Variations in technique exist between expert injectors in their approaches to the medial brow complex. Many inject using 20–30 units of Botox® distributed between five injection sites [19] Others treat this area with three injections, allowing diffusion to treat the adjacent areas. Differences in muscle mass affect the amount of toxin needed for relaxation of the glabellar complex, so each patient really needs to be treated based upon their individual anatomy. Patients with hypertrophic muscles in this area require higher doses of toxin, and men may require more units than women [28].

The most commonly utilized pattern for the glabella utilizes a range of doses in the five injection site technique: one injection for the procerus, one on each side of the medial corrugators, and one on each side of the lateral corrugators [27]. When injecting the lateral corrugators, care must be taken to inject at least 1 cm above the orbital rim in order to avoid potential inferior diffusion into the underlying levator palpebrae superioris muscle, which can result in eyelid ptosis.

Individual dosing adjustments are frequently required based on the prominence and distribution of the glabellar musculature. The adjustment for prominent "medial recruitment" of the orbicularis oculi along the vertical axis of the mid-pupillary line frequently can require 2–3 units of additional Botox® approximately 1.5 cm above the bony supraorbital rim. A more reliable landmark than the eyebrow (which can be tweezed and otherwise manipulated), the supraorbital rim should be used to identify locations for injections. Forceful injections in this area should also be avoided, as these may increase the risk of diffusion as well as increase the risk of bruising and headaches. When evaluating for the appropriate injection sites, observe the length and direction of the corrugator during frowning. Grasping the corrugators between one's noninjecting thumb and forefinger may help to isolate this muscle during the injection

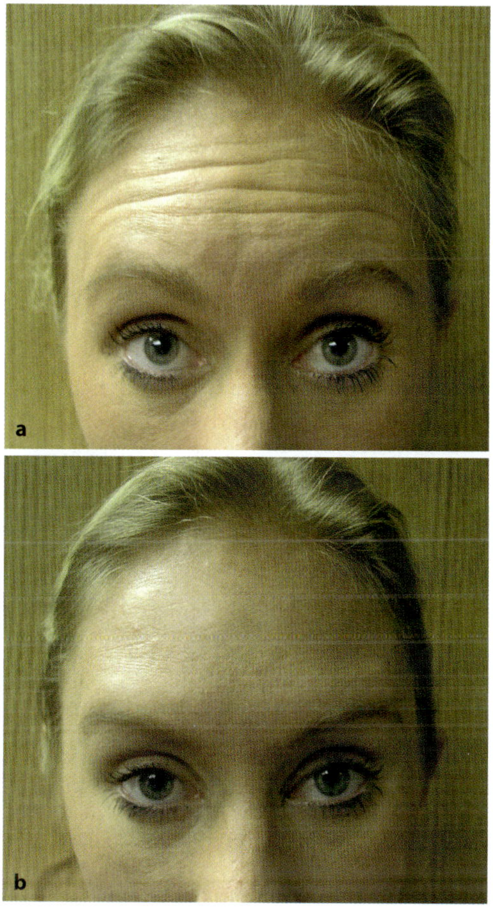

Fig. 4.3. **a** Before treatment of forehead. **b** Improvement in forehead wrinkles

itself. Again, if you follow a standard or recipe injection distribution, some patients will end up with significant pull medially at the mid-pupillary line. This is due to recruitment of the lateral corrugator and sometimes the orbicularis oculi, and may be treated with additional injections of small amounts of toxin as described above.

Forehead

Please refer to Figs. 4.3–4.6

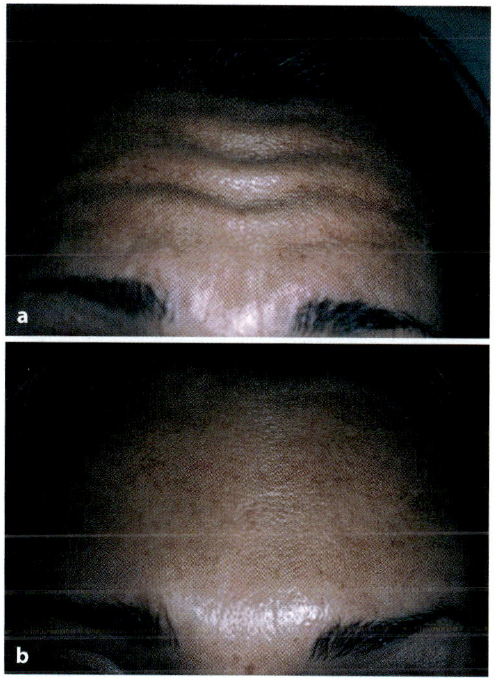

Fig. 4.4. **a** Before treatment of forehead. **b** Improvement in forehead wrinkles (photographs courtesy of David J. Goldberg, M.D)

Anatomy of the Forehead Musculature

The frontalis muscle has significant variability between individuals but, in general it is considered to be either a "V" shape or a uniform band. The vertical orientation of the frontalis muscle fibers allows it to function as a brow elevator. Knowledge of frontalis interaction with the musculature of the medial and lateral brow (described above), allows the skilled physician to tailor his or her technique to fit the goals and anatomy of each patient. Contraction of the frontalis muscle raises the brow, which results in transverse rhytides across the forehead. In order to visualize the function of the frontalis in a given patient, one can instruct the patient to elevate their brows maximally.

The superior aspect of the frontalis muscle is continuous with the galea aponeurotica of

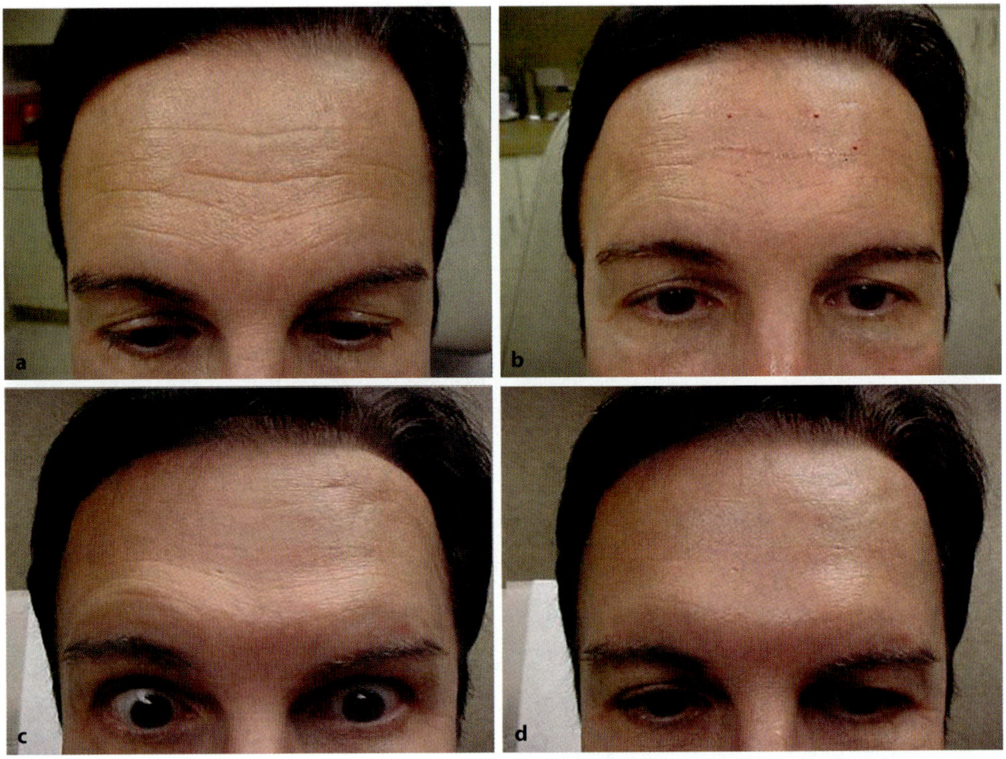

Fig. 4.5. **a** Forehead wrinkles before treatment. **b** Forehead wrinkles immediately after treatment with both botulinum toxin (BTX) and collagen filler injections. Note immediate improvement caused by filler. **c** Forehead wrinkles 1 week after treatment with both BTX and collagen filler injections. Further improvement induced by BTX injection. **d** Forehead wrinkles 2 weeks after treatment

the scalp. Inferiorly, the frontalis inserts into the skin of the brow. The lateral border of the frontalis muscle is the temporal fusion line. This fusion plane is the boundary between the frontal and temporal bones, and is easily palpated in most people. Inferior and lateral to the temporal fusion line, the downward pull from the lateral orbicularis muscle counteracts the upward pull of the frontalis. Understanding the interaction between these two opposing muscle groups is critical to creating a brow lift using BTXs [29].

Injection Technique for the Forehead

The injection technique for the frontalis muscle depends on the anatomy, gender, and goals of the individual being treated. The goal for some patients is to be entirely wrinkle-free. Except in rare instances, this should be avoided for several reasons. Eliminating every wrinkle of the forehead can increase the length of the forehead, and can neutralize the frontalis' baseline muscular contraction needed for the inherent brow elevation that can avoid sagging.

Preserving the arched brow in a female patient calls for a different injection technique than that use for a man with a horizontal

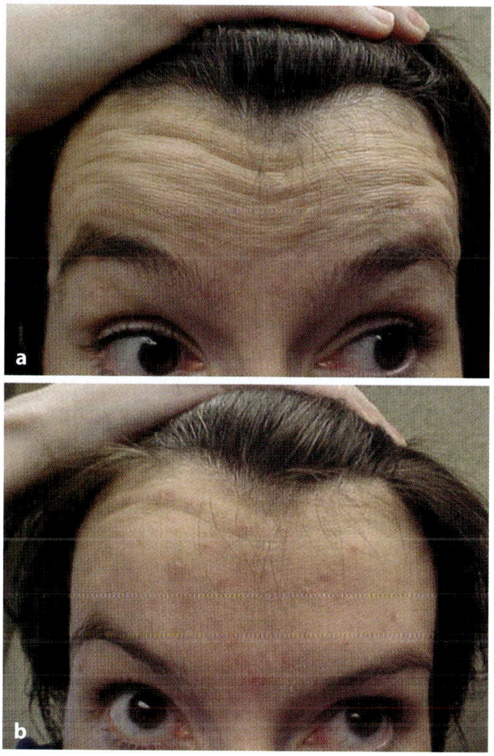

Fig. 4.6. **a** Before treatment of forehead. **b** Improvement in forehead wrinkles

brow. In a woman, avoiding injections near the temporal fusion plane allows residual frontalis pull upward and, thus the lateral brow to maintain an inherent degree of lift. In a man, injection of a small amount of BTX-A into the lateral aspect of the forehead is used to produce a horizontal brow. For men, the depressor component of the superior-lateral orbicularis oculi is usually not be injected as it will also contribute to a lateral brow lift. When injecting the forehead of older women, horizontally imprinted lines immediately above the lateral brow should not be injected as this musculature elevates the brow and compensates for redundant lateral brow/lid skin. Removing muscle activity from this area results in a "heavy" brow that may need to be manually suspended for makeup to be applied. Finally, for all forehead treatments, superficial injection is the preferred injection technique to avoid the discomfort associated with piercing the periosteum. Following injection, gentle pressure on the injection blebs may facilitate some mild diffusion to this large frontalis muscle.

When injecting a younger woman (25–40 years of age) with minimal skin laxity, several injections are made into the frontalis in a pattern that utilizes between five and nine injections. When treating women with wide or tall foreheads, adjustment of the injection sites must take their individual anatomy into account. Patients with tall foreheads may benefit from a second row of injections superior to the first one. Wider foreheads require more lateral injections to cover their increased expanse. Failure to extend the injections laterally in some patients can result in a "Mr. Spock" brow caused by untreated lateral frontalis musculature.

In most female patients, injection points should remain about 1.5 cm medial to the temporal fusion line. Medial injection points should be at least 3–3.5 cm above the brow. A 1- or 2-cm^3 dilution for Botox® will likely reduce the risk of spread to unintended areas of muscle. Treatment of the glabella may be accomplished concurrent with the frontalis treatment. Alternatively, injectors can first treat the glabella and have patients return 2 weeks later, frequently allowing lower overall dosages to be used in the forehead (secondary to spread from the glabellar complex to some of the inferior and medial frontalis fibers). Pretreatment marking of the muscles during animation will enable the physician to avoid injections that are placed too inferiorly. Average doses for frontalis treatments in women typically range from 10 to 18 units of Botox® (lower overall dosages than in years past in order to preserve a more "natural look"). Treatment of the frontalis in a man may require 20–40 units of Botox®. One study has shown that higher dosages of BTX-A used in the forehead are clearly associated with a longer duration of efficacy in this area [30].

4

Crow's Feet and Infraorbital Rhytides

Anatomy of the Periorbital Area and of the Eyelids

Variations in the patterns of the lateral crow's feet exist among patients, and they have been elegantly described by Kane [31]. The main muscle affecting the lateral orbital area is the orbicularis oculi, which is a thin band that surrounds the eye in a sphincter-like manner, constricting the skin surrounding the eye. Since it is a circular muscle, its actions are different in specific areas (related to the fiber direction in each segment of the muscle). For example, portions of the orbicularis inferior to the lateral brow function as brow depressors. Portions superior and lateral to the pupil may potentiate medial pull, and thus frowning. At times, this portion may be responsible for a patients' ability to frown following adequate injection of the glabella complex (the so called "medial recruitment" sometimes seen after patients have had multiple glabellar treatments and the adjacent musculature tries to take over some of the previous lateral corrugator muscular function). The pretarsal component of this muscle has important actions for maintaining the shape of the eye. Treatment of a thickened or hyperfunctional pretarsal orbicularis can not only soften a prominent band of muscle below the eye, but can also change an almond-shaped eye to a more rounded appearance [32]. In these patients with a bulging muscular pretarsal orbicularis band beneath the eye, low doses (1–2 units for each infraorbital area) can be used to soften this muscular bulge (but unfortunately the creping skin in this area will remain). This treatment should be reserved for patients with minimal lower eyelid laxity (ensured by checking a "snap test" in some patients). Higher doses injected into this site increases the risk of causing "festooning" of the fat beneath the atrophic muscle [33].

Injection Technique for the Periorbital Areas

The most popular indication for injection of the orbicularis muscle is to prevent and treat lateral canthal rhytides (more commonly known as crow's feet). Treatment of these evolving wrinkles is associated with a high patient satisfaction and is technically straightforward. Using between 8 and 15 units of Botox® on each side, three or four injections sites are treated [34]. Injections should be made at least 1 cm lateral to the orbital rim to avoid any unintended diffusion to the ocular muscles (which could produce diplopia). Since the orbicularis oculi is quite superficial, injections should be made by raising a wheal. At the inferior aspect of this treatment zone, care must be taken not to extend too close to the zygomatic arch by pursuing every inferior rhytide, as this may lead to toxin diffusion to the zygomaticus minor and major muscles (impairing the ability to raise the corners of the mouth and lips).

One of the most interesting and technically challenging injections is the nonsurgical/chemical lateral brow lift. This treatment involves injecting approximately 3–6 units of Botox® into the portion of the orbicularis that tugs the lateral brow down [3]. When done in conjunction with injection of the medial frontalis, an even more significant lateral brow elevation may be achieved. However, in severe cases of eyelid redundancy, surgical blepharoplasty is the treatment of choice.

Lateral Brow Lift

One of the hallmarks of a youthful feminine brow is lateral elevation, which tends to give the patient a more alert, open-eyed look. As the lateral brow drops with age, that wide-eyed appearance is replaced by one of fatigue. Precise injections of BTX-A into the superior and lateral aspect of a woman's orbicularis oculi can restore a more youthful arch to many brows. Locating the correct injection site to accomplish this is essential and requires that patients animate to elicit the injection-guiding musculature on each side. To do this, patients must first elevate their brows to find the temporal fusion plane (where the lateral frontalis ends). Next, they must close their eyes forcefully, so the physician can mark the site where the orbicularis oculi maximally pulls the lateral brow inward and downward. The physician may then inject 4–6 units just inferior to the point of maximal pull, making sure this point is at least 1.5 cm away (lateral and inferior) from the temporal fusion area elicited [3,29]. This technique, in some cases, can achieve a 2- to 3-mm elevation of lateral brow. For more significant cases of brow-lid redundant skin, small aliquots of fillers (such as Restylane, JuveDerm Ultra, or CosmoPlast) may be injected into the lateral aspect of the brow as well to help fill some of the redundant skin [35]. Combination therapy with BTX-A and filler may also increase the duration of response in this area, as has been documented in other sites of combination therapy such as the glabella [11].

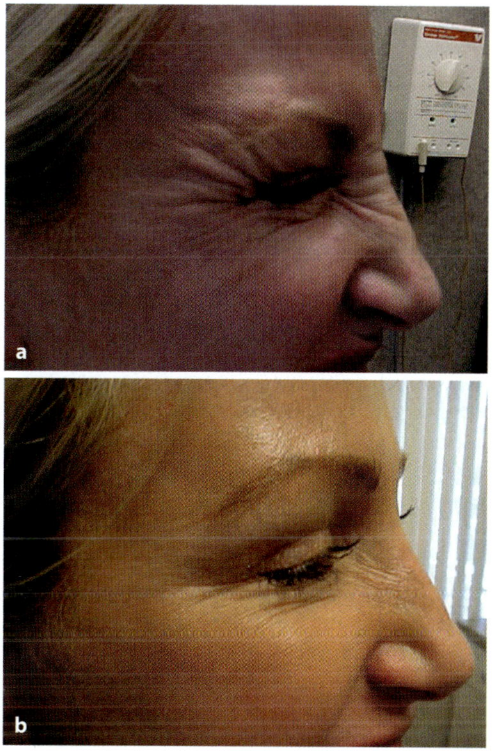

Fig. 4.7. **a** Before treatment of bunny lines. **b** Improvement in bunny lines after BTX injections

"Bunny Lines"

Please refer to Fig. 4.7

Anatomy/Injection

The upper nasalis muscle is responsible for the formation of "bunny lines" at the bridge of the nose that extend horizontally toward the medial canthus [36]. These lines may form a sharp contrast to a BTX-A treated smooth glabellar area, and thus may be considered a sign that someone has had the glabellar and crow's feet areas treated with BTX-A.

It is certainly a consideration that the nasalis be injected concurrently with the glabella. This muscle can be isolated for injection by having the patient scrunch their nose. The nasalis muscle is injected with approximately 3–5 units of Botox® superficially at each medial proximal nasal sidewall. Needle insertion should be superficial, and injections into the periosteal plane should definitely be avoided. Caution must also be exercised to avoid lateral placement of injections in this site, as this may affect the levator labii superioris aleque nasi (LLSAN), and cause elongation or drooping of the upper lip. To complete this cosmetic unit, it is best to also treat the procerus with 5–7 units of Botox® in order to complement the glabella and nasalis regions [37].

Lower Face

Anatomy of the Lower Face

The corners of the mouth are moved by two sets of opposing muscles: elevators and depressors. The major elevator of the lateral mouth and cheek is the zygomaticus major. Medial elevation is accomplished by the zygomaticus minor as well as the levator labii superioris.

4

The orbicularis oris is a sphincter-like muscle that surrounds the mouth. It is responsible for pursing the lips and the eventual formation of perioral rhytides. It is this pursing that frequently prompts complaints from women of lipstick "bleeding" into these vertical lines.

The position of the lips is also controlled by depressors (located inferiorly) that counteract the elevator muscles. In some individuals, the depressor anguli oris can cause the lateral aspects of the mouth to turn inferiorly over time. This may falsely impart a negative emotion for which patients frequently seek improvement.

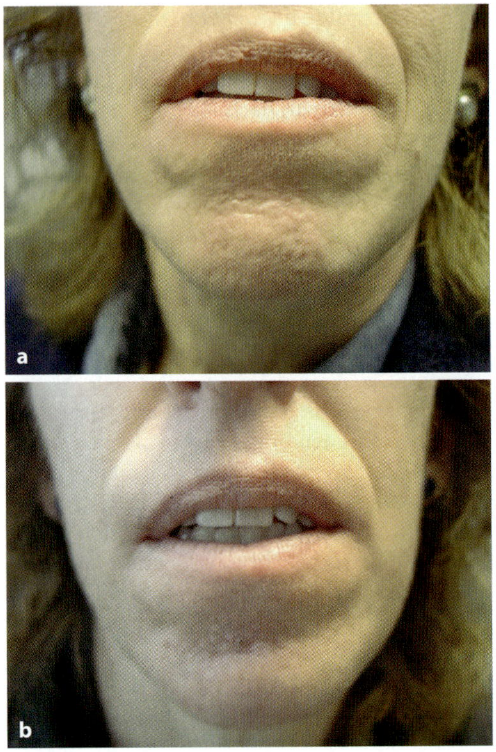

Fig. 4.8. **a** Dimpling of chin. **b** Improvement of chin dimpling after mentalis muscle injection

Injections of the Mentalis

Please refer to Fig. 4.8. At the most inferior portion of the central face lies the mentalis muscle. This muscle originates in the incisive fossa and inserts into the skin of the chin. It is responsible for the appearance of some of the subcutaneous imperfections in the chin area that are variously described as "pebbled chin," "apple dumpling chin," "golfball chin," or "peau d'orange chin". BTX-A treatment of this area relaxes the mentalis and can lead to significant improvement of the appearance of a chin with these types of small indentions [38].

The mentalis muscle may be triggered by asking the patient to push his or her lower lip upwards. Treatment of this area may be made with 4–8 units injected at the bony part of the chin (either as a single midline injection or as two medial injections approximately 1 cm apart). Caution should be taken as too lateral an injection can diffuse to depressor labii inferioris resulting in slurred speech. This treatment can also sometimes be used to soften the mental crease, but treatment of a prominent mental crease is best improved with filler substances.

Injection Technique for the Lips

Please refer to Figs. 4.9–4.11. Injection of the lips is generally more painful than other sites, and pretreatment with a topical anesthetic or ice may make this injection more tolerable. One common regimen employed for treatment in this area uses a more dilute solution of BTX-A. The total dose for treatment of this

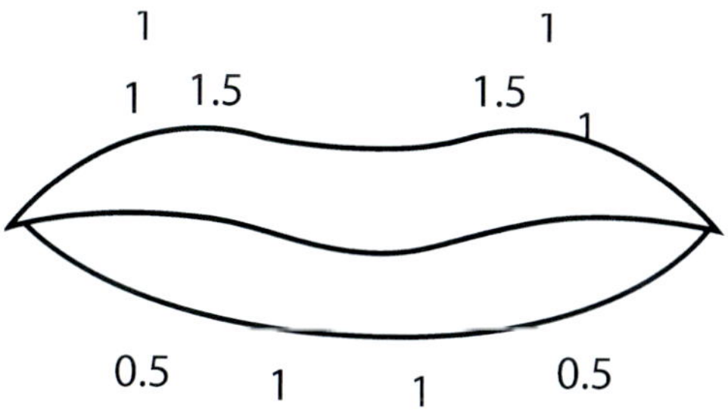

Fig. 4.9. BTX injection points for upper and lower lips

area is typically 6–10 units when the upper and lower lip vertical columns are treated simultaneously (which the authors recommend).

In the upper lip, two injection points on the vermillion border on each side of the upper lip spaced about 1.5 cm apart, as well as another more superior injection site between them 1 cm above the vermillion border. Maintenance of symmetry is critical to preservation of a midline philtrum. For the lower lip, injections should be placed along the vermillion border, using two sites on each side of the lip, also spaced about 1.5 cm apart. Following injection, pressure should be applied for a few minutes to enhance diffusion and reduce the risk of significant bruising in this highly vascular area.

Injection Technique for the "Gummy Smile"

A "gummy smile" refers to excessive showing of the gums above the maxillary teeth. This type of smile pattern can be treated by reducing the activity of the LLSAN muscle. This muscle may be also identified by asking the patient to "scrunch" the tip of his or her nose. Palpation of the pyriform aperture, which is adjacent to the alar groove, during this "scrunching" will facilitate site selection for this injection [39]. Injection of 1–3 units of Botox® should be placed in each superior medial nasolabial fold into the LLSAN. BTX-A

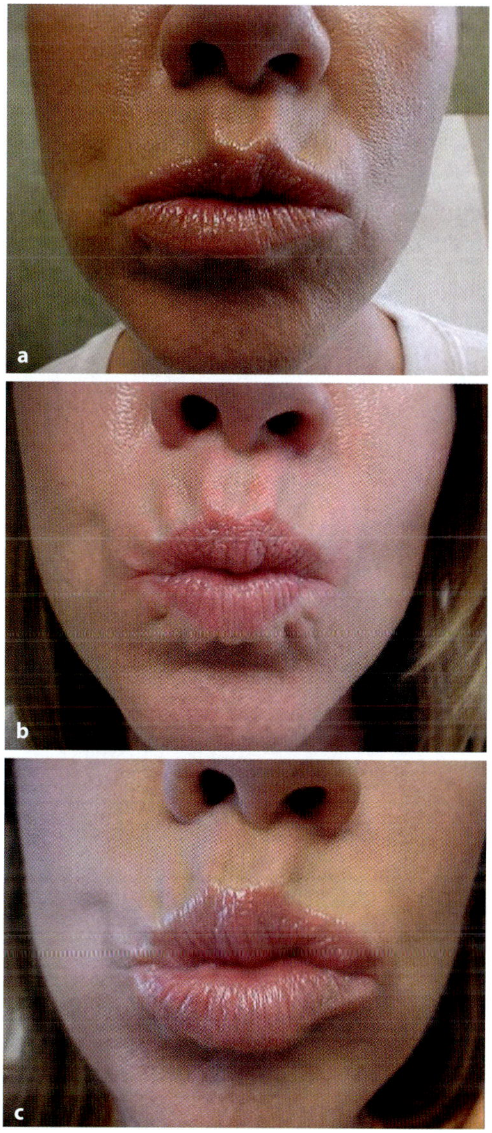

Fig. 4.10. **a** Lips before treatment. **b** Initial response to BTX injections. Touch-up treatment provided. **c** Asymmetry of the same patient improved after further injections provided

treatment of the area relaxes this muscle, causing the upper lip to mildly elongate and cover some of the previously exposed upper portion of the teeth. This treatment is best for younger patients with significant upper gum

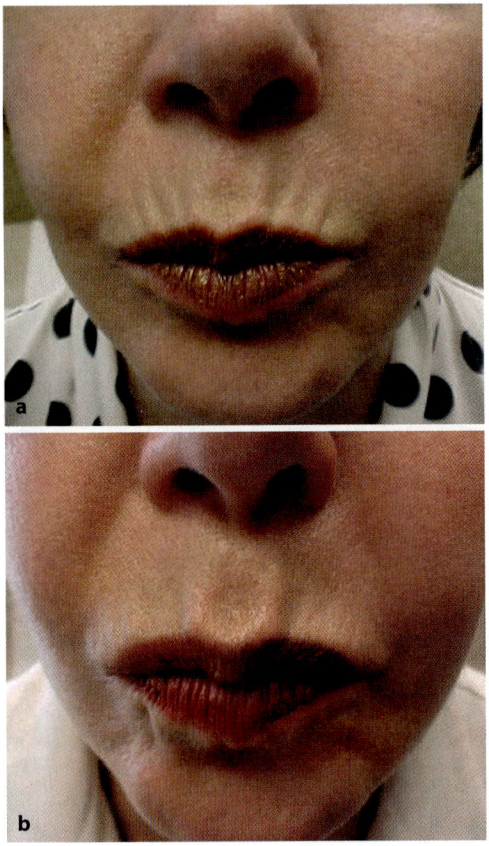

Fig. 4.11. **a** Vertical lip columns. **b** Improvement in vertical lip columns after botulinum toxin injections

show when smiling, sometimes called the "extreme canine smile." Caution should be exercised when treating older patients as BTX treatment of the LLSAN can cause an accentuation of mid-face flattening and cutaneous upper lip vertical elongation (which normally occurs to some extent with the normal aging process, and further accentuation of this elongation may be undesirable in those patients. Treatment of the LLSAN should be reserved for experienced physician injectors. Injection of this muscle is also sometimes performed in the case of patients with a very significant upper nasolabial fold, where a filler substance is used in combination.

Injection Technique for the "Downturned Smile"

A "downturned smile" can misrepresent emotions and impart a sad or concerned appearance. Treatment of a prominent depressor anguli oris and the associated downturned smile can result in a more neutral or horizontal smile. Usually 3–5 units of Botox® can be injected pointing laterally and aiming for the posterior aspect of the depressor anguli oris muscle. Injecting 1–2 mm above the mandible can be another helpful landmark to successfully treat this muscle and avoid unwanted diffusion medially toward the depressor labii inferioris (which would cause asymmetry and slurred speech). In some patients, however, the downward muscular prominence is so significant and accompanied by subcutaneous volume loss in the lateral lower oral commissure that a filler substance is also necessary to help achieve a softening of the downturned smile [23].

Injection Technique for Vertical Neck Bands

Surgical neck lift procedures, chin/neck liposuction, and less often the general aging process can result in prominent vertical neck bands that are a frequent source of patient concern. These hyperfunctional platysmal bands differ from horizontal lines, which are believed to be from prominence of the superficial musculoaponeurotic system. Vertical platysmal bands that are prominent at rest can be relaxed by experienced BTX-A injectors. As a word of caution, however, injections of the platysma may rarely (or at least theoretically with significant diffusion or higher doses) cause singers to have difficulty reaching high notes.

The specific injection sites are determined at rest. Typically, a total of 20–35 units of Botox® are used, with retreatment 2–3 weeks later if necessary. Injections of between 1 and

3 units per site of Botox® are spaced approximately 1.5 cm apart along the vertical band. The bands should be individually grasped between the nondominant thumb and forefinger, and each injection should be superficially placed. Deep injections or higher dosages could potentially relax the platysma enough to allow the elevators of the lower face to lift the neck and jowls. In addition, one report of severe dysphagia occurred following injection with 60 units of Botox® in this area [40]. This patient required nasogastric tube feedings for 6 weeks until the BTX-A effect wore off. Thus, caution should be exercised when treating the neck. If a patient complains of swallowing difficulties following a procedure they should be evaluated immediately. Treatment should consist of a prompt ear-nose-and-throat and gastroenterology evaluation. This procedure is best reserved for those with prominent resting vertical platysmal bands in patients with good skin tone as well as those who are post-submental liposuction or post-face/-necklift.

Adjunctive Uses of BTXs

One of the most interesting aspects of BTXs is their use in conjunction with other minimally invasive procedures such as injection of soft tissue augmentation products and with lasers and other light sources.

Use of Toxins with Fillers

The combination of fillers with BTXs is one that makes a great deal of sense as many patients desiring treatment of dynamic rhytides also require volume replacement. From a mechanistic perspective, the use of toxins can reduce the ability of muscles to "pump" soft tissue augmentation agents away from their initial sites of placement. Among the fillers used with BTXs are collagen, calcium hydroxylapatite (Radiesse), hyaluronic acids (Restylane and JuveDerm), and poly-L-lactic acid (Sculptra). Permanent fillers that may be used with toxins include silicone and Artefill.

In addition, many of the dynamic rhytides treated with BTXs will have some static component at the time of treatment. Despite adequate inhibition of muscle activity, these resting wrinkles persist. Fillers offer an additional opportunity to correct the static rhytides. Areas amenable to correction with nonpermanent fillers and toxins include the glabella, periorbital area, mentalis, perioral area, and in some cases, the nasolabial creases.

Materials used in conjunction with BTX in the glabella include collagens and hyaluronic acids. The collagens that are most frequently used for the glabella are those that are non-crosslinked (e.g., Zyderm I or II, and Cosmoderm I or II) and are placed superficially. The deeper-placed crosslinked collagens are not recommended for this area. Hyaluronic acid products potentially useful for this area include those that are animal derived (Hylaform) as well as those that are non-animal derived (Restylane, Captique, JuveDerm), although these are a bit more risky as they are placed deeper than the Zyderm and Cosmoderm products. Particle size is a consideration when selecting a filler for the glabella and it is prudent to avoid any of the fillers that have a large particle size (such as Hylaform Plus or Perlane). Injection of thicker products requires deeper placement and more pressure, which can increase the risk of necrosis of the skin in this midline watershed area between the supratrochlear vessels. In addition, the vascular plexus of the eye may be the unintended recipient of filler via retrograde flow. BTXs can enhance the duration and degree of filler correction in the glabella [11]. When treating the glabellar area with both fillers and BTX, the filler should be injected before the injection of the toxin. This can theoretically reduce the risk of untoward migration of the BTX-A from the typical gentle massage required after fillers are placed. In addition, the Zyderm and Cosmoderm products contain an anesthetic, which may decrease the discomfort of the subsequent BTX-A injection to this area.

The periorbital crow's feet area may also benefit from use of toxins with fillers. As with the glabellar area, fillers will help to alleviate the static component of the rhytide, while the BTX-A can prolong the duration of the soft-tissue correction by decreasing the muscular pumping action.

Collagens have long been used to treat the periorbital areas. The thin skin of this area mandates the use of a thinner collagen (such as Cosmoderm or Zyderm). Hyaluronic acids can also be helpful for adjunctive treatment of this area, especially if placed superficially in very small serial puncture aliquots using a 32-gauge needle.

Rhytides of the upper lip are one of the best places to use combinations of fillers and toxins. Patients that have static and dynamic perioral rhytides will greatly benefit from the synergistic effect of the two treatments. Fillers effective with BTXs include collagens and hyaluronic acids (particularly ones with small particle size and the use of a 32-gauge needle). Poly-L-lactic acid (Sculptra in the United States, NewFill in Europe), which is currently only FDA-approved for the treatment of HIV-related lipoatrophy, is not recommended for injection in this area, as it is likely to result in subcutaneous papule formation or hypertrophic scarring when placed superficially [41]. Silicone (Silkon 1000; currently only FDA-approved for retinal hemorrhage) is also a potential off-label choice for this area, provided that the microdroplet technique is utilized. Injection of the depressor anguli oris in conjunction with volume replacement of the marionette lines is another synergistic combination that is quite effective (see above section entitled "Injection Technique for the "Downturned Smile"). Treatment with BTX not only helps to reduce the depressor function (allowing for less filler to restore proper positioning of the corner of the mouth), but will also decrease the muscular pumping that tends to move fillers out of their intended locations. Fillers used for the marionette lines include collagens, hyaluronic acids, poly-L-lactic acid, silicone, and calcium hydroxylapatite. As with other locations, each has its relative risks and benefits.

Mentalis creases may also be treated with combinations of fillers and toxins. Depending on the degree of static rhytides, fillers may make the difference between a dissatisfied patient and one that is thrilled. The choice of filler for this area depends on the experience and preference of the physician and patient.

Treatment Care and Complications

Side Effects

Sequelae that can occur at any site after injection of BTX (or really most types of aesthetic injections) include pain, edema, erythema, ecchymosis, headache, and short-term hypesthesia. Generalized reactions that have occurred idiosyncratically include nausea, fatigue, malaise, flu-like symptoms, and rashes at sites distant from the injection [24]. Headaches precipitated by BTX-A injections can usually be treated with over-the-counter analgesics, and have been reported to have a similar incidence even when placebo is used [42]. In fact, when evaluating the actual incidence of complications other than headache (such as bruising, for example), these are also comparable to reactions seen with placebo. Most of these postinjection issues resolve spontaneously and require only patient reassurance. To date, there have been no long-term adverse effects or health hazards related to the cosmetic injection of BTX-A [24].

Aftercare

Following cosmetic BTX-A injections, it is recommended to instruct the patient to "exercise" the muscles treated for 1–2 h. Patients are also commonly recommended to avoid bending, lying down, going to sleep, or exercising for about 2 h after treatment to theoretically avoid potentiating the diffusion of the toxin to unintended areas. The basis for these recommendations is arguable, but seems to be at least substantiated to some extent by the fact that radiolabeling studies of BTX-A have shown protein migration and binding to take at least about 1 h [43].

Follow-up

Most experienced physicians do not routinely see patients back for posttreatment follow-up after BTX-A injections except when treating certain more challenging cosmetic areas such as the perioral area or the neck, and after first-time hyperhidrosis treatment sessions (where a starch-iodine test is often used to highlight residual "hot spots" requiring treatment). If a follow-up visit is done, it should be scheduled approximately 2 weeks after the injection.

Complications by Treatment Area

Please refer to Figs. 4.12 and 4.13

Glabella

Complications from injections of toxins to the brow area are rare. Potential complications include headache, respiratory infection, flu syndrome, temporary ptosis, and nausea [44]. Other problems that may more commonly occur include bruising or temporary periorbital edema (the incidence of which increases with increased volumes of injection).

Ptosis of the eyelid is the most unsettling complication seen with treatment of the glabellar complex and its management is subject to debate. Oculoplastic surgeons recommend treatment of eyelid ptosis with over-the-counter Naphcon A. A second-line agent, apraclonidine hydrochloride (Iopidine 0.5% ophthalmic solution), is an alpha adrenergic agonist that may also be helpful in the treatment of ptosis. Both products are believed to cause contraction of the adrenergically stimulated Muellers muscle, which can help to lift a ptotic lid upward despite a paralyzed levator palpebrae superioris muscle. Users of Iopidine need to be aware that its use could potentially unmask and exacerbate an underlying glaucoma, so use of this should be reserved for refractory cases [45]. Left untreated, the ptosis will resolve over the span of a few weeks.

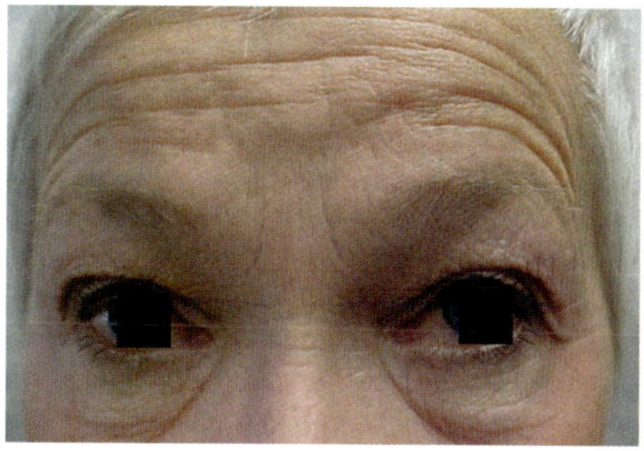

Fig. 4.12. Patient with dermatochalasis. BTX injections are contraindicated

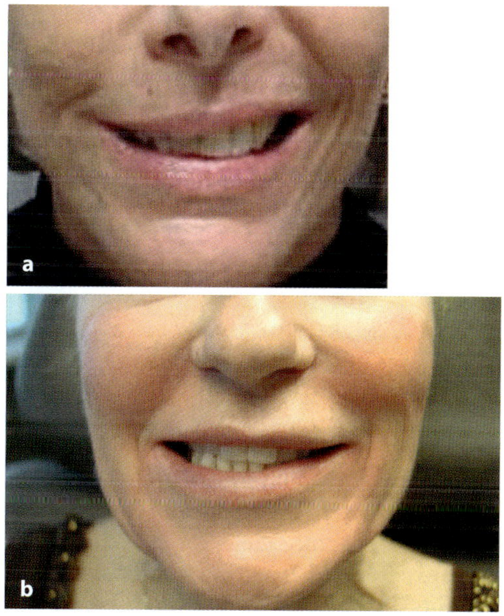

Fig. 4.13. **a** Asymmetry induced by improper injection technique by nonphysician BTX injector. **b** Asymmetry after injection

Forehead

Complications that can arise after injections of the frontalis include hematoma, brow ptosis, and headache. One problem that is encountered is the "Mr. Spock" brow that results when the lateral aspects of the frontalis elevate the lateral brow, producing a quizzical look. This situation is easily rectified with small dosages of 1–2 units placed in the residually functioning lateral frontalis. In those patients with at least moderate blepharochalasis, this "quizzical look" can alternatively sometimes be softened with about 2 units in the adjacent medial temporalis muscle.

Another situation unique to frontalis injections is an electrical shock sensation that occurs when the either the supratrochlear or supraorbital nerve is hit by the needle. Patients report a sharp pain that radiates along the distribution of the nerve toward the frontal scalp. This situation can often be avoided simply with superficial injections.

Orbital Area

The most common complication from injections in the periocular area are small hematomas and bruises. The rich vasculature of this area creates a minefield for injectors, and even experienced injectors will bruise some patients. It is helpful to wipe makeup off and have good lighting in order to try to avoid injury to these small vessels. More serious complications include ptosis, which occurs from injections that improperly placed and affect the levator palpebrae superioris. Injections placed too inferior on the zygomatic arch may lead to inability to raise the corners of the mouth or raise the lips, and this can be most unsettling for both physician and patient alike. Diplopia may occur from either direct injection or diffusion that brings toxin into contact with the extraocular musculature. Photophobia has also been reported [24].

Gummy Smile

Complications seen in this area may include asymmetry of the lips and too significant of an elongation of the upper lip

Platysma

There has been one report of diffusion of BTX (after 60 units of Botox®) to the swallowing apparatus musculature, with the patient requiring a nasogastric tube for several weeks [40].

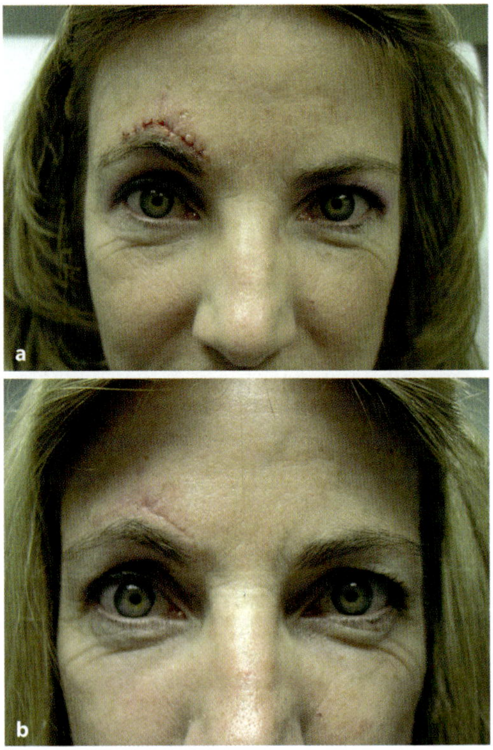

Fig. 4.14. **a** Asymmetry of forehead after surgery. **b** Improvement in asymmetrical surgical induced forehead lines after BTX injections

The Future

Please refer to Figs. 4.14 and 4.15. One of the most frequent uses of BTX is for cosmetic indications and this is likely to continue for the foreseeable future. Areas once thought not to be amenable to treatment are now routinely injected. Whereas Botox® is the only toxin currently available in the United States, there appear to be several on the horizon, Concomitant use of fillers, light sources, and BTXs have pushed the boundaries of nonsurgical rejuvenation, and it is likely that all of these modalities will continue to proliferate and improve over time. With experience, BTX injections are being used to treat wrinkles in more difficult locations, such as the nasolabial folds. Finally, BTX injections can be a wonderful adjunct to improve the cosmetic results seen after a variety of surgical procedures.

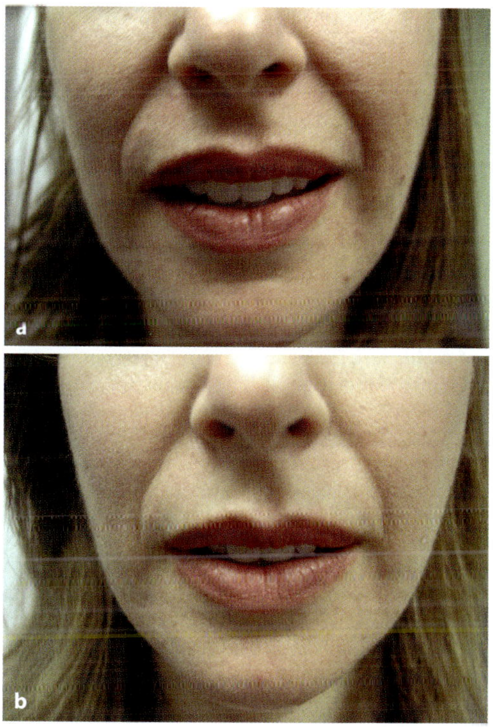

Fig. 4.15. **a** Prominent nasolabial folds. **b** Improvement in nasolabial folds after injection of miniscule amounts of BTX into each levator palpebrae superioris at the pyriform aperture

References

1. Carruthers JDA, Carruthers JA (1992) Treatment of glabellar frown lines with C. Botulinum exotoxin. J Dermatol Surg Oncol 18:17–21
2. American Society for Aesthetic Plastic Surgery http://www.surgery.org/press/statistics/php. Accessed September 21, 2006
3. Cohen JL, Dayan SH (2006) Botulinum toxin type a in the treatment of dermatochalasis: an open-label, randomized, dose-comparison study. J Drugs Dermatol 5:596–601
4. Carruthers J, Carruthers A, Zelichowska A (2000) The power of combined therapies: Botox® and ablative facial laser resurfacing. Am J Cosmet Surg 17:129–131
5. Brin MF, Binder W, Blitzer A, Schenroek L, Pogoda JM (2002) Botulinum type A Botox® for pain and headache. In: Brin MF, Hallett M, Jankovic J (eds) Scientific and Therapeutic Aspects of Botulinum Toxin. Lippincott Williams and Wilkins, Philadelphia, pp 233–250
6. Cohen JL, Solish N (2003) Treatment of hyperhidrosis with botulinum toxin. Facial Plast Surg Clin North Am 11:493–502
7. Solish N, Benohanian A, Kowalski JW; Canadian Dermatology Study Group on Health-Related Quality of Life in Primary Axillary Hyperhidrosis (2005) Prospective open-label study of botulinum toxin type A in patients with axillary hyperhidrosis: effects on functional impairment and quality of life. Dermatol Surg 31:405–413
8. Liu HT, Tsai SK, Kao MC, Hu JS (2006) Botulinum toxin A relieved neuropathic pain in a case of post-herpetic neuralgia. Pain Med 7.89–91
9. Charles Finn J, Cox SE, Earl ML (2003) Social implications of hyperfunctional facial lines. Dermatol Surg 29:450–455
10. Narurkar V, Cohen J, Flynn T, Hirsch R (2006) Analysis of complications by non-physicians in laser, light, RF devices, fillers and non-invasive procedures. Presented at the ASDS Annual Meeting, 29 October 2006, Palm Desert, California
11. Carruthers J, Carruthers A (2003) A prospective, randomized, parallel group study analyzing the effect of BTX-A (Botox®) and non-animal sourced hyaluronic acid (NASHA, Restylane) in combi-

nation compared with NASHA (Restylane) alone in severe glabellar rhytides in adult female subjects: treatment of severe glabellar rhytides with a hyaluronic acid derivative compared with the derivative BTX-A. Dermatol Surg 29:802–809
12. Alam M, Dover JS, Klein AW, Arndt KA (2002) Botulinum A exotoxin for hyperfunctional facial lines: where not to inject. Arch Dermatol 138:1180–1185
13. Semchyshyn N, Senglemann RD (2003) Botulinum toxin treatment of perioral rhytids. Dermatol Surg 29:490–495
14. Rohrer TE, Beer K (2005) Background to Botulinum toxin. In: Carruthers A, Carruthers J (eds) Botulinum Toxin. Elsevier Saunders, Philadelphia, pp 9–17
15. Scott AB (2004) Development of botulinum therapy. Dermatol Clin 22:131–133
16. Blitzer A, Brin MF, Keen MS, Aviv JE (1993) Botulinum toxin for the treatment of hyperfunctional lines of the face. Arch Otolaryngol Head Neck Surg 119:1018–1022
17. Alam M, Dover JS, Arndt KA (2002) Pain associated with injection of botulinum A exotoxin reconstituted using isotonic sodium chloride with and without preservative: a double-blind, randomized controlled trial. Arch Dermatol 138:510–514
18. Goodman G (2003) Diffusion and short-term efficacy of botulinum toxin A after the addition of hyaluronidase and its possible application for the treatment of axillary hyperhidrosis. Dermatol Surg 29:533–538
19. Hsu, TS, Dover JS, Arndt KA (2004) Effect of volume and concentration on the diffusion of botulinum exotoxin A. Arch Dermatol 140:1351–1354
20. Carruthers A, Carruthers J, Said S (2005) Dose-ranging study of botulinum toxin type A in the treatment of glabellar rhytides in females. Dermatol Surg 31:414–422
21. Flynn T, Carruthers JA, Carruthers A, Clark R (2003) Botulinum A toxin (Botox®) in the lower eyelid: dose-finding study. Dermatol Surg 29:943–950
22. Carruthers A, Carruthers J, Cohen J (2007) Dilution volume of botulinum toxin type A for the treatment of glabellar rhytides: does it matter? Dermatol Surg 33:S97–104
23. Cohen J, Hirsch R (2006) Challenge: correcting a downturned smile. Skin Aging 2:52
24. Cote TR, Mohan AK, Polder JA, Walton MK, Braun MM (2005) Botulinum toxin type A injections: adverse events reported to the US Food and Drug Administration in therapeutic and cosmetic cases. J Am Acad Dermatol 53:407–415
25. Klein AW (2003) Complications, adverse reactions, and insights with the use of botulinum toxin. Dermatol Surg 29:549–556
26. Moore P, Naumann M (2003) General and clinical aspects of treatment with botulinum toxin. In: Moore P, Naumann M (eds) Handbook of Botulinum Toxin Treatment, 2nd edn. Blackwell Science, Oxford, pp 28–75
27. Carruthers J, Fagien S, Matarasso S, for the Botox Consensus Group (2004) Consensus recommendations on the use of botulinum toxin type A in facial aesthetics. Plast Reconstr Surg 114:1S–22S
28. Carruthers JA, Lowe NJ, Menter MA, Gibson J, Nordquist M, Mordaunt J, Walker P, Eadie N; Botox® Glabellar Lines I Study Group (2002) A multicenter, double-blind, randomized, placebo-controlled study of the efficacy and safety of botulinum toxin type A in the treatment of glabellar lines. J Am Acad Dermatol 46:840–849
29. Glaich A, Cohen J, Goldberg L (2006) Achieving a lateral brow lift with botulinum toxin type A. J Cosmet Dermatol 19:121–123
30. Carruthers A, Carruthers J, Cohen J (2003) A prospective, double-blind, randomized, parallel group, dose-ranging study of Botox® in female subjects with horizontal forehead rhytides. Dermatol Surg 2003;29:462–467
31. Kane M (2003) Classification of crow's feet patterns among Caucasian women: the key to individualizing treatment. Plast Reconstr Surg 112:33S–39S
32. Flynn TC, Carruthers JA, Carruthers JA, Clark RE II (2003) Botulinum A toxin (Botox®) in the lower eyelid: dose-finding study. Dermatol Surg 29:943–951
33. Goldman M (2003) Festoon formation after infraorbital botulinum A toxin: a case report. Dermatol Surg 29:560–561
34. Lowe NJ, Ascher B, Heckmann M, Kumar C, Fraczek S, Eadie N; Botox® Facial Aesthetics Study Team (2005) Double-blind, randomized, placebo-controlled, dose–response study of the safety and efficacy of botulinum toxin type A in subjects with crow's feet. Dermatol Surg 31:257–262
35. Cohen J, Hirsch R (2006) Surgical insights: challenge: correcting low-lying brows. Skin Aging 14:30–31
36. Carruthers J, Carruthers A (2001) Botox® use in the mid and lower face and neck. Semin Cutan Med Surg 20:85–92
37. Tamura BM, Odo MY, Chang B, Cuce LC, Flynn TC (2005) Treatment of nasal wrinkles with botulinum toxin. Dermatol Surg 231:271–275
38. Beer K, Yohn M, Closter J (2005) A double-blinded, placebo-controlled study of Botox® for the

treatment of subjects with chin rhytids. J Drugs Dermatol 4:417–422

39. Kane MA (2003) The effect of botulinum toxin injections on the nasolabial fold. Plast Reconstr Surg 112:S66–72
40. Carruthers J, Carruthers A (1999) Practical cosmetic Botox® techniques. J Cutan Med Surg 3: S49–52
41. Beljaards RC, de Roos KP, Bruins FG (2005) NewFill for skin augmentation: a new filler or failure? Dermatol Surg 31:772–776; discussion 776
42. Naumann M, Jankovic J (2004) Safety of botulinum toxin type A: a systemic review and meta-analysis. Curr Med Res Opin 20:981–990
43. Hsu TS, Dover JS, Kaminer MS, Arndt KA, Tan MH (2003) Why make patients exercise facial muscles for 4 hours after botulinum toxin treatment? Arch Dermatol 139:948
44. Carruthers JA, Lowe NJ, Menter MA, Gibson J, Nordquist M, Morduant J, Walker P, Eadie N; Botox® Glabellar Lines I Study Group (2002) A multi-center, double-blind, randomized, placebo-controlled study of efficacy and safety of botulinum toxin type A in the treatment of glabellar lines. J Am Acad Dermatol 46:840–849
45. Fagien S (2004) Temporary management of upper lid ptosis, lid malposition, and eyelid fissure asymmetry with botulinum toxin type A. Plast Reconstr Surg 114:1892–1902

Chapter 5

Dermal Fillers

Derek Jones

5

> **Core Messages**
> - A variety of fillers are now available throughout the world.
> - Fillers vary mostly with regard to the biomaterial from which they are made and longevity.
> - Complications associated with longer-lasting fillers can be more persistent than those seen with shorter-acting fillers.
> - Fillers used for facial rejuvenation are ideally combined with the other modalities of treatment.

History

A substantial number of injectable dermal fillers are now available for soft-tissue augmentation. An ideal filler should be nontoxic, noncarcinogenic, nonteratogenic, nonallergenic, and long lasting. Furthermore, it should be simple to manufacture and store, easy to inject, and capable of producing an elegant and natural-appearing cosmetic correction with a low risk of adverse events. Attempts to augment soft tissue date to well over 100 years ago, when autologous fat grafts were employed to restore facial volume defects [1]. Paraffin was also first used as a bioimplant around 1900 to create a suitable testicular prosthesis [1]. However, its use as an injectable filler quickly fell into disfavor due to a high incidence of foreign-body reactions. Liquid silicone was first injected around 1950, and various forms were widely used over the next 30 years until the United States Food and Drug Administration (FDA) temporarily banned its use in 1982 over concerns of possible toxicity, foreign-body reactions, and migration. About this time, injectable bovine collagen became available in the United States, and today it remains the "gold standard" to which all newly available dermal fillers are compared. Recently, a variety of hyaluronic acid fillers have become FDA-approved, along with injectable forms of polylactic acid (PLA), calcium hydroxylapatite, and recombinant human collagen. The recent FDA approval of highly purified liquid silicone for ophthalmologic use has created resurgent interest in silicone as a permanent filler agent, while polymethylmethacrylate (PMMA) microspheres are soon poised to become the first FDA-approved permanent injectable filler. A list of currently FDA-approved dermal fillers is given in Table 5.1.

Fillers may be classified into biodegradable and nonbiodegradable products. The degradable material may be further classified into xenografts (derived from another species such as bovine collagen or hyaluronic acid of bacterial or avian origin), autografts (derived from the same person, such as autologous fat), and synthetic products (PLA and calcium hydroxylapatite). Another way to categorize this large number of fillers is to understand the types of defects each filler is capable of correcting. Conceptually, rhytides may be divided into three categories: superficial, medium and deep. Correspondingly, the level of volume loss in the skin is in the superficial dermis ("etched-in" rhytides), mid to deep dermis

Table 5.1. Currently available dermal fillers approved by the United States Food and Drug Administration

Bovine collagen	Zyplast, Zyderm (Allergan; Irvine,CA, USA)
Human collagen:	Cosmoderm, Cosmoplast (Allergan; Irvine, CA, USA)
Hyaluronic acid	Restylane, Perlane (Medicis; Scottsdale, AZ, USA) Captique, Hylaform, Hylaform Plus, Juvederm (Allergan- Irvine, CA, USA)
Polylactic acid	Scupltra (Dermik; Bridgewater, NJ, USA)
Calcium hydroxylapatite	Radiesse (BioForm; San Mateo, CA, USA)
Polymethylmethacrylate	Artefill (Artes; San Diego, CA, USA)
Liquid silicone	Silikon-1000 (Alcon- Fort Worth, TX, USA) *FDA approved for ophthalmic purposes*

(medium depth rhytides, such as nasolabial folds or oral commissures), or the subcutaneous plane (deeper contour defects such as facial lipoatrophy). The most appropriate fillers for each type of defect are listed in Fig. 5.1.

Currently Available Fillers and Potential Complications

Bovine and Bioengineered Collagen

Injectable bovine collagen was FDA-approved in 1981 as Zyderm collagen, which is 95% type 1 collagen and <5 % type 3 collagen, at a concentration of 35 mg/ml in a suspension of saline and 0.3% lidocaine [2]. The collagen is extracted from the skin of a United States herd of cattle that is kept quarantined to protect from them from possible prion contamination, which has been associated with mad cow disease (bovine spongiform encephalopathy). During manufacturing, the antigenic telopeptide regions of the molecule are removed to improve biocompatibility. Zyderm II collagen was introduced in 1983 at a higher concentration 65 mg/ml bovine collagen. Zyplast collagen, which became available in 1985, contains 35 mg/ml of bovine collagen, which is cross-linked with glutaraldehyde to improve longevity.

A disadvantage with bovine collagen is that 3% of individuals may display hypersensitivity. Double skin testing is now considered the standard of care, whereby a 0.1-ml aliquot of Zyderm collagen is injected into the dermis of the flexor forearm, with the skin test being repeated at 2–4 weeks. A positive skin test is manifest by redness, induration, tenderness, and/or pruritus at the injection site, which usually appears within 4 weeks postinjection. Injections may usually proceed safely if there is no reaction to the second skin test after 2 weeks. However, patients may rarely develop late-appearing hypersensitivity reactions. Skin tests are required for all patients naïve to bovine collagen or patients who have not received collagen within 1 year. Severe hypersensitivity reactions may be treated with topical, systemic, or intralesional cortisone, topical tacrolimus [3], or with immunosuppressants such as cyclosporine [4].

Cosmoderm and Cosmoplast are bioengineered injectable human collagen products that were FDA-approved 2003. Dermal fibroblasts are bioengineered from human foreskin using recombinant technology and then seeded and grown on a three-dimensional mesh network in cell culture. The final product is sterile and acellular, but otherwise identical to human dermis. The advantage is that no skin test is needed and hypersensitivity reactions are exceedingly rare. Cosmoderm, like Zyderm, consists of 35 mg/ml of collagen and is most useful for correcting fine "etched-in" lines. Cosmoplast, like Zyplast, consists of 65 mg/ml of collagen and is most useful for correcting middermal defects such as nasola-

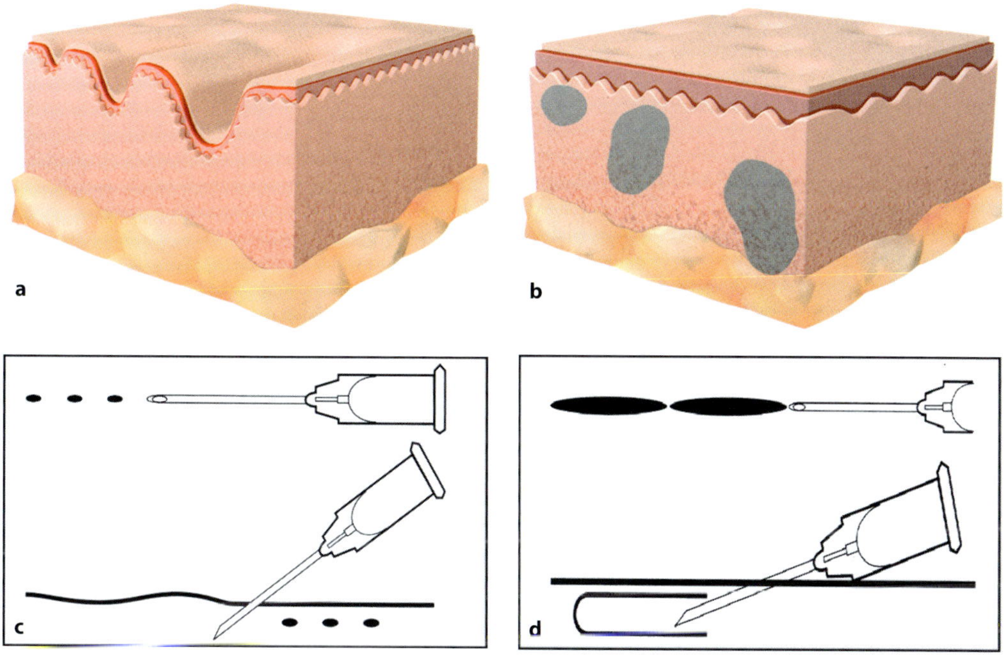

Fig. 5.1 a–d. **a** Schematic showing three different types of defect: *left* – fine lines; *middle* – moderate wrinkles; *right* – more prominent, pronounced defect. **b** Result of injections of appropriate filler product into the superficial dermis to treat fine lines (Cosmoderm or Zyderm), mid-dermis to treat moderate wrinkles (Zyplast, Cosmoplast, Hylaform, Captique, Restylane, or Juvederm), and deep dermis to treat more prominent, pronounced defects (Hylaform Plus, Perlane, Radiesse, Sculptra, or Silikon-1000). **c** Injection into dermis with serial puncture technique more commonly used with superficial fillers. **d** Injection into dermis

bial folds. With the recent advent of hyaluronic acids, collagen products have become less popular, as hyaluronic acids such as Restylane or Juvederm offer greater longevity of correction (5–6 months versus 2–3 months for collagen) [5]. However, there are indications for which collagen products may be the most appropriate filler. Among FDA-approved fillers, Zyderm and Cosmoderm are still the most useful for correcting very superficial dermal defects such as "etched-in" fine lines, where they are injected very superficially in the dermis using a serial puncture technique with about 50% overcorrection. Zyplast and Cosmoplast are also most useful for giving structure and crisp definition to the vermillion border of the lip, where hyaluronic acids may create too much volume and an overcorrected appearance. The author favors injecting Cosmoplast in the vermillion border of the lip to provide structure, and hyaluronic acid in conservative amounts in the pink of the lip to provide volume (Fig. 5.2).

Aside from rare hypersensitivity reactions, injection of collagen is generally well tolerated with few mild and transient side effects such as redness, tenderness, and edema. However, injection necrosis is a rare but important potential complication caused by interruption of the vascular supply of the area being injected by intravascular obstruction or extravascular compression from the injected material [6]. Unilateral blindness has been reported as a complication of inadvertent intravascular injection of fillers [7]. Injectable collagen products promote platelet aggregation, which compared to other fillers increases the risk of intravascular thrombosis and occlusion. The

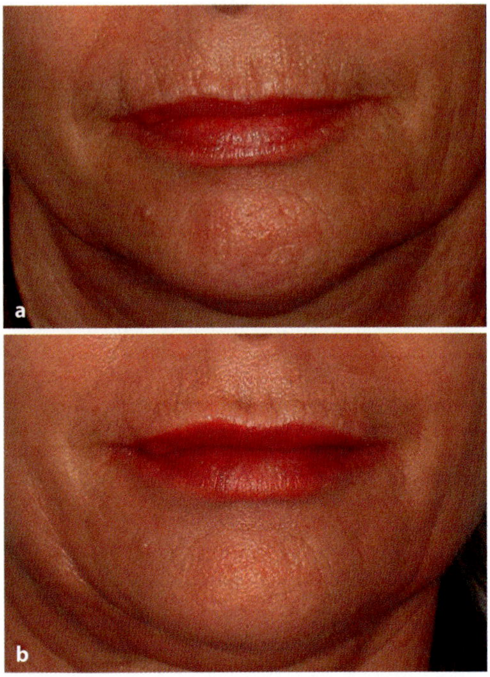

Fig. 5.2 a, b. Before (a) and 2 weeks after (b) injecting Cosmoplast to the vermillion border of the lip, Captique to the pink of the lip, and Cosmoderm to the superficial "etched in" rhytides of the upper lip. Overvolumizing the lip has been avoided

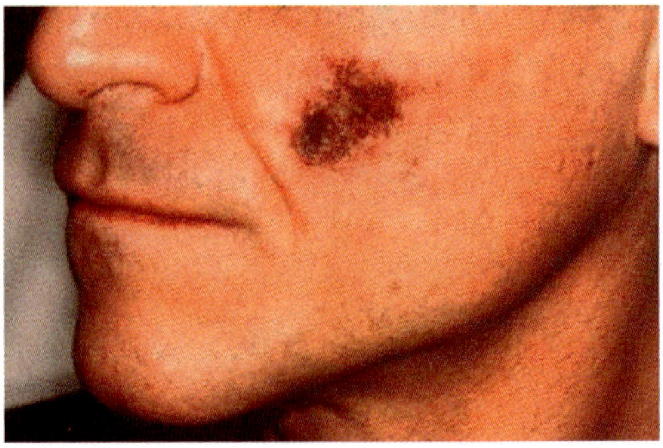

Fig. 5.3. Collagen necrosis subsequent to probable injection of a deep dermal arteriole. This healed with scar formation

glabella is a particularly high-risk area for injection necrosis, and the physician should have a good knowledge of the complex vascular supply of this area [6]. Zyplast and Cosmoplast, due to crosslinking and increased rigidity, are more often associated with injection necrosis than are Zyderm and Cosmoderm. Zyplast and Cosmoplast are associated with injection necrosis of the glabellar area most frequently, and are contraindicated in this site. Impending necrosis is immediately evident by persistent blanching at an area of injection, which subsequently turns dusky and then black within 1–3 days (Fig. 5.3). This is followed by eschar formation, skin sloughing, and frequent scar formation as the skin heals. Impending necrosis may be treated with massage and immediate application of heat and nitropaste [12]. Aspirating before injection, keeping injection volumes small and superficial to larger vessels, and avoidance of high-risk areas are important to avoid injection necrosis [12].

Hyaluronic Acids

There are several hyaluronic acid fillers now available, and the differences between the products often create substantial confusion. It is of utmost importance to understand the compositional properties of hyaluronic acids to understand their differences clinically. Hyaluronic acid exists as a naturally occurring carbohydrate chain or polymer consisting of alternating disaccharide subunits of sodium gluconorate and N-acetylglucosamine. Hyaluronic acid is an important component of human skin, and its most important property relative to a dermal filler is its propensity to bind and retain water [8,9]. Other functions of hyaluronic acid include aiding in cell motility, wound healing, and joint lubrication. The molecular structure of hyaluronic acid is essentially the same regardless of whether it is derived from an animal or bacterial source. The only difference between animal- and bacterially derived hyaluronic acid is the final length of the polymeric chain of repeating disaccharide subunits. Hyaluronic acids derived from streptococcal bacterial fermentation

(Restylane, Captique, Juvederm) have shorter chain lengths and a lower molecular weight (1.5–2.5 MDa), whereas avian (rooster comb)-derived hyaluronic acids (Hylaform, Hylaform Plus) have longer chain lengths and a higher molecular weight (4–6 MDa). These differences in chain length and molecular weight appear to have no clinical significance. There is no evidence to suggest that avian-derived hyaluronic acids are more antigenic than those derived from bacterial sources or are degraded more quickly in vivo. Chains of hyaluronic acid can be "free" or manipulated by molecular crosslinking or stabilizing the free polymers, whereby free chains of hyaluronic acid are molecularly attached or bonded to one another. Free polymers of hyaluronic acid that are not molecularly crosslinked have a very short residence time (only a few days) when injected into skin tissue. The residence time of crosslinked hyaluronic acid in the dermis is much longer (weeks to months). More heavily crosslinked products generally resist degradation from hyaluronidase in the body, and have longer tissue residence times. Furthermore, the more heavily crosslinked the hyaluronic acid, the more viscous the product. As the degree of crosslinking increases, a liquid will become a gel and then ultimately a solid. All currently available hyaluronic acid fillers consist of gels containing crosslinked hyaluronic acid derived from avian or bacterial sources. The bacterially derived products (Restylane, Perlane, Captique) and the avian-derived products (Hylaform and Hylaform Plus) are all gelatinous products that are pushed through screens during manufacturing, creating gel particle sizes of uniform shape, size, and consistency. Products made of larger gel particle sizes (Perlane, Hylaform Plus) are more resistant to degradation and are intended to correct deeper defects in the deep dermal or subcutaneous planes. Products made from smaller gel particle sizes (Restylane, Captique, Hylaform) are intended to correct middermal volume deficits. Very small particle sizes such as Restylane Fine Lines or Restylane Touch, which are not yet available in the United States, are intended for very superficial dermal defects ("etched-in" lines). By contrast, Juvederm utilizes Hylacross technology, whereby the solid gel of crosslinked hyaluronic acid is chopped up into random shapes and sizes, much like one might pulverize "jello" in a blender. Some suggest that such technology creates a more cohesive gel, which may favorably affect the smoothness of the implant in the dermis and increase longevity, although such claims remain to be proven in controlled studies.

A very important distinction between available hyaluronic acid fillers is the difference in concentration of hyaluronic acid and the degree to which each product is saturated with water. Remember that hyaluronic acid is hydrophilic (water loving), and will bind water up to a point of maximal saturation, at which point it no longer attracts more water. Hylaform, Hylaform Plus, and Captique each contain 5.5 mg/ml of hyaluronic acid and are maximally saturated with water. Conversely, Restylane contains 20 mg/ml hyaluronic acid, and Juvederm contains 24 mg/ml of hyaluronic acid. These higher-concentration hyaluronic acids are not maximally saturated with water and will continue to swell upon injection until they are maximally saturated. The difference clinically is that with the 5.5 mg/ml product (Hylaform, Hylaform Plus, Captique), what you see is what you get upon injection; there is very little swelling associated with these products. With the higher concentration 20- to 24-mg/ml products (Restylane, Juvederm), swelling is expected after injection and care must be taken not to overcorrect upon initial injection. The other main clinical difference between products of differing hyaluronic acid concentration is that clinical studies have proven that there is greater clinical persistence of correction with higher-concentration products as compared to the lower-concentration products.

The pivotal randomized, double-blind, multicenter comparison of the efficacy and tolerability of Restylane versus Zyplast for the correction of nasolabial folds was undertaken and results reported on in 2003 [5]. A cohort of 188 patients was treated with Restylane in one nasolabial fold and Zyplast on the contralateral side. A lower volume of Restylane was required for an "optimal result," and both patients and investigators judged this product to be more effective in maintaining cosmetic correction. Assessments using the investigator-based Wrinkle Severity Rating Scale and Global Improvement Aesthetic Improvement Scale at 6 months after baseline revealed that hyaluronic acid was superior in 56.9% and 62% of patients, respectively, while Zyplast was superior in 9.5% and 8.0% of patients, respectively.

Clinical phase 3 safety and efficacy studies of Hylaform were completed in 2002 and Hylaform was approved by the FDA in 2004. Over 300 patients were tested in a double-blinded, randomized study comparing Zyplast to Hylaform gel for the correction of nasolabial folds [9]. Results showed that Hylaform gel achieved at least equal results to Zyplast collagen at 4 months. There were no immunologic or allergic reactions, or significant adverse events, and the side effect profile was similar to Zyplast in terms of redness, swelling, bruising, and edema, which generally resolved within a few days.

Hylaform Plus is a variant of Hylaform, and has a similar concentration of hyaluronic acid but a larger particle size. It is intended for the correction of deeper folds. Hylaform Plus was approved by the FDA in 2004 following an FDA study showing that Hylaform Plus was comparable to Hylaform gel in correcting nasolabial folds at 12 weeks [9].

Hylaform, derived from rooster combs and having a lower concentration of hyaluronic acid (5.5 mg/ml), has also been compared in a clinical trial to Restylane, which is bacterially derived and has a higher concentration of hyaluronic acid (20 mg/ml) [10]. Eight female subjects were randomized to receive 0.7 ml Restylane in one nasolabial fold and 1.0 ml Hylaform to the contralateral side. High-quality digital photographs were compared at baseline and at 12 weeks after treatment by four blinded expert raters. Subjects also completed questionnaires to document tolerability and satisfaction. The average subject satisfaction score was 3.00 (out of 5) for Hylaform and 3.78 (out of 5) for Restylane. The blinded expert review panel rated an average improvement of 2.86 (out of 5) for Hylaform and 3.78 (out of 5) for Restylane. Restylane, therefore, displayed higher efficacy and subject satisfaction than Hylaform. The author has found that the duration of clinical efficacy with Hylaform is less than with Restylane. However, side effects such as swelling, pain on injection, and posttreatment erythema were less with Hylaform compared to Restylane. The same holds true for Captique, which is essentially identical to Hylaform in hyaluronic acid concentration and manufacturing process. The only difference that is clinically irrelevant is that Captique is manufactured from a bacterial fermentation process, while Hylaform is derived from avian rooster combs. In the author's practice, Hylaform or Captique are reserved only for patients who cannot tolerate the pain, swelling, erythema, and associated downtime associated with the use of Restylane.

Juvederm was FDA approved in June 2006 after having been available in Europe and Canada for several years. As mentioned previously, Juvederm, like Restylane, is manufactured from streptococcal bacteria, and contains a higher concentration of hyaluronic acid (24 mg/ml) and a higher amount of cross-linked hyaluronic acid than other currently available hyaluronic acid fillers. Unlike other available hyaluronic acid products, Juvederm is manufactured as a monophasic gel that appears to create a more cohesive product upon injection. A multicenter, double-blind, within-subject controlled study was undertaken to compare the safety and efficacy of three formulations of Juvederm (J30, J30HV, J24HV) compared to Zyplast collagen for nasolabial fold correction [11–14]. A cohort of 439 subjects was enrolled and 423 subjects completed the 24 week study (96%); 92% of subjects were female with an average age of 49 years (range 26–75 years) with a full range of Fitzpatrick skin types. Compared to Zyplast, all three formulations of Juvederm achieved a more sustained correction than Zyplast. A clinically significant (≥grade 1) improvement was maintained for 6 months in 80% (J24HV) and 90% (J30HV) of subjects. The majority of subjects achieved optimal correction with only one treatment. The subject preference ratings were significantly superior for all three Juvederm fillers over Zyplast at 6 months after last treatment. Juvederm was preferred over Zyplast by 88% (J24HV) and 84% (J30HV) of subjects. Juvederm will be available in the United States beginning January 1, 2007, with Juvederm 24HV and Juvederm 30HV being marketed under the trade names Juvederm Ultra and Juvederm Ultra Plus, respectively.

Serious adverse events with hyaluronic acid are rare. In a recent retrospective analysis of the safety of nonanimal, stabilized hyaluronic acid (Restylane, Perlane, Restylane Fine Lines; Q-Med, Uppsala Sweden) for soft-tissue augmentation, adverse events from Europe, Canada, Australia, South America, and Asia from 1999 and 2000 were reviewed [15]. Hypersensitivity reactions, including redness, swelling, localized granulomatous reactions, bacterial infection, and acneiform and cystic lesions, were the major adverse events and were often most likely secondary to impurities in bacterial fermentation. The incidence of hypersensitivity reactions appears to have substantially declined since the introduction in 1999 of a more purified hyaluronic acid raw material. The Tyndall effect is a bluish discoloration of the dermis that is caused by injecting hyaluronic acid too superficially within the dermis.

A unique advantage of hyaluronic acid is that rare granulomatous hyaluronic acid reactions (caused form rare allergy to the material or granulomatous foreign body reactions to protein contaminants) or unwanted hyaluronic acid placement can be easily treated and quickly resolved with an injection of hyaluronidase [15]. Hyaluronidase is an enzyme that dissolves hyaluronic acid when injected into the skin. It has been approved by the FDA for ophthalmologic use (Vitrase, Ista Pharmaceuticals, Irvine, CA, USA) but may be used off-label for dissolving exogenously injected dermal hyaluronic acid. Reports suggest that prompt dissolution of hyaluronic acid can be achieved with proper injection, with a paucity of adverse events. The availability of hyaluronidase should decrease the anxiety of both patient and physician should an adverse event occur.

Hyaluronic acids are truly versatile fillers and are indicated for volume enhancement of nasolabial folds (Figs. 5.4 and 5.5), oral commissures, infraocular grooves, cheek contouring (Figs. 5.6 and 5.7), and lipoatrophy. Combining hyaluronan fillers with Botox is considered the new minimally invasive rejuvenation paradigm, especially in the glabellar area [16,17].

Polylactic Acid

PLA is a synthetic biodegradable polymer that is resorbable. Injectable PLA (Sculptra) consists of microparticles of PLA suspended in a sodium carboxymethylcellulose gel. It is manufactured as a lyophilized powder that is reconstituted with sterile water shortly before injection. It is nonanimal in origin, and so no skin testing is required before injection. It should be injected strictly within the subcutis and is indicated for lipoatrophy in the cheeks or temple areas (Figs. 5.8 and 5.9). Much of the resulting soft tissue augmentation is delayed and occurs as a result of fibroplasia or neocollagenesis around the PLA microparticles. Injections of two vials should be undertaken at monthly intervals until optimal correction is achieved.

PLA was approved by the FDA in August 2004 specifically for the treatment of HIV-associated facial lipoatrophy. Interestingly, this product was granted fast-track approval for the unique needs of the HIV population with efficacy and safety based on published European data and two small physician sponsored investigational trails in the United States. The rigorous comparative and blinded FDA safety and efficacy studies usually required for other fillers were not performed. The most comprehensive study on PLA was the European

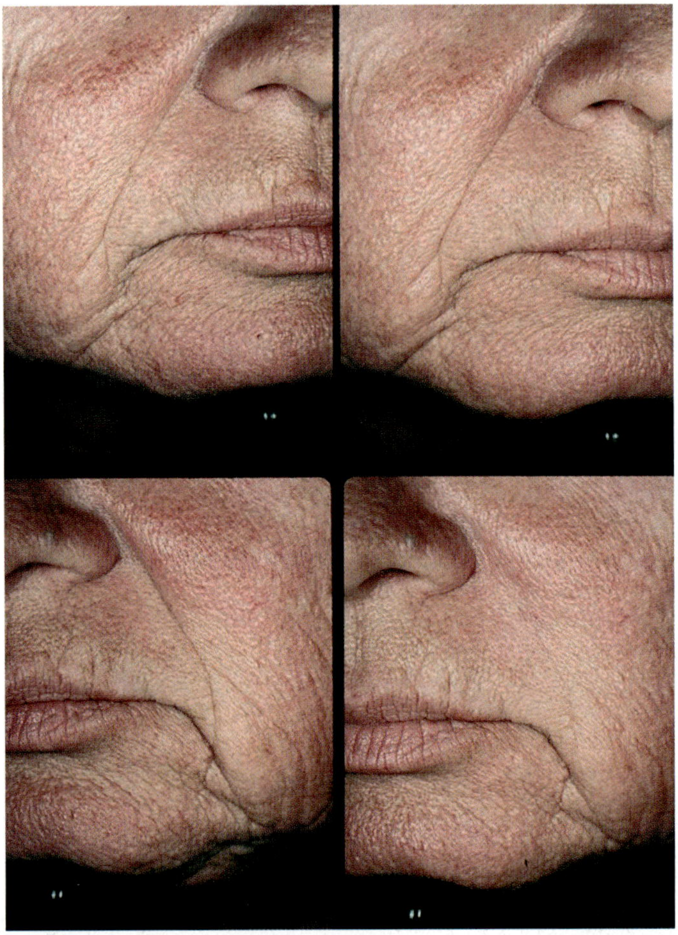

Fig. 5.4. Before (*top left*) and 6 months after Zyplast (*top right*), and before (*bottom left*) and 6 months after (*bottom right*) Restylane to the nasolabial folds

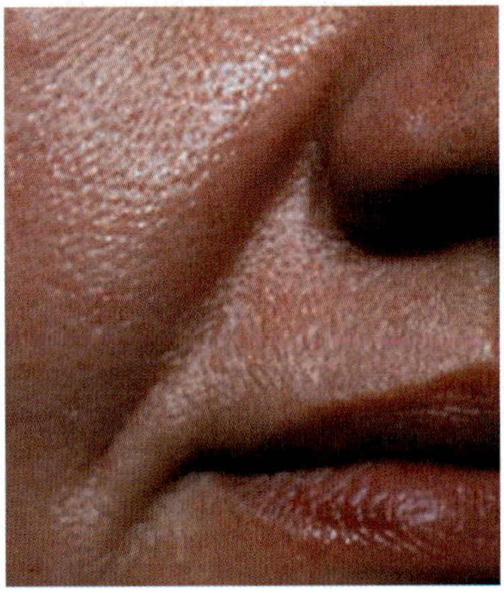

Fig. 5.5. Before Juvederm injection into the right nasolabial fold

VEGA study, which followed patients treated with PLA for 96 weeks [29]. Fifty patients with severe HIV-associated facial lipoatrophy received 4 sets of injections at day 0 and then every 2 weeks for 6 weeks. Patients were evaluated by clinical examination, facial ultrasonography, and photography at screening and at weeks 6, 24, 48, 72, and 96. At entry, the median facial fat thickness was 0 (range 0.0–2.1 mm). The median total cutaneous thickness increased significantly from baseline: +5.1 mm at week 6, +6.4 mm at week 24, +7.2 mm at week 48, +7.2 mm at week 72, and +6.8 mm at week 96 ($p<0.001$). No adverse events were observed. In 22 (44%) patients, palpable but nonvisible subcutaneous nodules were observed with a spontaneous resolution

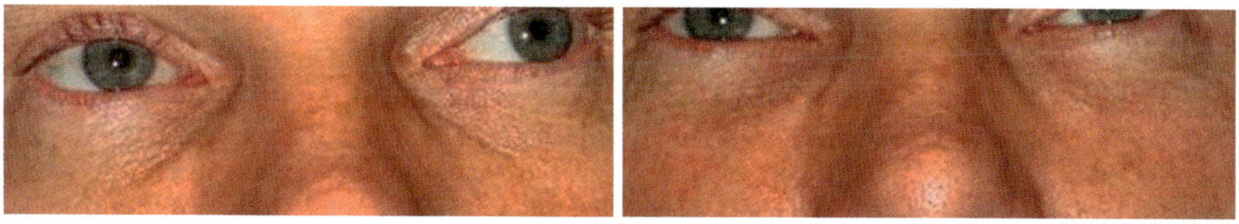

Fig. 5.6. Before (right) and after (left) Restylane to the infraocular groove. To obtain a good correction and avoid bruising, very small volumes should be injected in the avascular supraperiosteal plane immediately below the obicularis oculi

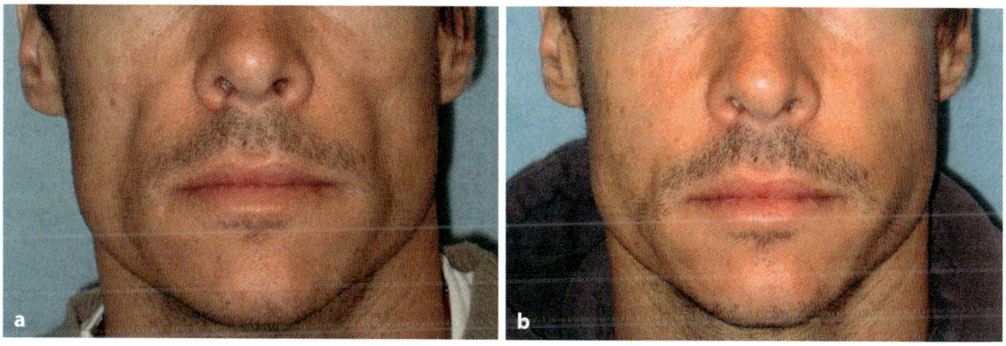

Fig. 5.7 a, b. Hyaluronic acid may be used for cheek contouring and to correct check hollows, as in this case of HIV facial lipoatrophy. **a** Before and **b** after Restylane. For this indication, hyaluronic acid is best injected deep to the dermis

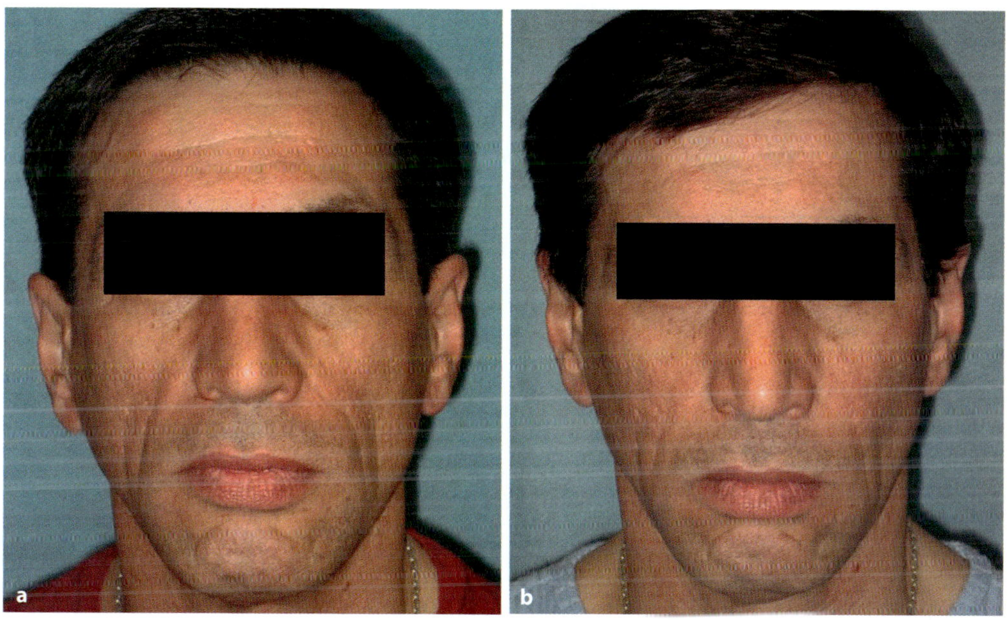

Fig. 5.8 a, b. **a** Pretreatment of facial lipoatrophy (non-HIV, age-related). **b** One month following the final treatment with eight vials of Sculptra injected in four treatment sessions over 3 months

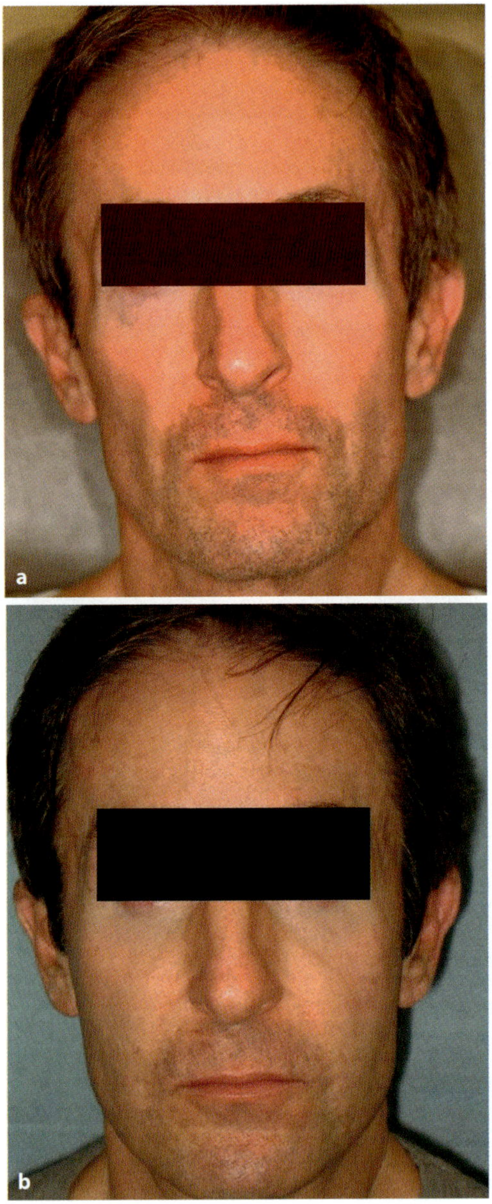

Fig. 5.9 a, b. **a** Pretreatment of facial lipoatrophy (non-HIV, age-related). **b** Eight months following five treatments with ten vials of Sculptra injected over 4 months

in 6 patients by week 96. It should be noted that the main efficacy end point in this study was the change in skin thickness as observed by ultrasound. The study did not rigorously measure whether or not optimal correction with complete restoration of cheek contours was achieved, as evidenced by ratings of pre- and posttreatment photographs by an objective, experienced physician not performing the treatment.

The safety and efficacy of PLA as an injectable filler is still a matter of controversy. Persistent granulomatous inflammatory responses caused by inadvertent intradermal injection of PLA have been observed (Fig. 5.10) [18]. Some physicians in the European Union believe that compared to other available fillers, the incidence of adverse events such as granulomatous reactions and subcutaneous lumps is too high to justify the routine use PLA as an injectable filler [19].

It is the author's belief that PLA is a good option for those individuals with panfacial stage 1 facial lipoatrophy, which is often seen not in cases of HIV, but as a consequence of the normal aging process in otherwise healthy, lean individuals. In these individuals, monthly injections of one to two vials strictly into the subcutis often achieve a subtle restoration of subcutaneous volume. Optimal correction of subcutaneous fat loss with PLA will often persist for 12–24 months, at which point patients often seek reinjection. The author finds that PLA is often not robust enough to treat more advanced cases of HIV facial lipoatrophy (stages 2–4).

The author has found that employing the following steps may help avoid complications. First, the product should be injected only into the subdermal space, which is the plane where the subcutaneous fat has atrophied. Dermal defects are best treated with a hyaluronic acid or collagen filler. The author employs a cross-hatched linear retrograde injection technique using a 2-inch, 25-gauge needle. Smaller needles often become clogged. Secondly, although the package insert recommends reconstitution of each vial of PLA with 3 ml of sterile water, the author finds that subcutaneous lumps are avoided if each vial is reconstituted with 5 ml of sterile water, or 4 ml of sterile water and 1 ml of 1% lidocaine without epineph-

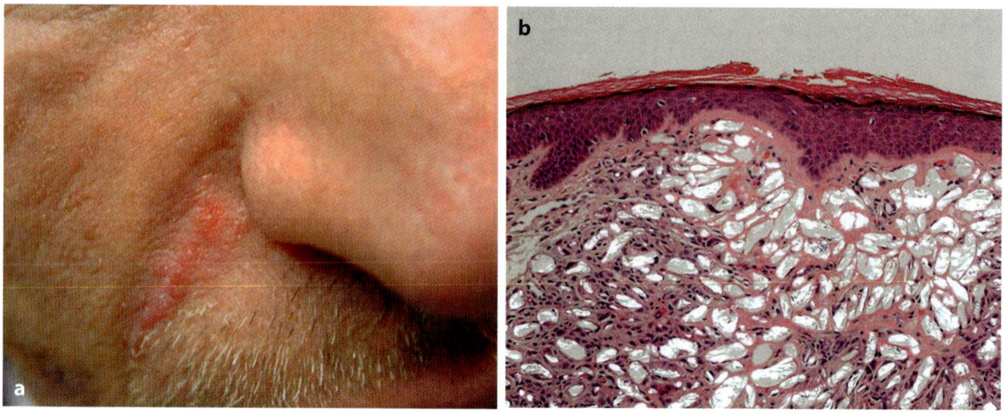

Fig. 5.10 a, b. a Persistent inflammatory papules from superficial dermal injection of polylactic acid. b Histology shows a granulomatous reaction to polylactic acid within the high dermis. This product should not be injected intradermally

rine, at least 24 h prior to injection. Third, the reconstituted vial should be vigorously shaken immediately prior to transfer into the syringe. Finally, patients should be instructed to frequently massage the treated area in the days to weeks following the procedure to prevent the formation of lumpy fibroplasia. Some advocate the "rule of fives," whereby the patient massages the area for 5 min, 5 times daily, for 5 days after the injection.

Calcium Hydroxylapatite

Radiesse is a synthetic product made of calcium hydroxylapatite suspended in a gel carrier. It is FDA approved as a soft-tissue marker for radiologic procedures and as an implant for injection laryngoplasty. Skin testing is not required. The product may legally be injected as a soft-tissue filler according to FDA rules governing off-label use of a device. Radiesse has recently emerged as a longer-lasting injectable soft-tissue filler with durability of correction lasting 6 months or longer.

A recent study evaluated 82 patients who were injected with Radiesse mostly into the nasolabial folds (e.g., Fig. 5.11) [20]. Results were evaluated by physicians and patients at 3 and 6 months. There average rating as to a "positive" look and feel of correction was 4.6 on a scale of 1–5 at 3 months, with similar findings at 6 months. No serious adverse events were noted. Clinical, histological, and electron microscopic findings after injection of Radiesse have been performed by Goldberg et al. [21]. Results have shown that calcium hydroxylapatite particles are persistent on biopsy of the injection site at 6 months, with evidence of new collagen formation being seen.

The author finds Radiesse most useful in patients with very deep nasolabial folds who do not respond to three or more syringes of hyaluronic acid. In should be injected in small amounts using multiple passes with a linear retrograde injection technique into the deep dermis or immediate subcutaneous plane. Overcorrection should be avoided. It is also useful treatment for HIV- (Fig. 5.12) and non-HIV-associated facial lipoatrophy, where it should be injected into the subcutaneous plane using a linear retrograde, crosshatched technique. Palpable lumpiness and swelling often occurs with injections of larger volumes, but often resolves within several days to a few weeks. Radiesse has recently undergone FDA studies for the treatment of nasolabial folds and HIV-associated lipoatrophy. The FDA advisory panel has recently voted in favor of

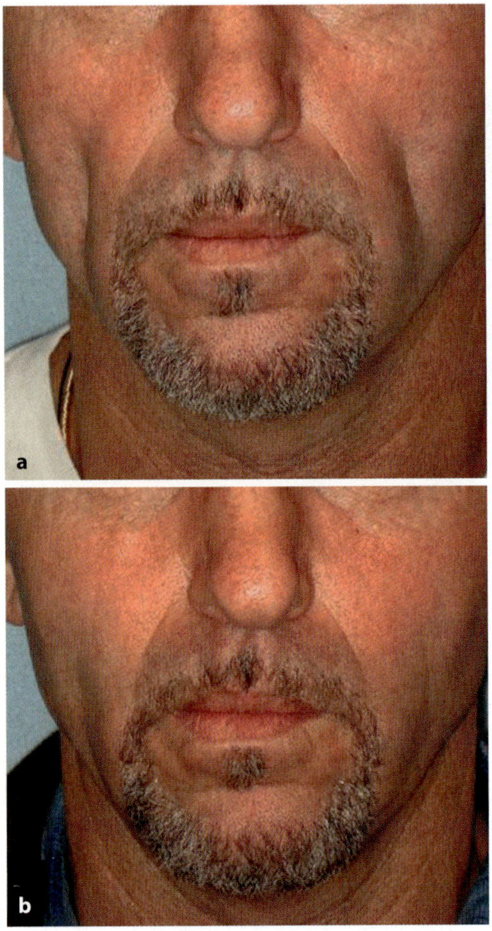

Fig. 5.11 a, b. Before (**a**) and after Radiesse (**b**) for non-HIV facial lipoatrophy

FDA approval for these indications, although formal FDA approval is pending at this time.

Complications with Radiesse often manifest as persistent lumps or nodules that are most common with a too-superficial injection technique or with injection into the lips (Fig. 5.13) or areas were the overlying dermis is very thin, such as in the periocular region. A high incidence of lip nodules after Radiesse injection has led many to include lip augmentation as a contraindication.

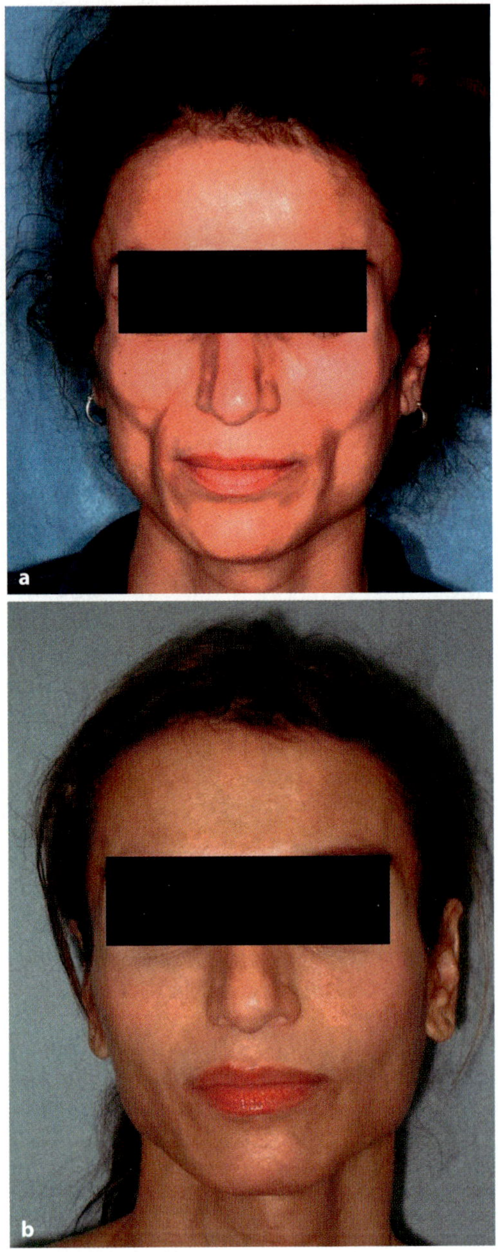

Fig. 5.12 a, b. HIV facial lipoatrophy pre- (**a**) and posttreatment (**b**) with Radiesse. Very large volumes, up to 8 cm^3 or more may be required for large volume loss. Palpable and visible lumpiness often results with large-volume correction, but improves with time. In the author's opinion, the cosmetic result with Radiesse for large-volume loss as seen in HIV is not as good as results obtained with liquid injectable silicone [22]

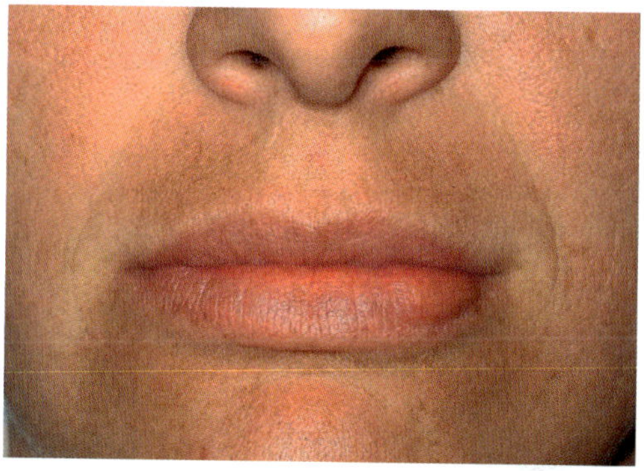

Fig. 5.13. Lip nodule that persists 15 months after injection of Radiesse in to lip

Liquid Injectable Silicone

Before collagen injectable fillers were approved by the FDA in the early 1980s, liquid injectable silicone (LIS) was the injectable filler of choice owing to its superb feel, long-lasting results, and apparent ease of use. Cases of granuloma formation and migration eventually made this filler less popular and it fell completely into disfavor in the early 1990s when all forms of silicone for cosmetic implantation purposes were banned by the FDA over concerns over possible toxicity and systemic reactions due to silicone breast implants [23].

The tide once again turned in the late 1990s after two forms of liquid silicone (Silikon-1000, Adatosil-5000) were FDA approved (in 1994 and 1997, respectively) as an injectable intraocular implant to treat retinal detachment. Concurrently in 1997, the FDA Modernization Act was passed, which allowed FDA-approved injectable devices (such as injectable fillers) to be used under the same off-label provisions previously applicable only to drugs. The FDA has further clarified that under these guidelines, off label injection of FDA-approved liquid silicone for soft-tissue augmentation is legal, as long as the physician does not advertise for such use and bases such treatment on the unique needs of individual patients. Currently, LIS is the only truly permanent filler that can be legally employed in the United States. Although its off-label use is considered legal by the FDA, it is important to note that liability carriers have varied policies regarding the off-label use of LIS. Silikon-1000 and Adatosil-5000 are highly purified injectable silicones. The composition of these FDA-approved silicones in many instances is much different than for the "medical-grade" silicone oils that were frequently injected for cosmetic purposes from the 1960s through the early 1990s, when practitioners often obtained silicone from multiple sources, including clandestine and noncommercial sources. An analysis of a variety of these previously injected silicone oils revealed unacceptable levels of elemental and low-molecular-weight impurities that may unfavorably affect biocompatibility [23].

Currently, LIS is employed for soft-tissue augmentation amidst controversy, with advocates and critics using anecdotal data to argue their case [24]. Critics claim that LIS is inherently unpredictable, with adverse events such as migration or granuloma formation, which may present as indurated, inflamed papules or nodules, appearing months to years following injection (Fig. 5.14). Advocates cite a wealth of anecdotal data to argue that the optimal and safe correction of a variety of atrophic defects can be routinely achieved as long as the following three rules are followed:

Rule 1

Inject only highly purified FDA approved LIS. Currently the only product that should be injected off-label is Silikon-1000. Adatosil-5000, which is also FDA-approved, is far too viscous to be easily injected through small-gauge needles.

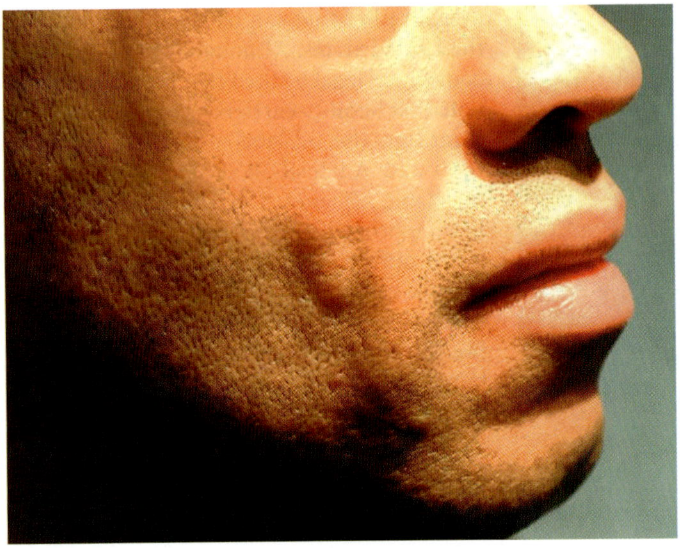

Fig. 5.14. A persistent nodule from intradermal injection of liquid silicone

Rule 2

Employ the microdroplet serial puncture technique, defined as 0.01 ml or less injected through a 27-G needle, into the immediate subdermal plane at 2- to 4-mm intervals. Intradermal injection should be assiduously avoided, as it may create intradermal papules. The one exception to this rule is atrophic dermal acne scars, where very small microdroplets (0.001 ml) should be injected into the deep dermis. The microdroplet technique also avoids the potential of migration, which may occur when large a bolus of LIS in injected all at once.

Rule 3

Inject very small volumes at monthly intervals or longer. Undercorrection is the immediate goal. Optimal correction occurs slowly over time as fibroplasia ensues around the microdroplets, creating further tissue augmentation and anchoring each microdroplet into place, which obviates the risk of migration.

Much has been written recently in the scientific literature regarding LIS [23]. The physician interested in this modality should become thoroughly acquainted with this literature before injecting, and seek appropriate training. In the author's opinion, the best indication for employing LIS exists for disfiguring acne scarring and HIV lipoatrophy, where other fillers often are not capable of achieving the affordable, sustained and cosmetically superior result as can be achieved with LIS (Fig. 5.15). Recently, Jones et al. reported on the use of Silikon-1000 to treat HIV-associated facial lipoatrophy [24]. To date, over 1200 patients with HIV-associated facial lipoatrophy have been treated with Silikon-1000 at 4 centers. The protocol employs 2 ml of Silikon-1000 injected with microdroplet serial puncture technique into the subdermal plane at monthly intervals until optimal correction is achieved. The results of this ongoing pilot trial reveal that the majority of patients achieve a superior and cosmetically pleasing and sustained correction with an average number of three treatments for each stage of lipoatrophy. No serious adverse events have been noted with up to 5 years of follow up in many. Barnett has also recently reported on his 30 years

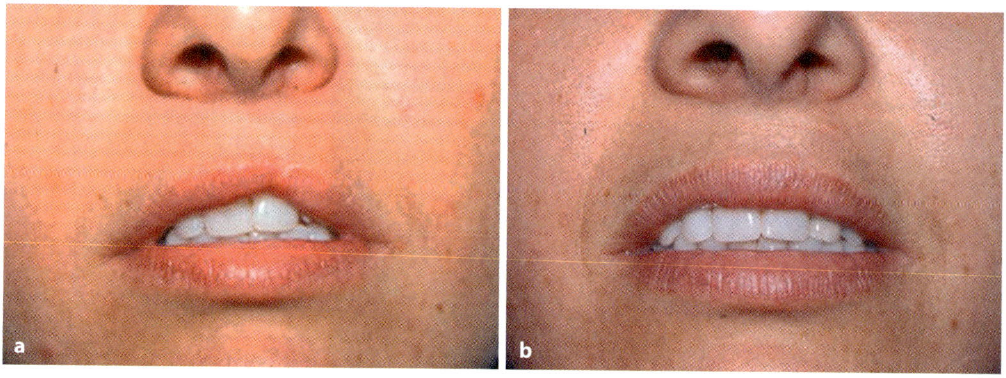

Fig. 5.15 a, b. Before (a) and after (b) liquid injectable silicone for correction of a lip scar. Courtesy of Doris Hexsel, MD (Brazil)

of experience in using LIS to treat acne scarring [25].

Polymethylmethacrylate

Artefill consists of 20% volume of PMMA smooth microspheres suspended in 80% volume bovine collagen [26]. When injected into the subdermal plane, the microscopically smooth microspheres stimulate fibroblasts to encapsulate each individual one of the estimated six million microspheres contained in 1 ml of Artefill, which further contributes to tissue augmentation by way of fibroplasia, in much the same way as fibroplasia occurs with liquid silicone or PLA.

Although the collagen vehicle is absorbed, the PMMA is truly permanent and is not reabsorbed by the body. Artefill has undergone rigorous FDA study and has recently received FDA approval. The physician should undertake careful training in the proper injection technique. As with all permanent fillers, mistakes may not be easily reversible. Like LIS, only small volumes should be employed and overcorrection should be avoided. It should be injected using the linear threading technique into the deep dermis or deeper. Several granulomatous reactions have been noted in the European and Canadian experience with this product (Fig. 5.16) [27]. Most of these reactions can be avoided with the proper injection technique and successfully treated with the use of intralesional cortisone. This product should not be used for lip augmentation. With careful use, physicians should be able to achieve excellent results, particularly for very deep nasolabial folds and oral commissures (Fig. 5.17).

Consent

A variety of consent forms are used for patients receiving fillers. Addendum 5.1 represents a reasonable consent to be used prior to the injection of nonpermanent fillers.

Personal Approach

Fillers are generally injected through small-gauge needles (23–32 G), and most fillers are injected through 30-G needles. Thicker fillers, such as Radiesse, Silikon-1000, and Sculptra are injected through larger-bore needles (27 G or larger). Either serial puncture or linear threading techniques should be employed at the level of skin (superficial dermis, mid-dermis, deep dermis) or subcutaneous plane that

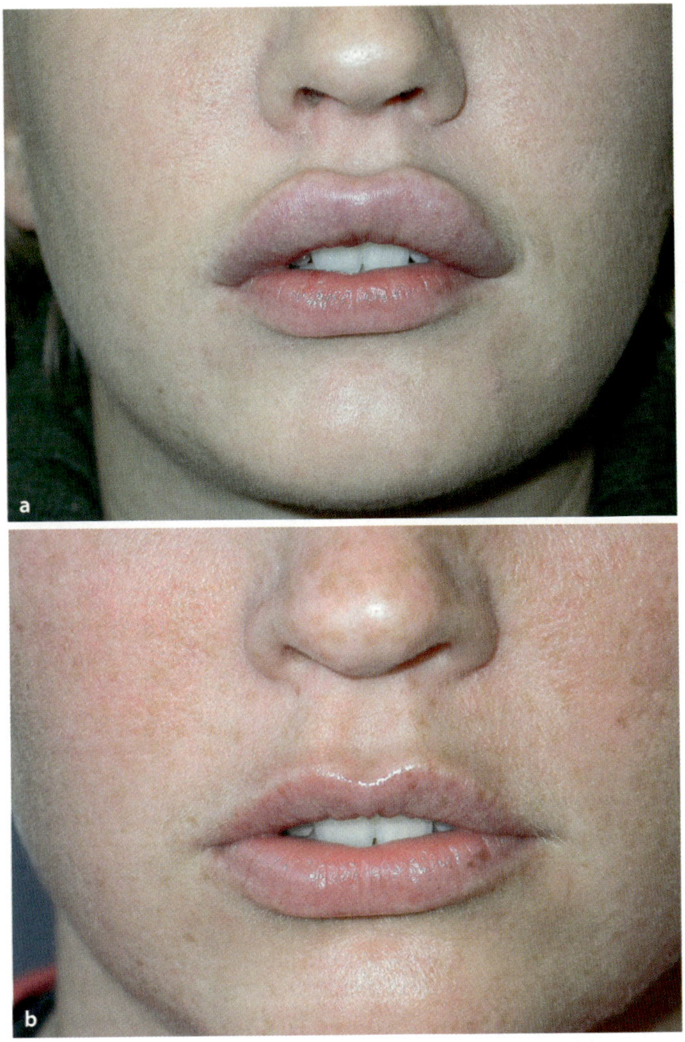

Fig. 5.16 a, b. Granulomatous reaction secondary to Artefill in the upper lip (**a**). Complete resolution was achieved by treating with intralesional cortisone 40 mg/cm^3 intralesionally on two occasions (**b**). Courtesy of Alastair Carruthers, MD

is most appropriate for each filler. The fanning technique and crosshatching techniques are variations on the linear threading technique whereby multiple linear threads are injected in a radial fashion (fanning) through a single puncture site, while cross hatching involves injecting linear threads at 90° angles to each other to create a grid pattern. Linear threading may be either antegrade or retrograde, where the filler is injected as the needle is advanced (antegrade) or where the needle is completely inserted into the appropriate plane and the filler injected as the needle is withdrawn (retrograde). Different techniques are employed depending on the filler being injected, and the nature and location of the volume deficit. The author usually favors variations on the linear threading technique for the majority of injectable fillers, with the exception of Cosmoderm or Cosmoplast, which should be injected with the serial puncture technique into the very high dermis to treat superficial "etched-in" lines, and Silikon-1000, which should be injected exclusively

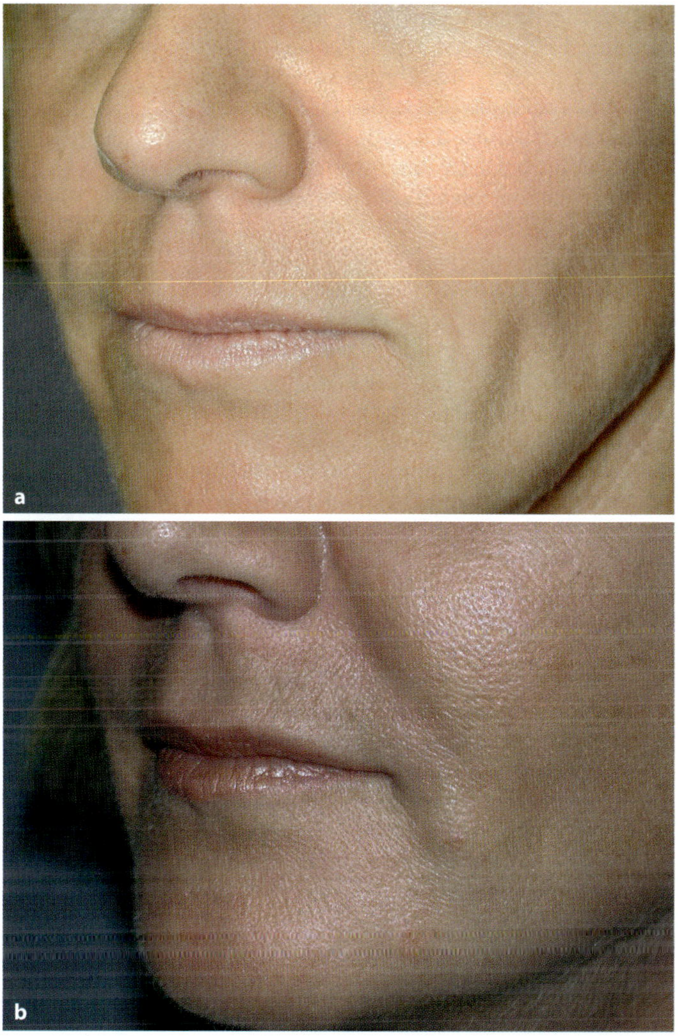

Fig. 5.17. Before (**a**) and after (**b**) Artefill for nasolabial fold correction. Over-correction should be avoided. Courtesy of Alastair Carruthers, MD

with the serial puncture technique into the immediate subdermal plane or deeper. Furthermore, the author favors the retrograde approach with linear injection, as there may be greater risk with the antegrade approach of accidentally injecting into a blood vessel and causing vascular injury or occlusion with potential tissue ischemia. Other comments about specifics to my approach are described above.

The Future

To predict the future of fillers in the United States, one should look at the fillers currently available in Europe [28–31]. It is much easier to bring an injectable filler to market in Europe, as fillers are required to undergo much less rigorous clinical testing before being allowed for general use within the European Union. Therefore, there are many fillers that are currently widely used in Europe but which are only now undergoing FDA testing. At least two new hyaluronic acid fillers are now undergoing FDA clinical trials: Puragen (Mentor) and Belotero (Merk). Also scheduled for FDA trials is Evolence (ColBar Life Sciences), which is a crosslinked porcine-derived collagen that purportedly has greater longevity than currently available collagen products in the United States.

A novel concept in fillers is the so called injectable "endoprosthesis," which includes Aquamid (Aquamid, Ferrosan, Copenhagen, Denmark) and Bio-Alcamid (Bio-Alcamid, Polymekon, Italy). These nonbiodegradable fillers are composed of 97% water and 3% synthetic polymer. In the case of Aquamid, the polymer is polyacrylamide, whereas with Bio-Alcamid the polymer is the molecularly similar polyalkylamide. Both are intended for large-volume augmentation, as may be necessary in hemifacial lipoatrophy (Romberg's disease) or HIV-associated lipoatrophy. The implants are injected into the subcutaneous space in a bolus form. Fibroplasia ensues around the periphery of the balloon-like implant creating an injectable "prosthesis." Recent reports have documented the success of Bio-Alcamid for the treatment of HIV-associated facial lipoatrophy [28]. However, the author has treated numerous patients who have traveled to Tijuana, Mexico to be treated with Bio-Alcamid for HIV-associated lipoatrophy and who have developed late-appearing bacterial abscesses or palpable disfiguring lumpiness. In the majority of cases, the balloon-like implants can be partially removed with an incision-and-drainage (I and D) procedure. Late-appearing abscesses, which are usually caused by streptococcal bacteria, can be treated by I and D in combination with oral antibiotics. Delayed inflammatory reactions have also been noted recently in patients who have received Aquamid [29]. Both products are scheduled for FDA clinical trials.

References

1. Amin S, Marmur E, Goldberg D (2004) Complications from injectable polyacrylamide gel, a new nonbiodegradable soft tissue filler. Dermatol Surg 30:1507–1509
2. Barnett J, Barnett C (2005) Treatment of acne scars with liquid silicone injections: 30-year perspective. Dermatol Surg 31:1542–1549
3. Baumann L, Kaufman J, Saghari S (2006) Collagen fillers. Dermatol Ther 19:134–140
4. Baumann L, Kerdel F (1999) Treatment of bovine collagen allergy with cyclosporine. Dermatol Surg 25:247–249
5. Baumann L, Shamban A, Lupo M (2006) Comparison of hyaluronic acid-based fillers and cross-linked bovine collagen: a double-masked, multicenter, randomized within-subject study. Poster #203 presented at the Academy 2006 meeting of the American Academy of Dermatology, 26–30 July, San Diego, USA
6. Bowman P, Narins RS (2005) Hylans and soft tissue augmentation. In: Carruthers J, Carruthers A (eds) Procedures in Cosmetic Dermatology: Soft Tissue Augmentation. WB Saunders, Philadelphia, pp 33–54
7. Brody H (2005) Use of hyaluronidase in the treatment of granulomatous hyaluronic acid reactions or unwanted hyaluronic acid misplacement. Dermatol Surg 31:893–897
8. Carruthers A, Carruthers J (2005) Polymethylmethacrylate microspheres/collagen as a tissue augmenting agent: personal experience over 5 years. Dermatol Surg 31:1561–1565
9. Carruthers J, Carruthers A (2003) Deep resting glabellar rhytides respond to BTX-A and Hylan B. Dermatol Surg 29:539–544
10. Coleman KR, Carruthers J (2006) Combination therapy with BOTOX and fillers: the new rejuvenation paradigm. Dermatol Ther 19:177–188
11. Friedman P, Mafong E, Kauvar A, Geronemus R (2002) Safety data of injectable nonanimal stabilized hyaluronic acid gel for soft tissue augmentation. Dermatol Surg 28:491–494
12. Glaich A, Cohen J, Goldberg L (2006) Injection necrosis of the glabella: protocol for prevention and treatment after use of dermal fillers. Dermatol Surg 32:276–281
13. Grimes P, Thomas J, Murphy D (2006) Efficacy and safety of novel hyaluronic acid-based fillers and crosslinked bovine collagen in Caucasians and persons of color. Poster #204 presented at the Academy 2006 meeting of the American Academy of Dermatology, 26–30 July, San Diego, USA

14. Jones D (2005) HIV facial lipoatrophy: causes and treatment options. Dermatol Surg 31:1519–1529
15. Jones D, Carruthers A, Orentreich D, Brody H, Lai M, Azen S, Van Dyke G (2004) Highly Purified 1000-cSt silicone oil for treatment of human immunodeficiency virus–associated facial lipoatrophy: an open pilot trial. Dermatol Surg 30:1279–1286
16. Klein A, Elson M (2000) The history of substances for soft tissue augmentation. Dermatol Surg 26:1096–1105
17. Lemperle G, Romano J, Busso M (2003) Soft tissue augmentation with Artecoll: 10-year history, indications, techniques, and complications. Dermatol Surg 29:573–587
18. Lowe N, Maxwell A, Rickie P (2005) Adverse reactions to dermal fillers: review. Dermatol Surg 31:1626–1633
19. Marmur E, Phelps R, Goldberg D (2004) Clinical, histologic and electron microscopic findings after injection of a calcium hydroxylapatite filler. J Cosmet Laser Ther 6:223–226
20. Monheit G, Thomas J, Murphy D (2006) Photographic documentation from a double-blind randomized multicenter study comparing new hyaluronic acid-based fillers with crosslinked bovine collagen. Poster #202 presented at the Academy 2006 meeting of the American Academy of Dermatology, 26–30 July, San Diego, USA
21. Moody B, Sengelmann R (2001) Topical Tacrolimus in the treatment of bovine collagen hypersensitivity. Dermatol Surg 27:789–791
22. Narins R, Brandt F, Leyden J, Lorenc P, Rubin M, Smith S (2003) A randomized, double-blind, multicenter comparison of the efficacy and tolerability of Restylane versus Zyplast for the correction of nasolabial folds. Dermatol Surg 29:588–595
23. Monheit GD, Coleman KM (2006) Hyaluronic acid fillers. Dermatol Ther 19:141–150
24. Prather C, Jones D (2006) Liquid injectable silicone for soft tissue augmentation. Dermatol Ther 19:159–168
25. Rao J, Genevieve C, Goldman M (2005) Clinical comparison between two hyaluronic acid-derived fillers in the treatment of nasolabial folds: Hylaform versus Restylane. Dermatol Surg 31:1587–1590
26. Roy D, Sadick N, Mangat D (2006) Clinical trial of a novel filler material for soft tissue augmentation of the face containing synthetic calcium hydroxylapatite microspheres. Dermatol Surg 32:1134–1139
27. Smith S, Jones D, Thomas J, et al (2006) Efficacy and safety following repeat treatments for a new family of hyaluronic acid-based fillers. Poster #202 presented at the Academy 2006 meeting of the American Academy of Dermatology, 26–30 July, San Diego, USA
28. Treacy P, Goldberg D (2006) Use of a biopolymer polyalkylimide filler for facial lipodystrophy in HIV-positive patients undergoing treatment with antiretroviral drugs. Dermatol Surg 32:804–808
29. Valantin MA, Aubron-Olivier C, Ghosn J, Laglenne E, Pauchard M, Schoen H, Bousquet R, Katz P, Costagliola D, Katlama C (2003) Polylactic acid implants (New-Fill) to correct facial lipoatrophy in HIV-infected patients: results of the open-label study VEGA. AIDS 17:2471–2477
30. Vleggaar D (2005) Facial volumetric correction with injectable poly-L-lactic Acid. Dermatol Surg 31:1511–1518
31. Wildemore J, Jones D (2006) Persistent granulomatous inflammatory response induced by injectable poly-L-lactic acid for HIV lipoatrophy. J Dermatol Surg 32.1407–1409

Chapter 6

Chemical Peeling

6

Ross M. Campbell and Gary D. Monheit

Core Messages

- Superficial, medium, and deep chemical peels vary based on their active ingredients and their depth of dermal damage.
- Peeling procedures are easy to learn and generally inexpensive to perform.
- There are few absolute contraindications to peel procedures.
- There are an increasing number of materials available for the performance of superficial, medium, and deep chemical peels.

History

Chemical peels have been a pillar of facial rejuvenation since its inception. Patients' enthusiasm for the effects of peels has grown tremendously over the last 20 years, as has the general public's interest in acquiring a youthful appearance by rehabilitating photoaged skin. Advertising has further heightened the public's interest for cosmetic agents, over-the-counter chemicals and treatment programs that have entered the general market of products meant to rejuvenate skin and erase the marks of sun damage and age. Physicians must be able to analyze the patient's skin type and the degree of photoaging, and prescribe the correct facial rejuvenation procedure. This should be the procedure or combination of procedures that will give the greatest benefit for the least risk factors and morbidity. Chemical peeling has been the tried and true basic procedure.

Chemical peeling involves the application of a chemical exfoliant to wound the epidermis and dermis for the removal of superficial lesions and improve the texture of skin. Various acidic and basic chemical agents are used to produce the varying effects of light to medium to deep chemical peels through differences in their ability to destroy skin. The level of penetration, destruction, and inflammation determines the level of peeling. Light superficial peels stimulate epidermal growth through the removal of the stratum corneum without necrosis. Through exfoliation, it thickens the epidermis with qualitative regenerative changes. Full superficial chemical peels destroy the epidermis and thus induce the regeneration of new epidermis. Medium depth peels further destroy the epidermis and induce inflammation within the papillary dermis. Finally, a deep chemical peel extends the inflammatory response to the deep reticular dermis and induces new collagen production and ground substances [1]. These have now been well classified and usage has been categorized for various degenerative conditions associated with photoaging skin based on levels of penetration. The physician thus has tools capable of solving problems that may be mild, moderate, or severe with agents that are very superficial, superficial, medium-depth, and deep peeling chemicals.

The use of exfoliating agents to peel the epidermis and superficial dermis date back to ancient Egypt. Sour milk baths were used by ancient Egyptian women to sooth the skin.

Alabaster, salt, brimstone, pumice stone, and various animal oils were once used to exfoliate the skin and produce a more cosmetically elegant appearance. Fire was once used by the Turks to lightly singe the skin causing exfoliation and an improved aesthetic glow [2].

In the early 20th century, phenol was introduced as the premier peeling agent for postacne scarring [3]. Paraprofessionals were the first to use phenol, resorcinol, and other acid emollients for exfoliation. Various formulations of phenol peels were tried, both with and without occlusion; however, its use was limited due to severe facial scarring and cardiac toxicity. Baker and Gordon first learned the safe use of a dilute phenol preparation from a Hungarian aesthetician and promoted the present formula written in the literature today

Between 1940 and 1970, a variety of exfoliating agents were introduced, some of which were combined to cause a deeper dermal injury. Examples include sulfur, resorcinol pastes, salicylic acid, and solid carbon dioxide (CO_2).

In the 1950s and 1960s, trichloracetic acid (TCA) became the agent of choice for superficial, medium, and deep peeling. The use of 50% and greater TCA, though, led to scarring and pigmentary complications that became common among dermatologists and plastic surgeons. The need for safer medium and deep peeling agents led to the search for combination products that would improve efficacy. Brody first combined solid CO_2 ice with 35% TCA, which produced a deeper resurfacing procedure [4]. This was followed by Monheit's combination of Jessner's solution with 35% TCA. Other combinations were to follow.

The need for deeper dermal injury to improve contour deformities due to acne scarring led to the concept of chemabrasion [5]. Chemabrasion, introduced in the 1970s, is the combined process of performing a full or partial face chemical peel followed by dermabra-

Table 6.1. Classification of chemical skin resurfacing methods. *TCA* Trichloracetic acid, *YAG* yttrium aluminum garnet

Level of resurfacing required	Method
Superficial–very light	Low-potency formulations of glycolic acid or other alpha-hydroxy acid 10–20% TCA (weight-to-volume formulation) Jessner's solution (Table 6.4) Tretinoin Salicylic acid
Superficial–light	70% glycolic acid Jessner's solution 25–30% TCA
Medium-depth	88% phenol 35–40% TCA Jessner's – 35% TCA 70% glycolic acid – 35% TCA Solid CO_2 – 35% TCA Conservative manual dermasanding Erbium:YAG laser resurfacing Conservative CO_2 laser resurfacing
Deep	Unoccluded or occluded Baker-Gordon phenol peel TCA in concentrations >50%

sion on the same day. Chemical peeling today is often combined with other mechanical resurfacing modalities including laser resurfacing and dermasanding.

Current Available Technology

Many new "peels" have come to market in recent years, including over-the-counter peels and spa or physician "proprietary" peels that demand physicians to remain abreast of new products. Fortunately, since all peeling agents, superficial, medium-depth and deep, are derived from basic chemicals known to cause exfoliation, destruction and/or inflammation of skin in a controlled manner, the clinician must ask what is new and better about the particular product (Table 6.1). Peeling agents, regardless of their "proprietary" new name, fall into chemical families. The clinical evaluation of these generic agents is well documented in the medical literature as to efficacy, technical care, and safety.

Superficial chemical peeling is truly an exfoliation of the stratum corneum or the entire epidermis to encourage regrowth with less photodamage and a more youthful appearance. It usually takes repetitive peeling sessions to obtain maximal results. These agents have been broken down into very superficial chemical peels that will remove the stratum corneum only, and superficial chemical peels that will remove stratum corneum and damaged epidermis. It is to be noted that the effects of superficial peeling on photoaging skin is subtle and will not produce a prolonged or very noticeable effect on dermal lesions such as wrinkles and furrows. Agents used include: TCA 10–20%, Jessner's solution, glycolic acid 40–70%, salicylic acid (betahydroxy acid) 20–30%, and tretinoin. Each of these agents has its own characteristics and methodology, and a physician must be thoroughly familiar with the chemicals, methods of application, and the nature of healing. The usual time for healing is from 1 to 4 days depending on the chemical and its strength. Very light peeling agents include low concentrations of glycolic acid, 10% TCA, and salicylic acid, a betahydroxy acid.

Medium-depth chemical peeling is defined as controlled damage from a chemical agent to the papillary dermis, resulting in specific changes that can be performed in a single setting. Agents currently used include combination products: Jessner's solution, 70% glycolic acid, and solid CO_2 with 35% TCA. The hallmark for this level peel was 50% TCA. It has traditionally achieved acceptable results in ameliorating fine wrinkles, actinic changes, and preneoplasia. However, since higher-dosage TCA itself is an agent more likely to be fraught with complications, especially scarring, in strengths of 50% or higher, it has fallen out of favor as a single-agent chemical peel. It is for this reason that the combination products along with a 35% TCA formula have been found equally effective in producing this level of control damage without the risk of side effects.

Brody first developed the use of solid CO_2 applied with acetone to the skin as a freezing technique prior to the application of 35% TCA [4]. This appears to break the epidermal barrier for a more even and complete penetration of the TCA. Monheit then demonstrated the use of Jessner's solution prior to the application of 35% TCA [6]. The Jessner's solution was found to be effective in destroying the epidermal barrier by breaking up individual epidermal cells. This allowed deeper penetration of the 35% TCA and a more even application of the peeling solution. Similarly, Coleman has demonstrated the use of 70% glycolic acid prior to the application of 35% TCA [7]. Its effect has been very similar to that of Jessner's solution.

Deep chemical peeling induces inflammation to the deep reticular dermis. This entails the use of either TCA at concentrations above 50%, or the Gordon-Baker phenol peel [8]. Laser resurfacing can also be used to reliably reach this level of damage. For this reason, it is not included as a standard treatment for deep chemical peeling. The Baker-Gordon phenol peel has been used successfully for over 40 years for deep chemical peeling and produces reliable results.

The approach to photoaging skin has expanded beyond a one-stage procedure to now include preparatory medical therapy and posttreatment cosmeceutical topical therapy to maintain results and prevent further photodamage. Thus, the dermatologist's office has become not only a surgical treatment session, but also an educational setting for skin protection and care and a marketplace for the patient to obtain the necessary topicals for skin protection. It is up to the dermatologist, cosmetic surgeon, or plastic surgeon to fully understand the nature of skin and sun damage, protective techniques available, and active agents that work as cosmeceutical preparations. Having available multiple procedures to solve these problems will make their patients better candidates for the right procedure to restore and rehabilitate their skin.

Advantages

Chemical peeling has several distinct advantages over other facial rejuvenation procedures. It is a relatively simple procedure that is fairly easy to learn, yet may be technique-sensitive. If performed properly on the correctly chosen patient, the procedure will reliably produce what the physician predicts. Superficial peels are used for minimal damage with little downtime, while deep peels have significant downtime and morbidity to produce more dramatic and longer-lasting results. Finally, the price of most chemicals is far more economical than the lasers or light-source tools on the market.

Disadvantages

Disadvantages of chemical peeling are usually related to the learning curve needed to choose the correct peel for each patient. Application of the peel is technique-sensitive, while monitoring and caring for the healing patient requires experience in recognizing the normal appearance of the wound for each level of peel at different time intervals.

Indications

The chief indications for chemical peeling are associated with the reversal of actinic changes such as photodamage, rhytides, actinic growths, pigmentary dyschromias, and acne scars [9]. The physician thus can use classification systems to quantitate and qualitate the level of photodamage and prescribe the appropriate chemical peeling combination.

Superficial chemical peels are indicated in the management of acne and its postinflammatory erythema, mild photoaging, epidermal growths such as lentigines and keratoses, as well as melasma and other pigmentary dyschromias. The medium-depth chemical peel thus has five major indications: (1) destruction of epidermal lesions (actinic keratoses), (2) resurfacing the level II moderate photoaging skin, (3) pigmentary dyschromias, (4) mild acne scars, and (5) blending photoaging skin with laser resurfacing and deep chemical peeling.

Actinic Keratoses

This procedure is well suited for the male with epidermal lesions such as actinic keratoses that have required repeated removal with either cryosurgery or chemoexfoliation (5-fluoruracil). The entire face can be treated as a unit or subfacial cosmetic unit such as the forehead, temples, and cheeks, and can be treated independently. Active lesions as well as incipient growths as yet undetected will be removed as the epidermis is sloughed. Advantages for the male patient include a limited recovery period (7 days) with little postoperative erythema after healing. There is little risking of pigmentary changes, either hypopigmentation or hyperpigmentation, thus the patient can return to work after the skin has healed.

Moderate Photoaging Skin

Glogau level II damage responds well to this peeling combination with removal of the epidermal lesions and dermal changes that will freshen sallow, atrophic skin and soften other rhytides. This also is an excellent peel for the male patient in that it will heal in 10 days with minimal risk of textural or color complications.

Pigmentary Dyschromias

Although color change can be treated with repetitive chemical peeling, the medium-depth peel will be a single treatment preceded and followed by the use of bleaching agents and retinoic acid. In most cases, the pigmentary problems are resolved with this single treatment program.

Mild Acne Scars

The medium-depth peel may improve the slight contour abnormalities and pigmentary abnormalities that are often associated with mild acne scars.

Blending Other Resurfacing Procedures

In a patient in whom there are advanced photoaging changes such as crow's feet and rhytides in the periorbital area with medium-depth changes on the remaining face, a medium-depth peel can be used to integrate these procedures together. That is, laser resurfacing or deep chemical peeling can be performed over the periorbital and perioral areas that may have more advanced photoaging changes, while the medium-depth chemical peel is used for the rest of the face. This will blend the facial skin as a unit so that the therapeutic textural changes will not be restricted to one area.

Deep chemical peels are indicated for severely photoaged skin. It has been demonstrated to improve deep perioral and periorbital rhytides, crow's feet, forehead lines and wrinkles, as well as the other textural and lesional changes associated with the more severe photoaging process.

Analyzing the patient with photoaging skin must take into account skin color and skin type as well as the degree of photoaging. Various classification systems are available to help the physician define the right program or therapeutic procedure for his or her patient. The Fitzpatrick skin type system classifies degrees of pigmentation and ability to tan using a grading system (I–VI; Table 6.2). It prognosticates sun sensitivity, susceptibility to photodamage, and ability for facultative melanogenesis (one's intrinsic ability to tan) [10]. In addition, this system classifies skin as to its risk factors for complications during chemical peeling. Fitzpatrick divides skin types I–VI, taking into account both color and reaction to the sun. Skin types I and II are pale white and freckled with a high degree of potential to burn with sun exposure. Three and

Table 6.2. Fitzpatrick's classification of skin types

Skin type	Color	Reaction to sun
I	Very white or freckled	Always burns
II	White	Usually burns
III	White to olive	Sometimes burns
IV	Brown	Rarely burns
V	Dark Brown	Very rarely burns
VI	Black	Never burns

Table 6.3. Glogau's classification of photoaging groups

Group	Subgroup description
I. Mild (typically age 28–35 years)	A. Little wrinkling or scarring B. No keratoses C. Requires little or no make-up
II. Moderate (age 35–50 years)	A. Early wrinkling; mild scarring B. Sallow color with early actinic keratoses C. Little make-up
III. Advanced (age 50–65) years	A. Persistent wrinkling or moderate acne scarring B. Discoloration with telangiectasias and actinic keratoses C. Wears make-up always
IV. Severe (age 60–75 years)	A. Wrinkling: photoaging, gravitational and dynamic B. Actinic keratoses with or without skin cancer or severe acne scars C. Wears make-up with poor coverage

four can burn but usually is an olive to brown coloration. Five and six are dark brown to black skin that rarely ever burns and usually does not need sunscreen protection. The patient with type I or II skin with significant photodamage needs regular sunscreen protection prior to and after the procedure. Fortunately, there is little risk for hypopigmentation or reactive hyperpigmentation after a chemical peeling procedure with type I or II skin. In contrast, the patient with type III through VI skin has a greater risk for pigmentary dyschromia – hyper or hypopigmentation, after a chemical peel and may need pre- and posttreatment with both sunscreen and bleaching to prevent these complications [11]. Pigmentary risks are generally not a great problem with very superficial and superficial chemical peeling, but may become a problem with medium and deep chemical peeling. It can also be a significant risk when regional areas such as the lips and eyelids are peeled with deep peeling or a pulsed CO_2 laser, creating a significant color change in these cosmetic units from the rest of the face. The physician must inform the patient of this potential problem, the "alabaster look" seen after taped deep chemical peels in regional areas, especially if they are of skin types III–VI. The benefits of the procedure must outweigh these risks and, in addition, plans should be made for appropriate techniques to prevent these unwanted changes in color.

The Glogau system classifies the severity of photodamage, taking into account the degree of epidermal and dermal degenerative effects [12]. The categorization is I–IV, ranging from mild, to moderate, advanced, and severe photodamaged skin (Table 6.3). These categories are devised for therapeutic intervention. Category I in young individuals, or minimal degree photodamage should be treated with light chemical peeling and medical treatment. Categories II and III would entail medium-depth chemical peeling, and category IV would need those modalities listed plus cosmetic surgical intervention for gravitational changes.

Monheit and Fulton have devised a system of quantitating photodamage and have developed numerical scores that would fit into corresponding rejuvenation programs (Table 6.4) [13]. In analyzing photodamage, the major categories include epidermal color with skin lesions and dermal with textural changes. Dermal changes include wrinkles, cross-hatched lines, sallow color, leathery appearance, crinkly thin parchment skin, and the white nodules of milia. Each of these is classified, giving the patient a point score, 1–4. In

Table 6.4. Monheit and Fulton's index of photoaging. *AKs* actinic keratoses, *SKs* seborrheic keratoses

Texture Changes	Points				Score
Wrinkles – dynamic	1	2	3	4	
(% of potential lines)	<25%	<50%	<75%	<100%	
Wrinkles – photoaging	1	2	3	4	
(% of potential lines)	<25%	<50%	<75%	<100%	
Crosshatched lines – fine lines	1	2	3	4	
(% of potential lines)	<10%	<20%	<40%	<60%	
Sallow color and dyschromia	1	2	3	4	
	Dull	Yellow	Brown	Black	
Leathery appearance	1	2	3	4	
Crinkly (thin and parchment)	1	2	3	4	
Pebbly (deep whitish nodules)	2	4	6	8	
(% of face)	<25%	<50%	<75%	<100%	
Pore number and size	2	4	6	8	
	<25%	<50%	<75%	<100%	
Lesions	Points				Score
Freckles – mottled skin	1	2	3	4	
(number present)	<10	<25	<50	<100	
Lentigenes (dark/irregular) and SKs	2	4	6	8	
(size)	<5mm	<10mm	<15mm	<20mm	
Telangiectasias – erythema flush	1	2	3	4	
(number present)	<5	<10	<15	>15	
AKs and SKs	2	4	6	8	
(number present)	<5	<10	<15	>15	
Skin cancers	2	4	6	8	
(number present – now or by history)	1 ca	2 ca	3 ca	>4 ca	
Senile comedones	1	2	3	4	
(in cheekbone area)	<5	<10	<20	>20	
Total Score					

addition, the number and extent of lesions are categorized from freckles, lentigines, telangiectasias, actinic and seborrheic keratoses, skin cancers, and senile comedones. These are also added in a classification system of 1–4, and the final score results are tabulated. A total score of 1–4 would indicate very mild damage and the patient would adequately respond to a five-step skin-care program including sunscreen protection, retinoic acid, glycolic acid peels, and selective lesional removal. A score of 5–9 would include all of the above plus a repetitive superficial peeling agents program such as glycolic acid, Jessner's solution, or lactic acid peels. A score of 10–14 would include medium-depth chemical peeling, and a score of 15 or above would include deep chemical peeling or laser resurfacing. This enables the patient to understand during the consultation their degree of photodamage and the necessity for an individualized peeling program.

Contraindications

The preoperative consultation is important in identifying at-risk patients who are best avoided or who necessitate an extra cautious approach, as well as in selecting patients who are ideal candidates for intervention. The dermatologist must evaluate the prospective patient and his or her skin condition carefully to determine if a chemical resurfacing procedure is indicated. When resurfacing is deemed appropriate, selection of the proper procedure for each patient is critical to assure that the desired results are achieved in a safe and effective manner. In general, the degree of skin surface irregularities is proportional to the depth of the injury that must be created by resurfacing in order to achieve significant improvement.

There are relatively few absolute contraindications for chemical resurfacing, but certain patients are more susceptible to complications and, with foresight, can be educated more specifically regarding their prospective risks and perhaps cause the physician to choose a more superficial procedure (Table 6.5). The preoperative consultation is essential for the physician to assess the expectations and mental preparedness of the patient. If it is determined that the patient is not prepared or has unrealistic expectations, or the physician–patient relationship is strained, then the procedure should be strongly reconsidered. The general health and nutritional status of the patient must be deemed appropriate to undergo the depth of procedure planned. Isotretinoin therapy within the last 6 months is an absolute contraindication for medium-depth or deep resurfacing procedures to avoid the excessive granulation observed in some patients undergoing systemic retinoid therapy. Resurfacing procedures should also be avoided in patients with active infection or open wounds.

Caution is advised in patients with other underlying skin disease. The peeling agent is a chemical eshcarotic that damages the skin in

Table 6.5. Contraindications to chemical skin resurfacing

Absolute	Poor physician–patient relationship
	Lack of psychological stability and mental preparedness
	Unrealistic expectations
	Poor general health and nutritional status
	Isotretinoin therapy within the last 6 months*
	Complete absence of intact pilosebaceous units on the face
	Active infection or open wounds (such as herpes, excoriations, or open acne cysts)
Relative	Medium-depth or deep resurfacing procedure within the last 3–12 months*
	Recent facial surgery involving extensive undermining, such as a rhytidectomy*
	History of abnormal scar formation or delayed wound healing
	History of therapeutic radiation exposure
	History of certain skin diseases (such as rosacea, seborrheic dermatitis, atopic dermatitis, psoriasis, and vitiligo) or active retinoid dermatitis
	Fitzpatrick skin types IV, V, and VI*

* These contraindications apply only to medium-depth and deep resurfacing procedures

a therapeutic manner. It is important that the physician understand the patient's skin and its ability to withstand this damage. Certain skin types withstand the damage to a greater degree than others, and particular skin disorders have a greater tendency to produce side effects and complications from chemical peels. Patients with extensive photodamage may require stronger peeling agents and repeated applications of medium-depth peeling solutions to obtain therapeutic results. Patients with skin disorders such as atopic dermatitis, seborrheic dermatitis, psoriasis, and contact dermatitis may find their disease exacerbated in the postoperative period or even develop problems with postoperative healing such as prolonged healing, posterythema syndrome, or contact sensitivity during a postoperative period. Rosacea is a disorder of vasomotor instability in the skin and may develop an exaggerated inflammatory response to the peeling agents. Other important factors include any history of abnormal scar formation or history of radiation therapy to the proposed facial skin as chronic radiation dermatitis decreases the body's ability to heal properly. A general rule of thumb is to examine the facial hair in the area treated by radiation and if it is intact, there are enough pilosebaceous units to heal the skin properly after medium or even deep chemical peeling. This, though, is not absolute and one should find in the patient's history the dates of radiation treatment and how many rads were used for each individual treatment. Some patients with the greatest amount of radiation dermatitis had treatments that were given for acne in the mid 1950s, and over the years the skin developed the resultant degenerative changes for which they now seek physician assistance [14].

Herpes simplex reactivation can be a postoperative problem with significant morbidity. Patients susceptible should be pretreated with antiherpetic agents such as acyclovir or valcyclovir to prevent herpetic activation. These patients can be identified in the preoperative consultation and placed on appropriate therapy at the time of the chemical peel. All antiherpetic agents act by inhibiting viral replication in the intact epidermal cell. The significance of this in chemical peeling is that the skin must be reepithelialized before the agent has its full effect. Thus, the antiviral agent must be continued in deep chemical peeling for the entire 2 weeks, or in medium-depth peeling for at least 10 days [15]. Antiviral agents are rarely needed for light or superficial chemical peeling, as the injury pattern usually is not enough to activate the herpes simplex virus.

Informed Consent

After the patient is deemed a good candidate for resurfacing, a thorough preoperative discussion is needed to obtain informed consent. The patient should understand that chemical resurfacing procedures cannot reliably reduce pore size and that their ability to improve lax skin and deeper wrinkles and scars is limited depending on the type of intervention being performed. The patient must fully understand the potential benefits, limitations, and risks of the procedure, and an informed consent must be signed. A test spot may be useful in some patients to assess their suitability for resurfacing and may be particularly helpful when there is a great deal of concern about the chances of postoperative pigmentary dyschromias [16]. Although a favorable test spot result does not guarantee a positive outcome following full-face resurfacing, an unfavorable test spot result is useful to identify high-risk patients. If the dermatologist feels any uncertainty about the patient's suitability or the likelihood of a favorable result, then the procedure should not be performed.

Personal Approach

Prior to the application of peeling solutions, the surgeon must vigorously cleanse the skin surface to remove residual oils, debris, and excess stratum corneum. The face is initially scrubbed with 10 cm×10 cm gauze pads containing 0.25% Irgasan (Septisol, Vestal Laboratories, St. Louis, Missouri, USA), then rinsed with water and dried. Because of the defatting and degreasing properties of acetone, gauze pads moistened in an acetone preparation are then used to cleanse the skin even further. Finally, the cleansed skin is palpated immediately prior to peeling in order to check for the presence of residual oil, and if any is felt, the process is repeated. The importance of cleansing in the peeling procedure cannot be overemphasized. A thorough and evenly distributed cleansing and degreasing of the face assures uniform penetration of the peeling solution and leads to an even result without skip areas [17].

Superficial Chemical Peeling

Superficial chemical peels can be used for comedonal acne and postinflammatory erythema or pigmentation from acne, treatment for mild photoaging skin – Glogau I and II, and the treatment of melasma.

Multiple peels on a repeated basis are usually necessary to obtain optimal results with superficial chemical peels. The frequency of peels and degree of exposure to the peeling agent may be increased gradually as necessary. Results are enhanced by medical or cosmeceutical therapy including a retinoid and, if necessary, a bleaching agent. All superficial chemical peels share the advantages of only mild stinging and burning during application as well as minimal time needed for recovery.

A TCA concentration of 10–20% will produce a light whitening or frosting effect on the skin with a result of sloughing of the upper one-half to one-third of the epidermis. The TCA is applied evenly with either a saturated 5 cm×5 cm gauze, or a sable brush, and it usually takes 15–45 s for the frosting to become evident. This would be categorized as a level I frosting with the appearance of erythema and streaky whitening on the surface (Fig. 6.1). Levels II and III frosting are seen in medium-depth and deeper peels. Level II frosting is defined as white-coated frosting with erythema showing through (Fig. 6.2). A level III frosting, which is associated with penetration to the reticular dermis, is solid white enamel frosting with no background of erythema.

The patient experiences stinging and some burning during the procedure, but very rapidly this subsides and the patient then can resume normal activities. There is erythema and resulting desquamation, which can last anywhere from 1 to 3 days. Sunscreens and light moisturizers are permitted and care is minimal in this superficial chemical peel.

Jessner's solution is a combination acid-escharotic that has been used for over 100 years in the treatment of hyperkeratotic skin disorders (Table 6.6). It has been used as part of acne treatment for the removal of comedones and inflammatory acne activity. Its use as a superficial peeling agent performs as an intense keratolytic agent. The application is similar to superficial TCA application with wet gauze, sponges, or a sable brush, producing an erythema with blotchy frosting. Tentative applications are done on an every-other-week basis and the levels of Jessner's solution coatings can be increased with repetitive applications. The visual endpoint produces a predictable outcome with epidermal exfoliation and regrowth. This usually occurs within 2–4 days and is treated with mild cleansers, moisturizing lotion, and sunscreen protection. Salicylic acid, a beta-hydroxy acid that is one of the ingredients in Jessner's solution, can also be used alone in superficial chemical peeling [18]. It is a preferred therapy for comedonal acne as it is lipophilic and concentrates in the pilosebaceous apparatus. It is quite effective as an adjunctive therapy for open and closed comedones and resolving postacne erythema because it is a relatively noninflammatory compound and is useful with other agents as a peeling agent for postinflammatory hyperpigmentation.

Alphahydroxy acids, specifically glycolic acid, became the wonder drug of the early 1990s with promises of skin rejuvenation with home use and topical therapy. Hydroxy acids

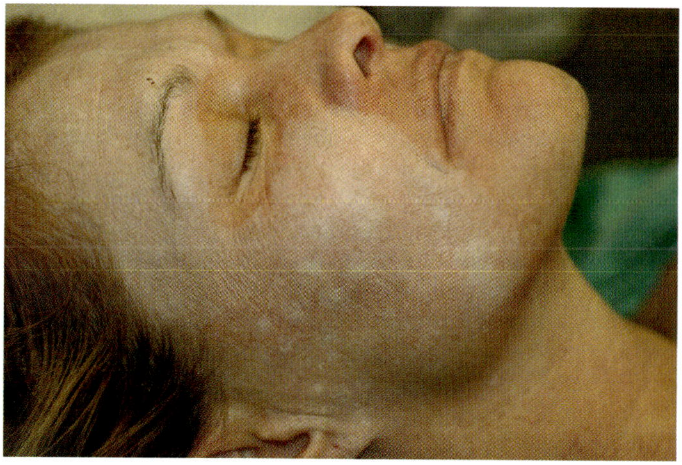

Fig. 6.1. Photograph of level 1 frosting with Jessner's solution – 35% trichloracetic acid (TCA) peel demonstrating erythema and streaky whitening on the surface of the right cheek

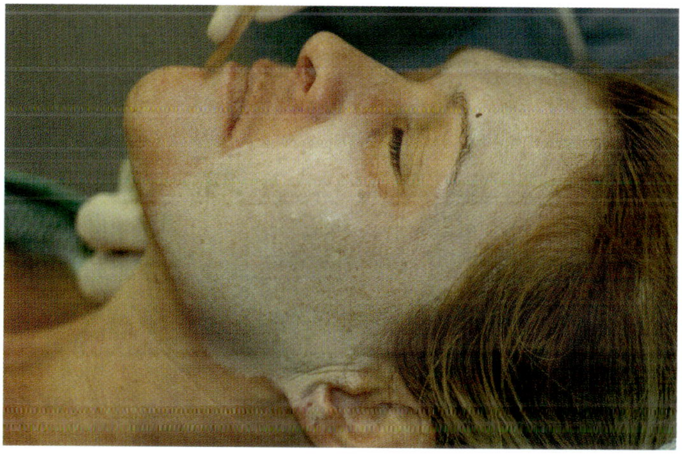

Fig. 6.2. Photograph of level 2 frosting with Jessner's solution – 35% TCA peel demonstrating a white-coated frosting with some erythema showing through on the surface of the left cheek

are found in foods such as glycolic acid as naturally present in sugar cane, lactic acid in sour milk, malic acid in apples, citric acid in fruits, and tartaric acid in grapes. Lactic acid and glycolic acid are widely available and can be purchased for physician use. Glycolic acid is found in unbuffered concentrations of 50 70% for use as a chemical peel. Weekly or every other week applications of 40–70% unbuffered glycolic acid treatments have been used for wrinkles by applying the solution to the face with a cotton swab, a sable brush, or saturated 5 cm×5 cm gauze. The time of application is critical for glycolic acid, as it must be rinsed off with water or neutralized with 5% sodium bicarbonate after 2–4 min. Mild erythema may occur for 1 h with slight stinging and minimal scaling. Wrinkle reduction and removal of benign keratoses have been report-

Table 6.6. Jessner's solution (Combes' formula)

Resorcinol	14 g
Salicylic acid	14 g
85% lactic acid	14 g
95% ethanol	100 ml

ed from repeated applications of these peeling solutions.

Retinoic acid has been classified as a cosmoceutical agent that produces minimally superficial chemical peeling and pharmacologic changes on the epithelium. Rather than its application as a peeling agent, it is used in a homecare program to enhance the effects of a chemical peel on the skin. It is used in combination with a sunscreen and/or moisturizing program as a supplement to most peeling regimens. Chronic use of retinoic acid has been demonstrated to change degenerative photodamage effects in the epidermis [19]. The thickened basket-weave stratum corneum, the atrophic Malpighian layer, and the dysplastic cells in the epidermis have been shown to change to a more normal or youthful epidermis with chronic applications. It is also been demonstrated that the use of retinoic acid prior to peeling, dermabrasion, or laser resurfacing, will speed epidermal healing [20,21]. Specifically with chemical peeling, it also enhances the depth of the peel by decreasing the thickness of the stratum corneum [22].

Most preparatory programs for superficial, medium, and deep chemical peels include the daily use of retinoic acid up to 6 weeks prior to the peeling event. There are various strengths of retinoic acid available on the market, and one must use a weaker formulation for sensitive skin and a stronger formulation for significantly photodamaged skin. Retinoid dermatitis may ensue 1 or 2 weeks after initiation of the agent. One should not perform a peeling procedure with retinoid dermatitis present as the inflamed skin may develop problems with healing or even postoperative complications. The dermatitis should subside by decreasing treatment so that the skin does not appear inflamed when the chemical peel is performed.

To treat melasma effectively, the skin must be pre- and posttreated with sunscreen, hydroquinone 4–8%, and retinoic acid. Hydroquinone is a pharmacologic agent that blocks the enzyme tyrosinase from developing melanin precursors for the production of new pigment. Its use essentially blocks new pigment as the new epidermis is healing after a chemical peel. It is thus necessary to use when peeling for the treatment of pigmentary dyschromias and also when using chemical peels in types III–VI Fitzpatrick's skin, the skin type most prone to developing pigmentary problems.

Prior to the initial treatment with a superficial peel, both patient and physician must understand the limitations, especially on photoaging, to avoid future disappointment. First, the net effect of repetitive superficial chemical peels never approaches the beneficial effect obtained with a single medium-depth or deep peel. The improvements in photoaged skin following superficial peels are usually subtle because there is little to no effect on the dermis. These peels thus cannot produce an appreciable effect on textural changes such as deep wrinkles and furrows that originate within the dermis. Nevertheless, their ease of use and minimal downtime makes these "lunch-time" peels rewarding for patients with realistic expectations and are a favorite among the busy baby-boomers.

Medium-Depth Chemical Peeling

Combining TCA with solid CO_2, Jessner's solution, or 70% glycolic acid have been proven more effective and safer than the use of 50% TCA alone for medium-depth chemical peeling. The application and frosting are more controlled with the combination so that the "hot spots" with higher concentrations of TCA, which can produce dyschromias and scarring, are not a significant problem with lowered concentration TCA as used in this combination medium-depth peel. The Monheit version of the Jessner's solution–35% TCA peel is a relatively simple and safe combination. The technique is used for mild-to-moderate photoaging including pigmentary changes, lentigines, epidermal growths, dyschromias, and rhytides. It freshens sallow, atrophic skin and softens fine rhytides with minimal risk of textural or pigmentary complications. Collagen remodeling occurs for as long as 3–4 months postoperatively, during which there is continued improvement in texture and rhytides. Deep furrows, however, are not eliminated with this peel. It is a single procedure with a healing time of 7–10 days. It is useful also to remove diffuse actinic keratoses as an alternative to chemical exfoliation with topical 5-fluorouracil chemotherapy. It reduces the morbidity significantly and gives the cosmetic benefits of improved photoaging skin.

The procedure is usually performed with mild preoperative sedation and nonsteroidal anti-inflammatory agents. The patient is told that the peeling agent will sting and burn temporarily and aspirin is given before the peel and continued through the first 24 h if the patient can tolerate the medication. Its inflammatory effect is especially helpful in reducing swelling and relieving pain. If given before surgery, it may be all the patient requires during the postoperative phase. For full-face peels, though, it is useful to give preoperative sedation (diazepam 5–10 mg orally) and mild analgesia, meperidine 25 mg (Demerol; Winthrop, New York, USA), and hydroxyzine hydrochloride 25 mg intramuscularly (Vistaril; Lorec, New York, USA). The discomfort from this peel is not long lasting, so short-acting sedatives and analgesics are all that are necessary.

The Jessner's solution is applied evenly with either cotton-tip applicators or 5 cm×5 cm gauze, usually in one coat to achieve a light but even frosting. The frosting achieved with Jessner's solution is much lighter than that produced by TCA and the patient is usually not uncomfortable. A mild erythema appears with a faint tinge of frost evenly over the face. Even strokes are used to apply the solution to the unit area covering the forehead to the cheeks to the nose and chin. The eyelids are treated last, creating the same erythema with blotchy frosting.

The TCA is then applied evenly with one to four cotton-tipped applicators that can be applied over different areas with light or heavier doses of the acid. Four cotton-tipped applicators are applied in broad strokes over the forehead and also on the medial cheeks. Two mildly soaked cotton-tipped applicators can be used across the lips and chin, and one damp cotton-tipped applicator on the eyelids. Thus, the dosage of application is technique-dependent on the amount used and the number of cotton-tipped applicators applied. The cotton-tipped applicator is useful in quantitating the amount of peel solution to be applied.

The white frost from the TCA application appears on the treated area in a few moments. Even application should eliminate the need to go over areas a second or a third time, but if frosting is incomplete or uneven, the solution should be reapplied. TCA takes longer to frost than Baker's formula or straight phenol, but a shorter period of time than the superficial peeling agents do. The surgeon should wait at least 3–4 min after the application of TCA to ensure the frosting has reached its peak. He then can analyze the completeness of a frosted cosmetic unit and touch up the area as needed. Areas of poor frosting should be retreated carefully with a thin application of TCA. The physician should achieve a level II–III frosting. A deeper level III frosting should be restricted only to areas of heavy actinic damage and thicker skin. Most medium-depth chemical peels use a level II frosting and this is especially true over eyelids and areas of sensitive skin. Those areas with a greater tendency to scar formation, such as the zygomatic arch, the bony prominences of the jawline, and chin, should only receive up to a level II frosting. Overcoating TCA will increase its penetration so that a second or third application will penetrate deeper, creating further damage. One must be careful in overcoating only areas in which the take up was not adequate or the skin is much thicker.

Anatomic areas of the face are peeled sequentially from forehead to temple to cheeks, and finally to the lips and eyelids. The white frosting indicates keratocoagulation and at that point the reaction is complete. Careful feathering of the solution into the hairline and around the rim of the jaw and brow conceals the line of demarcation between peeled and nonpeeled areas. The perioral area has rhytides that require a complete and even application of solution over the lip skin to the vermilion. This is accomplished best with the help of an assistant who stretches and fixates the upper and lower lips while the peel solution is applied (Fig. 6.3).

Certain areas and skin lesions require special attention. Thicker keratoses do not frost evenly and thus do not pick up peel solution. Additional applications rubbed vigorously into the lesion may be needed for peel solution penetration. Wrinkled skin should be stretched to allow an even coating of solution into the folds and troughs. Oral rhytides require peel solution to be applied with the wood portion of a cotton-tipped applicator and extended into the vermilion of the lip. Deeper furrows such as expression lines will not be eradicated by peel solution and thus should be treated like the remaining skin.

Eyelid skin must be treated delicately and carefully. A semidry applicator should be used to carry the solution within 2–3 mm of the lid margin. The patient should be positioned with the head elevated at 30° and the eyelids closed. Excess peel solution on the cotton tip should be drained gently on the bottom before application. The applicator is then rolled gently on the lids and periorbital skin. Never leave excess peel solution on the lids because the solution can roll into the eyes. Dry tears with a cotton-tipped applicator during peeling because they may pull peel solution to the puncta and eye by capillary attraction (Fig. 6.4). There is an immediate burning sensation as the peel solution is applied, but this subsides as frosting is completed. Cool saline compresses offer symptomatic relief for a peeled area as the solution is applied to other areas (Fig. 6.5). The compresses are placed over the face for 5–6 min after the peel until the patient is comfortable. Unlike the compresses in glycolic acid peels, the saline following a TCA peel simply provides relief and does not "neutralize" the acid. The burning subsides fully by the time the patient is ready to be discharged. At that time, most of the frosting has faded and a brawny desquamation is evident. After completing the peel, the skin should be well lubricated and instructions given for postoperative care (Fig. 6.6).

The medium-depth peel is dependent on three components for therapeutic effect: (1) degreasing, (2) Jessner's solution, and (3) 35% TCA. The amount of each agent applied creates the intensity and thus the effectiveness of this peel. The general outline of the procedure is detailed in Table 6.7. The variables can be adjusted according to the patient's skin type and the areas of the face being treated. It is thus the workhorse of peeling and resurfacing as it can be individuated for most patients.

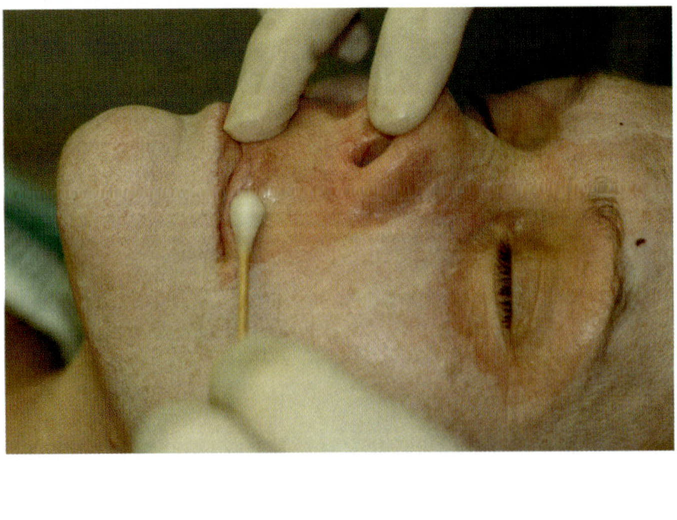

Fig. 6.3. Photograph demonstrating the application of the peel to the perioral region with an assistant stretching and fixating the upper and lower lips

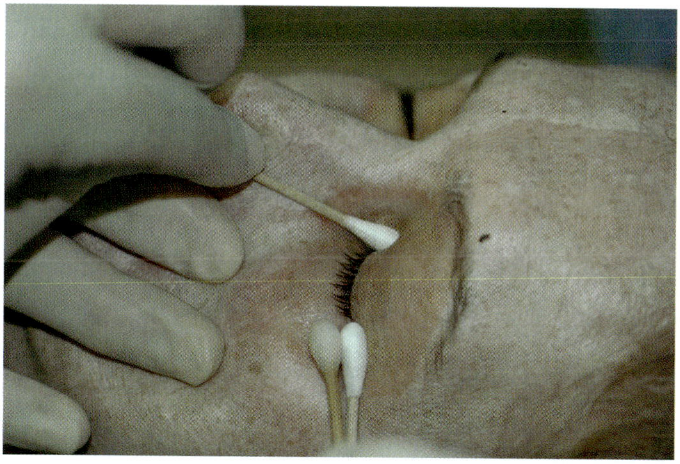

Fig. 6.4. Photograph demonstrating the use of cotton tip applicators to prevent wicking of peel solution into the eye

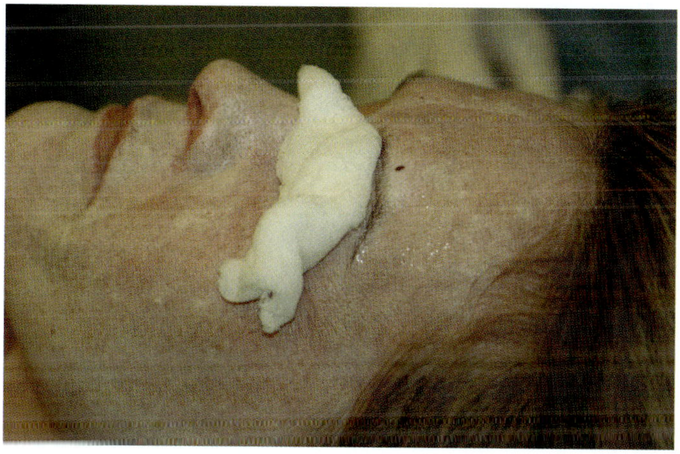

Fig. 6.5. Photograph demonstrating the application of cool saline compresses after completing the chemical peel

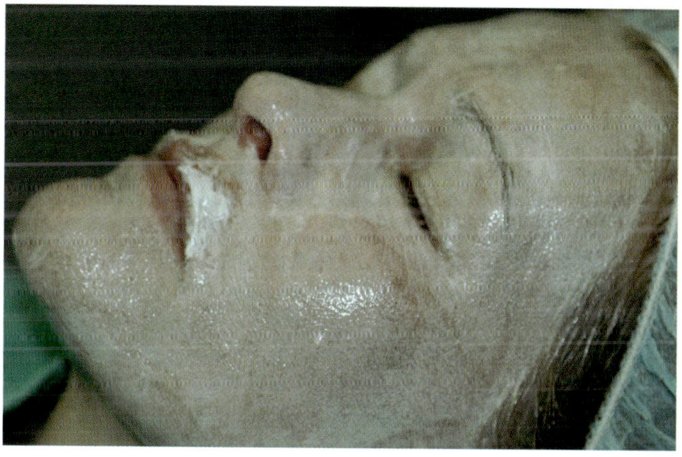

Fig. 6.6. Photograph demonstrating the application of emollients after completing the chemical peel

Table. 6.7. Outline of the Jessner's-35% TCA medium-depth chemical peel procedure

Stage	Procedure
1	The skin should be cleaned thoroughly with Septisol to remove oils
2	Acetone or acetone/alcohol is used to further debride oil and scale from the surface of the skin
3	Jessner's solution is applied
4	TCA (35%) is applied until a light frost appears
5	Cool saline compresses are applied to neutralize the solution
6	The peel will heal with 0.25% acetic acid soaks and a mild emollient cream

Deep Chemical Peeling

The patient undergoing deep chemical peeling must recognize the significant risk factors, the increased morbidity, and possible complications involved in this procedure so that the benefits can be weighed positively against these particular factors. In the hands of those that do this technique regularly, it is a reliable and safe method of rejuvenating advanced to severely photoaged skin including deeper perioral rhytides, periorbital rhytides and crow's feet, forehead lines and wrinkles, as well as the other textural and lesional changes associated with the more severe photoaging process.

There are two modalities for deep chemical peeling, Baker's formula phenol unoccluded, and Baker's formula phenol occluded. Occlusion is accomplished with the application of waterproof zinc oxide tape. The tape is placed directly after the phenol is applied to each individual cosmetic unit. Tape occlusion increases the penetration of the Baker's phenol solution and is particularly helpful for deeply lined "weather-beaten" faces. A taped Baker's formula phenol peel creates the deepest damage in midreticular dermis and this form of chemical peeling should only be performed by the most knowledgeable and experienced cosmetic surgeons who understand the risks of overpenetration and deep damage to the reticular dermis. These complications include hyper- and hypopigmentation, textural changes such as the "alabaster skin," and the potential for scarring.

Table 6.8. The Baker–Gordon formula

88% liquid phenol, USP	3 ml
Tap water	2 ml
Septisol liquid soap	8 drops
Croton oil	3 drops

The Baker-Gordon formula for this peel was first described in 1961, and since then has been used successfully for over 25 years (Table 6.8). The Baker-Gordon formula penetrates further into the dermis than full-strength undiluted phenol because full-strength phenol allegedly causes an immediate coagulation of epidermal keratin proteins and self-blocks further penetration. Dilution to approximately 50–55% in the Baker-Gordon formula causes keratolysis and keratocoagulation, resulting in greater penetration. The liquid soap, hexachlorophene, is a surfactant that reduces skin tension, allowing a more even penetration. Croton oil is a vesicant epidermolytic agent that enhances phenol absorption. The freshly prepared formula is not miscible, and must be stirred in a clear glass medicine cup immediately before application to the patient. Although the mixture can be stored in an amber glass bottle for short periods, this is usually unnecessary and should be reformulated on a regular basis.

Deep chemical peeling is a labor-intensive procedure that must be taken seriously as all major surgical procedures are. The patient requires preoperative sedation with an intravenous line and preoperative intravenous hydration. Usually 1 l of fluid is given preoperatively and a further 1 l is given during the procedure. Phenol is both a cardiotoxin and a hepatotoxin, and is nephrotoxic. For this reason, one must be concerned with the serum concentration of phenol through cutaneous absorption. Methods to limit this include:

1. Intravenous hydration prior to and during the procedure to flush the phenol products through the serum.
2. Extending the time of application for a full-face peel over 1 hour. Cosmetic units are applied for the 15-min wait in between each unit. That is, the forehead, cheeks, chin, lips, and eyelids are each given a 15-min period of time for a total of 1–1.5 h for the procedure.
3. All patients are monitored and if there is any electrocardiography abnormality (i.e. premature ventricular contraction or premature atrial contraction), the procedure is stopped and the patient is watched carefully for other signs of toxicity.
4. Many physicians believe that oxygen given during the procedure can be helpful in preventing arrhythmic complications.
5. Any patient with a history of cardioarrhythmia, hepatic or renal compromise, or on medications that give a propensity for arrhythmias, should not undergo the Baker-Gordon phenol peel.

Before the administration of anesthesia, the patient's face is marked in seated position, noting landmarks such as the mandibular angle, the chin, the preauricular sulcus, the orbital rim, and the forehead. This is done to extend the peel thoroughly throughout the limits of the face and slightly over the mandibular rim to blend any color change. This peel does require sedation. An intravenous combination such as fentanyl citrate (Sublimaze) and midazolam (Versed) can be administered intravenously by an anesthetist while the patient is monitored and given intravenous sedation. It is helpful to use local nerve blocks along the supraorbital nerve, infraorbital nerve, and mental nerve with Marcaine, which should provide some local anesthesia for up to 4 h.

The patients should arrive having taken nothing by mouth, and having shaved and cleansed their face the morning of surgery. The face then is cleansed and degreased with a keratolytic agent such as hexachlorophene with alcohol over the entire face, with emphasis placed on oily areas such as the nose, the hairline, and midfacial cheeks.

Chemical agent is then applied to six individual aesthetic units: forehead, perioral, right and left cheeks, nose, and periorbital areas. Each cosmetic area takes 15 min for application, allowing 60–90 min for the entire procedure. Cotton-tipped applicators are used with a similar technique as discussed for the medium-depth Jessner–35% TCA peel. Less agent is used because frosting becomes evident much quicker. An immediate burning sensation is present for 15–20 s and subsides quickly, but pain returns in 20 min and persists for 6–8 h. The last area for the peel is the periorbital skin, on which the chemical is applied with only damp cotton-tipped applicators. Care must be used to keep the drops away from the eye and keep tears off the skin. Tearing may allow the peel solution to reach the eye by capillary attraction. It is important to remember that water dilution of a chemical may increase the absorption; therefore, if the chemical does get into the eye, these should be flushed with mineral oil rather than water.

Following the full application of peel solution, the frosting becomes evident and the tape can be applied for an occluded peel. Ice packs can be applied at the conclusion of the peel for comfort, and if this is an untaped peel, petrolatum is used. A biosynthetic dressing has been described such as Vigilon or Flexzan for the first 24 h. The patient is usually seen in 24 h to either remove the tape or the biosynthetic dressing and monitor the healing. It is at this time the patient is again reinstructed to methods of compresses and occlusive ointments or dressings. It is important to keep the skin crust-free.

Postoperative Care and Complications

Superficial chemical peels have the simplest postoperative care. Mild cleansers and moisturizers, as well as sunscreens are generally all that is needed to keep patients comfortable and prevent complications.

Medium-depth peels will have edema, erythema, and desquamation postoperatively. With periorbital and even forehead peels, eyelid edema can be severe enough to close the lids. For the first 24 h, the patient is instructed to soak four times a day with a 0.25% acetic acid compress made of 1 tablespoon of white vinegar in 1 pint of warm water. A bland emollient is applied to the desquamating areas after soaks. After 24 h, the patient can shower and clean gently with a mild nondetergent cleanser. The erythema intensifies as desquamation becomes complete within 4–5 days. Healing is completed within 7–10 days. At the end of 1 week, the bright red color has faded to pink and has the appearance of sunburn. This can be covered by cosmetics and will fade fully within 2–3 weeks.

The four stages of wound healing are apparent after a deep chemical peel. They include: (1) inflammation, (2) coagulation, (3) reepithelialization, and (4) fibroplasia. At the conclusion of the chemical peel, the inflammatory phase has already begun with a brawny, dusky erythema that will progress over the first 12 h. This is an accentuation of pigmented lesions on the skin as the coagulation phase separates the epidermis producing serum exudation, crusting, and pyoderma. It is during this phase that it is important to use debridant soaks and compresses as well as occlusive salves. These will remove the sloughed, necrotic epidermis and prevent the serum exudate from hardening as crust and scab. The 25% acetic acid soaks found in the vinegar/water preparation are antibacterial, especially against pseudomonas and Gram-negative bacteria. In addition, the mildly acidic nature of the solution is physiologic for the healing granulation tissue, and mildly debridant, as it will dissolve and cleanse the necrotic material and serum. Bland emollients and salves such as petrolatum, or Eucerin or Aquaphor (Beiersdorf, Wilton, CT, USA), are preferred as the skin can be monitored carefully day by day for potential complications.

Reepithelialization begins on day 3 and continues until days 10–14. Occlusive salves promote faster reepithelialization and fewer tendencies for delayed healing. The final stages of fibroplasia continue well beyond the initial closure of the peeled wound and continue with neoangiogenesis and new collagen formation for 3 or 4 months. Prolonged erythema may last 2–4 months in unusual cases of sensitive skin or with contact dermatitis. New collagen formation can continue to improve texture and rhytides for a period up to 4 months during this last phase of fibroplasia.

Many of the complications seen in peeling can be recognized early during healing stages. The cosmetic surgeon should be well acquainted with the normal appearance of a healing wound and its time frame for both medium and deep peeling. Prolongation of the granulation tissue phase beyond 7–10 days may indicate delayed wound healing. This could be the result of viral, bacterial, or fungal infections, contact dermatitis interfering with wound healing, or other systemic factors. This red flag should alert the physician to careful investigation, and prompt treatment should be instituted to forestall potential irreparable damage that may result in scarring.

Complications can be caused either intraoperatively or postoperatively. The two inherent errors that lead to intraoperative complications are (1) incorrect peel pharmacology and (2) accidental solution misplacement. It is the physician's responsibility to know the solution and its concentration is correct. TCA concentrations should be measured weight by volume, as this is the standard for measuring depth of peel. Glycolic acid and lactic acid solutions as well as Jessner's solution must be checked for expiration date as the potency decreases with time. Alcohol or water absorption may inappropriately increase the potency, so one must assure the shelf life is appropriate. The peel solution should be applied with cotton-tipped applicators, and in medium and deep peels, it is best to pour the peel solution into a secondary container rather than apply the solution spun around the neck of the bottle. Intact crystals may give the solution a higher concentration as it is taken directly from its container. One should be careful to apply the solution to its appropriate location and not to pass the wet cotton-tipped applicator directly over the central face where a drop may inadvertently reach sensitive areas such as the eyes. Saline and bicarbonate of soda should be available to dilute TCA or neutralize glycolic acid if they are placed inappropriately. Likewise, mineral oil should be present for Baker's phenol peels. Postoperative complications most commonly result from local infection or contact dermatitis. The best deterrent for local infection is the continuous use of soaks to debride crusting and necrotic material. Streptococcal or staphylococcal infection can occur under biosynthetic membranes or thick occlusive ointments. The use of 0.25% acetic acid soaks seems to deter this, as well as the judicious removal of the ointment with each soak. *Staphylococcus*, *Escherichia coli*, or even *pseudomonas* infection may result from improper care during healing and should be treated promptly with the appropriate oral antibiotic.

Frequent postoperative visits are necessary to recognize the early onset of a bacterial infection. It may present itself as delayed wound healing, ulcerations, build up of necrotic material with excessive scabbing, crusting, purulent drainage, and odor. Early recognition will peel the skin and prevent the spread of infection and scarring. Additionally, if the patient was not placed on antiviral therapy before the procedure, the physician must be keenly aware of the early signs of herpetic infection and appropriate therapy begun immediately and continued until resolution of infection and reepithelialization is complete.

Delayed wound healing and persistent erythema are signs that the peel is not healing normally. The cosmetic surgeon must know the normal timetable for each of the healing events to occur so that he or she may recognize at what time healing is delayed or the erythema is not fading adequately. Delayed wound healing may respond to physician debridement and appropriate antibiotics if an infection is present, corticosteroids if due to contact allergic or contact irritant dermatitis along with the change of the offending contact agent, or protection with a biosynthetic membrane such as Flexzan or Vigilon. When this diagnosis is made, these patients must be followed daily with dressing changes and a close watch on the healing skin.

Persistent erythema is a syndrome whereby the skin remains erythematous beyond what is normal for the individual peel. A superficial peel loses its erythema in 15–30 days, a medium-depth peel within 60 days, and a deep chemical peel within 90 days. Erythema and/or pruritus beyond this period of time are considered abnormal and fit this syndrome. It may be contact dermatitis, contact sensitization, exacerbation of prior skin disease, or a genetic susceptibility to erythema, but may also indicate a sign of potential scarring. Erythema is the result of the angiogenic factors stimulating vasodilation, which also includes the phase of fibroplasia, which is being stimulated for a prolonged period of time. For this reason, it can be accompanied by skin thickening and scarring. It should be treated promptly and appropriately with topical steroids, systemic steroids, intralesional steroids if thickening is occurring, and skin protection that would eliminate the factors of irritancy and allergy. If thickening or scarring becomes evident, other measures that may be helpful include the daily use of silicone sheeting and the pulsed dye laser to treat the vascular factors. With prompt intervention, scarring can be averted in many cases.

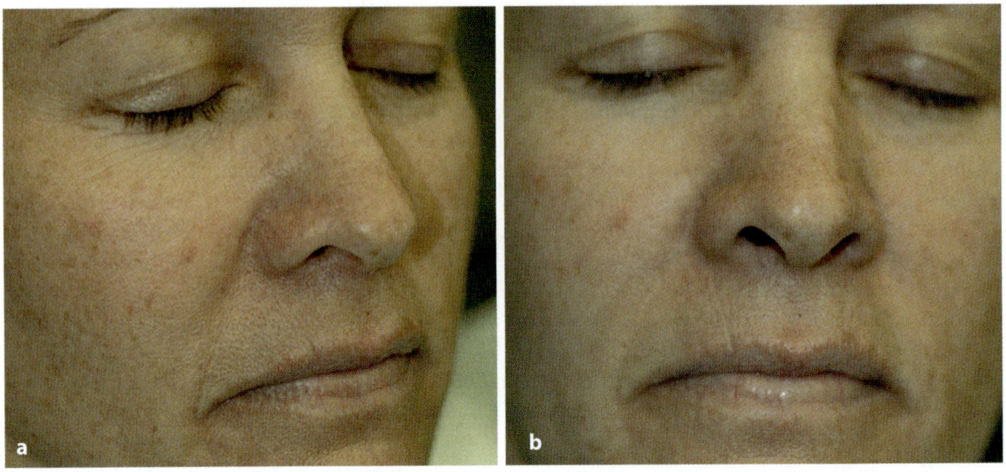

Fig. 6.7. **a** Preoperative photograph, right frontal view. **b** Preoperative photograph, frontal view

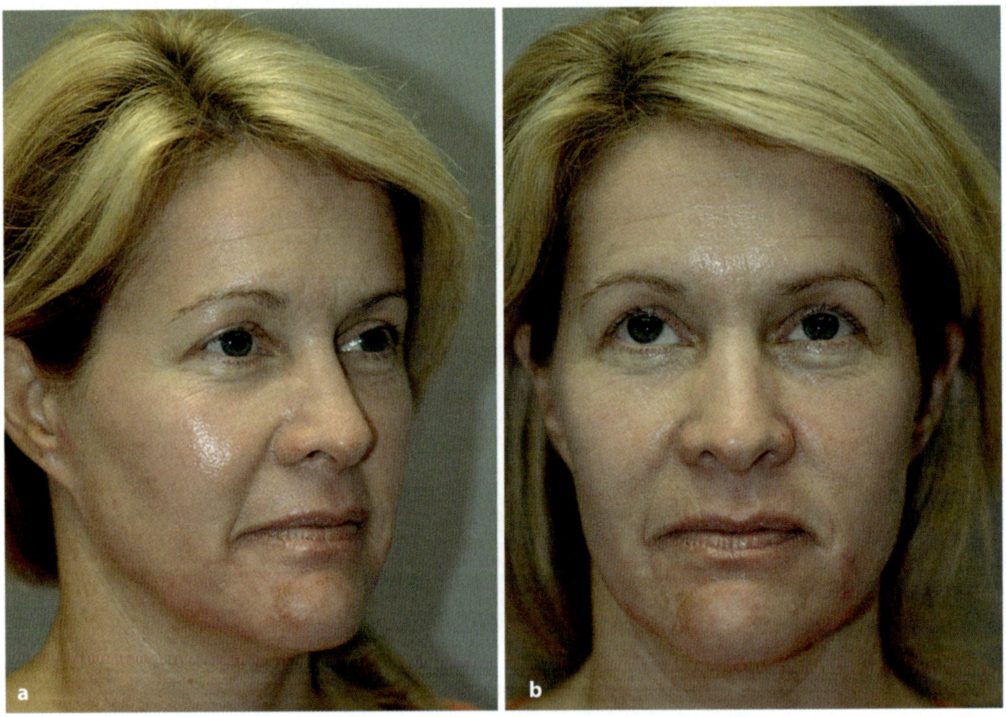

Fig. 6.8. **a** Postoperative photograph, right frontal view, 7 days after application of Jessner's solution-35% TCA medium-depth chemical peel. **b** Postoperative photograph, frontal view, 7 days after application of Jessner's solution-35% TCA medium-depth chemical peel

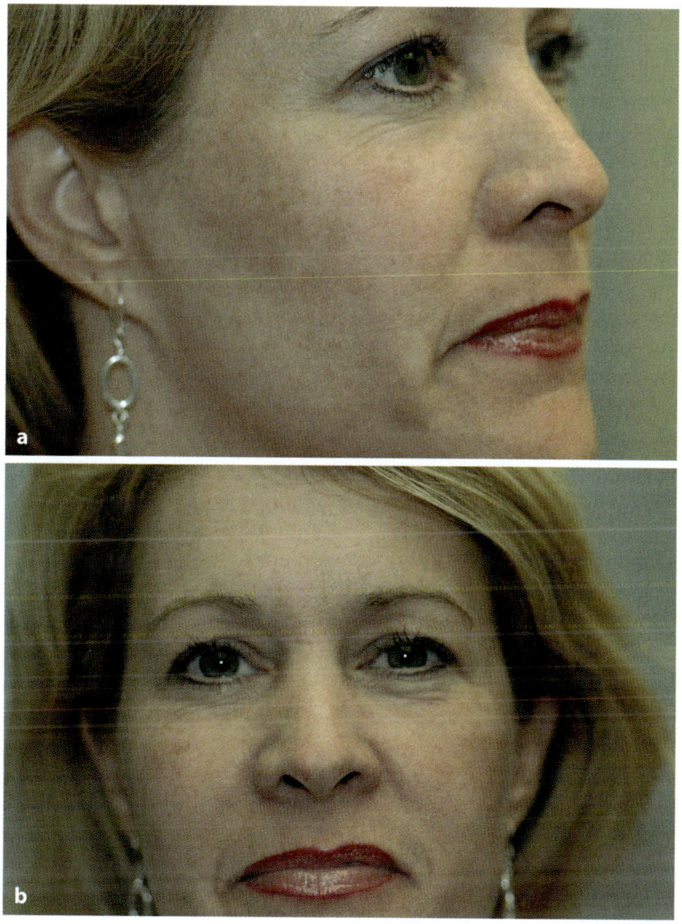

Fig. 6.9. **a** Postoperative photograph, right frontal view, 14 days after application of Jessner's solution-35% TCA medium-depth chemical peel. **b** Postoperative photograph, frontal view, 14 days after application of Jessner's solution-35% TCA medium-depth chemical peel

Results and Photographs

Figures 6.7–6.9 demonstrate the typical results of the Jessner's solution–35% TCA peel preoperatively (Fig. 6.7), 1 week postoperatively (Fig. 6.8), and 2 weeks postoperatively (Fig. 6.9). Of note, this patient also underwent dermasanding of her upper cutaneous lip for deep rhytides. At week 1, the epidermis has exfoliated and new epidermis is present (Fig. 6.8). At week 2, the patient has healed completely and is very satisfied with results (Fig. 6.9). The patient had notable improvement of pigmentary dyschromias and her moderately photoaged skin.

The Future

Chemical peels have been a mainstay in the treatment of photoaging. Knowledge of the the mechanisms and chemicals used in chemical resurfacing allows the physician the ability to adapt the most appropriate treatment for each patient. The physician has the responsibility of choosing the correct modality to treat skin conditions such as photoaging skin, scars, dyschromias, and the removal of skin growths. There are many agents available including the three levels of chemical peels reviewed herein. It is the responsibility of the physician to have thorough knowledge of all of these tools to give each patient the most appropriate treatment for their condition.

References

1. Stegman SJ (1982) A comparative histologic study of the effects of three peeling agents and dermabrasion on normal and sun-damaged skin. Aesthetic Plast Surg 6:123–125
2. Brody HJ, Monheit GD, Resnick SS, Alt TH (2000) A History of chemical peeling. Dermatol Surg 26:405–409
3. Mackee GM, Karp FL (1952) The treatment of post-acne scars with phenol. Br J Dermatol 64:456–459
4. Brody HJ (1989) Variations and comparisons in medium depth chemical peeling. J Dermatol Surg Oncol; 15:953–963
5. Stagnone JJ (1977) Chemabrasion, a combined technique of chemical peeling and dermabrasion. J Dermatol Surg Oncol 3:217–219
6. Monheit GD (1989) The Jessner's + TCA peel: a medium depth chemical peel. J Dermatol Surg Oncol 15:945–950
7. Coleman WP III, Futrell JM (1994) The glycolic acid trichloroacetic acid peel. J Dermatol Surg Oncol 20:76–80
8. Baker TJ, Gordon HL (eds) (1986) Chemical Face Peeling. Surgical Rejuvenation of the Face. Mosby, St. Louis
9. Glogau RG (1994) Chemical peeling and aging skin. J Geriatr Dermatol 2:30–35
10. Fitzpatrick TB (1988) The validity and practicality of sun-reactive skin types I through VI. Archiv Dermatol 124:869–871
11. Monheit GD (1995) Chemical peeling for pigmentary dyschromias. Cosmetic Dermatol 8:10–15
12. Glogau RG (1994) Chemical peeling and aging skin. J Geriatr Dermatol 2:30–35
13. Monheit GD (1999) Chemical Peeling. Presented at the American Academy of Dermatology Annual Meeting, 25 March, New Orleans, LA
14. Wolfe SA (1982) Chemical face peeling following therapeutic irradiation. Plastic Reconstr Surg 69:859–862
15. Monheit GD (1995) Facial resurfacing may trigger the herpes simplex virus. Cosmet Dermatol 88:9–16
16. Swinehart JM (1990)Test spots in dermabrasion and chemical peeling. J Dermatol Surg Oncol 16:557–563
17. Monheit GD (1996) Skin preparation: an essential step before chemical peeling or laser resurfacing. Cosmet Dermatol 9:13–14
18. Kligman DE, Sadiq I, Pagnoni A, Stoudemayer T, Kligman AM (1998) High-strength tretinoin: a method for rapid retinization of facial skin. J Am Acad Dermatol 39:S93–97
19. Kang S, Bergfeld W, Gottlieb AB, Hickman J, Humeniuk J, Kempers S, Lebwohl M, Lowe N, McMichael A, Milbauer J, Phillips T, Powers J, Rodriguez D, Savin R, Shavin J, Sherer D, Silvis N, Weinstein R, Weiss J, Hammerberg C, Fisher GJ, Nighland M, Grossman R, Nyirady J (2005) Long-term efficacy and safety of tretinoin emollient cream 0.05% in the treatment of photodamaged facial skin: a two-year, randomized, placebo-controlled trial. Am J Clin Dermatol 6:245–653
20. Mandy SH (1986) Tretinoin in the preoperative and postoperative management of dermabrasion. J Am Acad Dermatol 15:879–879
21. Hevia O, Nemeth AJ, Taylor JR (1991) Tretinoin accelerates healing after trichloroacetic acid chemical peel. Arch Dermatol 127:678–682
22. Humphreys TR, Werth V, Dzubow L, Kligman A (1996) Treatment of photodamaged skin with trichloroacetic acid and topical tretinoin. J Am Acad Dermatol 34:638–644

Chapter 7

Mesotherapy and Injectable Lipolysis

7

Adam M. Rotunda

Core Messages

- Mesotherapy describes a diverse array of cutaneous injection techniques that utilizes medications and other compounds proposed to have a therapeutic effect on local medical or cosmetic conditions.
- Injectable lipolysis refers to a treatment using biologically active detergents to cause focal ablation of adipose tissue.
- The active ingredient used in injectable lipolysis is deoxycholate.
- Injectable lipolysis may become a relatively safe and efficacious method to treat submental and mandibular fat and jowls.
- Mesotherapy may have as yet unproved potential to enhance the appearance of facial skin.

History

Mesotherapy

Despite its popularity, "mesotherapy" remains an enigma to both physicians and patients due to confusion in terminology and history, inadequate peer review, and nonstandardization of ingredients and treatment protocols [1]. Despite these limitations, there appears to be a growing interest in mesotherapy [1–3] driven by its potential application to a number of cosmetic and medical conditions (Table 7.1).

Table 7.1. Some of the more common medical and cosmetic conditions purported to benefit from traditional mesotherapy

Cosmetic	Medical
Cellulite	Acne
Hypertrophic or keloid scars	Allergies
Melasma	Arthritis
Photoaging	Asthma
Rhytides	Cancer pain
Striae distensae (stretch marks)	Carpal tunnel syndrome
Telangiectasias	Eczema
Vitiligo	Gout
	Headache
	Hearing loss
	Hepatitis
	Herpetic neuralgia
	Lower back pain
	Lymphedema
	Oral pain (dental work)
	Osteophytes ("bone spurs")
	Peripheral vascular disease
	Reflex sympathetic dystrophy
	Pruritus
	Psoriasis
	Sports injuries (i.e., sprains, strains, tears, bursitis, tendonitis, plantar fasciitis, calcium deposits)
	Temporal-mandibular pain syndrome
	Tinnitis
	Vertigo
	Vitiligo

A relatively new treatment that uses deoxycholate (DC), a natural detergent, along with phosphatidylcholine (PC), a natural phospholipid, has been mislabeled as mesotherapy. This treatment has been more rigorously investigated than traditional mesotherapy and may have significant potential to treat localized collections of adipose tissue.

Although the colloquial definition of mesotherapy (seen commonly in local advertisements and made popular by the popular media) describes a method to reduce cellulite, treat fat, or "refresh" the aging face, the original use of traditional mesotherapy, as described in 1952 by French physician, Michel Pistor, was for medical, rather than cosmetic, conditions [1,4]. As mesotherapy was increasingly accepted in Europe, its applications were broadened by European research and clinical experience in the decades that followed. Eventually, mesotherapy was recognized by the French Academy of Medicine in 1987 as a distinct medical specialty. In time, the technique evolved to address several dermatologic and cosmetic conditions, such as cellulite, alopecia, acne scarring, and "facial rejuvenation" [1].

Dr. Pistor theorized that injections of numerous medications and other compounds into various levels of the skin could maximize their therapeutic effects locally, while significantly reducing adverse effects systemically. This theory apparently translated well clinically for pain relief in dental care, musculoskeletal disease, and cancer, where local injections of anesthetics, anti-inflammatory medications, and vasodilators became standard regimens [5]. Less apparent was whether numerous other pharmacologically active substances (i.e., tretinoin, hyaluronic acid, antioxidants) injected in a similar manner would yield a clinically significant cosmetic improvement.

Mesotherapy employs several novel injection techniques in an attempt to deposit medication mixtures at the exact anatomical site of the target problem (Table 7.2). It can be reasoned that intralesional triamcinolone, used for decades by United States dermatologists for numerous inflammatory conditions, and the most popular cosmetic injectable treatments (botulinum toxin, soft-tissue fillers) are akin to mesotherapy.

Mesotherapy was introduced prominently into the United States popular media after being headlined by singer Roberta Flack, who cited mesotherapy (and a calorie-restricted diet) as being significantly responsible for her dramatic weight loss. Traditional European, "body-contouring" mesotherapy incorporates agents purported to stimulate lipolysis and treat cellulite [1,6]. The media attention created a transient stir by glamorizing this novel "fat-melting method," but the medical community remained skeptical. In policy statements, both the American Society for Dermatologic Surgery and the American Society of Plastic Surgeons chose not to endorse meso-

Table 7.2. Traditional mesotherapy injection techniques

Technique	Depth	Needle (mm)	Condition
Intraepidermic Rapid and superficial (Tremor)	Epidermis	1–4	Facial rejuvenation
Superficial intradermic, similar to a PPD wheal (multipricking)	Dermis	4, 6	Cellulite
Deep intradermic (point-per-point)	Dermis	4	Arthritis, tendonitis
Intrahypodermic	Subcutaneous	13	Lower back pain (musculoskeletal)

therapy until controlled research into its safety and efficacy were performed [3,7].

To date, there are no published reports demonstrating that common "traditional mesotherapy" ingredients have any clinical effects on cellulite or fat [6]. However, two recent peer-reviewed reports have focused on melasma and facial rejuvenation [8,9].

A study from Korea describes the effect of traditional mesotherapy on melasma in a prospective, open-label clinical series [8]. The investigators treated the cheeks of 89 women with superficial injections of 0.05 ml tranexamic acid (0.4%), a plasminogen inhibitor that acts downstream to inhibit tyrosinase, a key enzyme in melanogenesis. After 12, weekly treatments, the investigator noted a significant improvement in the Melasma Area and Severity Score at weeks 8 and 12, but only 9.4% and 76% of patients graded their improvement as "good" and "fair," respectively. Although promising, without blinding and long term follow-up, no conclusions can be drawn at this time. It is conceivable that superficial injections of other conventional topical bleaching agents used in the United States, such as hydroquinone, kojic acid, and retinoic acid, may have therapeutic utility alone or in combination for melasma.

Goldberg's group recently reported their experiences with traditional mesotherapy techniques to increase facial elasticity, and to reduce erythema, fine lines, and dyspigmentation [9]. The authors treated the faces of ten patients with superficial injections of a locally compounded multivitamin solution mixed with nonconjugated hyaluronic acid (in contrast to the popular crosslinked, conjugated, hyaluronic acid dermal fillers). Approximately 0.01 ml of the solution was injected with a 1.15-mm adjustable hub needle (Fig. 7.1) at 1-cm intervals on the full face, resulting in over 200 injections each session. Patients were treated four times at monthly intervals and were followed up at 2 months for a final evaluation.

Treatment was evaluated clinically and histologically. The authors performed a temporal sequence method that allowed a blinded

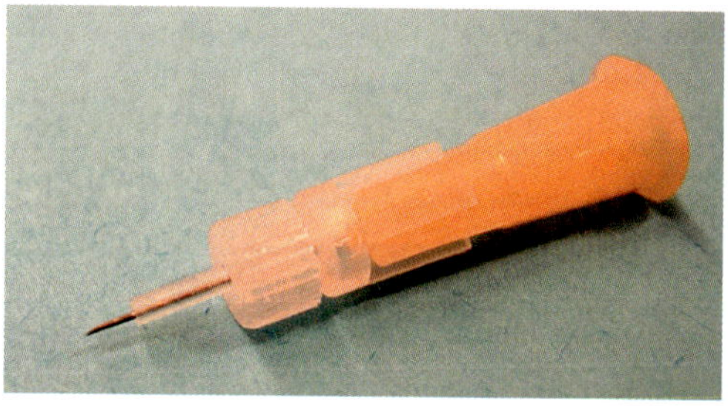

Fig. 7.1. Adjustable hub mesotherapy needle (photograph courtesy of David J. Goldberg, MD)

physician to note any difference between before and after photographs. Individual parameters of facial rejuvenation pre- and post-treatment were also compared. There were no significant differences noted by the evaluating physicians or patients (Fig. 7.2). Histologic examination by a blinded dermatolopathologist using conventional hematoxylin and eosin stain also revealed no significant changes 6 months after beginning the treatment. Collagen fiber diameter decreased in size from 59 to 48 nm on electron microscopy, suggesting the presence of new collagen.

The authors theorized that the superficial mechanical injury from numerous micropunctures, rather than the ingredients themselves, created a "repair zone" of new collagen. Side effects were transient and included pinpoint bleeding and erythema (Fig. 7.3). Two patients experienced upper lip urticaria. Although four out of ten patients self-reported a short (1-week) period of improved skin tone and smoothness (likely due to transient edema), there were no tong-term tactile benefits. The authors conclude that nonspecific inflammation as a consequence of the injection trauma, rather than the ingredients, was respon sible for neocollagenesis. It is anticipated that additional studies, using other agents, may lead to greater degree of improvement.

Rigorous investigation in the future will determine whether "traditional mesothera py" is accepted into mainstream medicine simply becomes an unsubstantiated fad. The rest of this chapter will focus on injectable lipolysis for the utility of facial contouring.

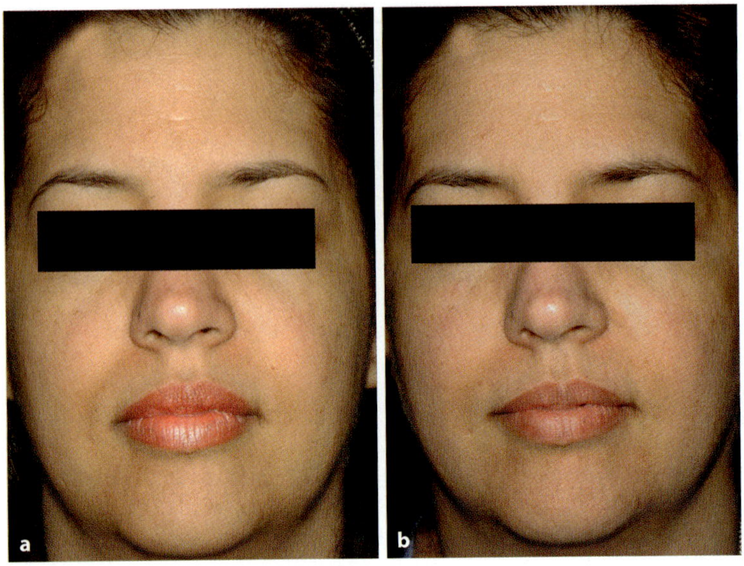

Fig. 7.2 a, b. Patient before (*left image*) and 2 months after (*right image*) four, monthly facial mesotherapy treatments. No significant changes were noted by the patient or the evaluating physician (photographs courtesy of David J. Goldberg, MD)

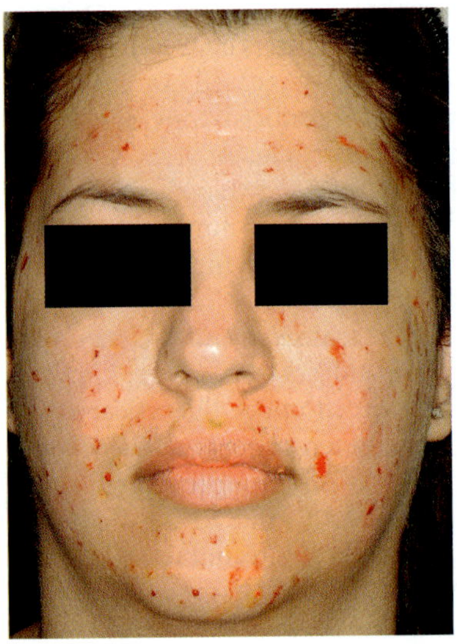

Fig. 7.3. Pinpoint bleeding immediately after superficial mesotherapy injections (photograph courtesy of David J. Goldberg, MD)

Injectable Lipolysis

In distinction to "traditional mesotherapy," a new treatment using PC for localized fat reduction has emerged after Sergio Maggiore presented his experience using PC for xanthelasma in 1988 [10]. PC is a lecithin (soy)-derived phospholipid comprising approximately 40% of the mammalian cell membrane mass forming the lipid bilayers that separate the insides of cells from their environment [11]. PC is insoluble in water, and thus aqueous (intravenously, injectable) PC solutions require a detergent (traditionally DC) to solubilize them. Russian investigations noted that intravenous injections of PC/DC combinations were useful for fat embolism [12]. Lipostabil was introduced by Natterman International GMBH in Europe as a solution consisting of primarily PC (5%) and DC (2.5%), with relatively small amounts of vitamin E, sodium hydroxide, and ethanol, in sterile water. The PC formulation is currently legally available in several European countries as Lipostabil N (Sanofi-Aventis) and is approved for intravenous administration for dyslipidemia, fat emboli, and as an anticirrhotic because of its lip-

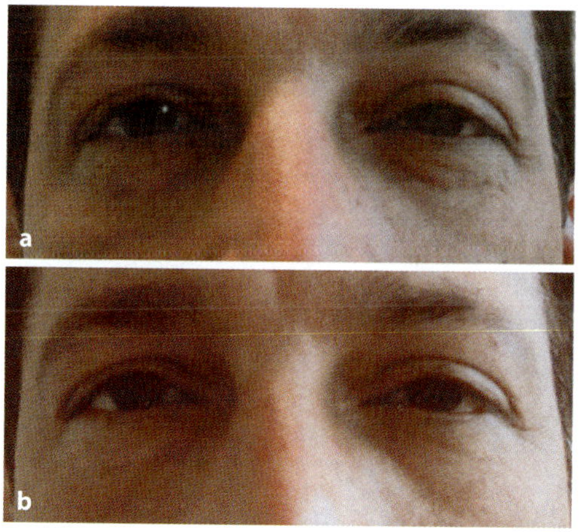

Fig. 7.4 a, b. Patient before (*top*) and after (*bottom*) five infraorbital phosphatidylcholine injections

id-reducing, antifibrotic, and antioxidant effects [12–14].

Maggiore used the PC formulation off-label to treat localized fat deposits with the assumption that its antilipid effects in serum could similarly act subcutaneously. This theory held fast for many years (and is still maintained by some) until recent laboratory investigations isolated the medication's individual components [15]. Numerous published reports describe the use of Lipostabil and compounded PC/DC combinations (Lipostabil is unapproved in the USA) to "dissolve" fat in sites traditionally treated with liposuction [16–20]. Although not as dramatic as liposuction, the results from these preliminary studies suggest that these relatively easily performed injections may be effective at reducing small collections of fat.

Patricia Rittes, MD, a dermatologist in Sao Paolo, Brazil, was the first to publish her experiences using Lipostabil for infraorbital fat herniation [16]. According to the report, "all" of the 30 treated patients had some degree of improvement (extent unspecified). Most patients had one or two treatments, although a couple of patients had up to four treatments. An unblinded physician in a similar study [21] noted significant improvement in seven of ten patients (Fig. 7.4). Half of the treated patients reported persistence of results an average of 9 months after the last treatment. These reports were additionally corroborated by a recent open-label series from Ireland [22]. In this study, 21 patients were similarly treated with bilateral injections of 0.4 ml of Lipostabil subcutaneously into the infraorbital fat pads. Treatments were every 6 weeks. Seventy-six percent of patients had significant improvement (evaluated by patients at each follow-up visit and by physicians after treatment using digital photography). Interestingly, seven patients (one-third) thought their improvement was significant (>75%) after just one treatment, although five patients had "no response" after two treatments and subsequently discontinued. Aside from the anticipated marked swelling and erythema for 3–5 days, findings consistent with the previous reports, there were no adverse events at a 6-month follow-up.

Several authorities in the cosmetic arena have expressed concern about infraorbital PC treatments due to potentially significant post-treatment swelling, unknown long-term effects, and unregulated status [23,24]. Despite an alarming animal study performed in Brazil [24], which describes liver failure in pigs treated with a PC-based formulation, there have thus far been no reports of liver damage in humans, and it is possible that extrapolating these animal studies to humans is misguided [1]. Numerous reports describe the use of PC/DC formulations for lipomas, "buffalo" humps, jowls, submental, truncal, and extremity fat in humans with no significant systemic or organ-specific toxicity (Fig. 7.5) [16–21,25]. Numerous weekend-long courses have become popular for physicians seeking hands on demonstration of the published injection techniques. While instructive, these case series and unblinded nonrandomized, retrospective, and prospective studies need to be corroborated by large, randomized, double-blind studies.

A positive corollary of these reports are formal laboratory investigations that have isolated the active PC ingredient and provided a

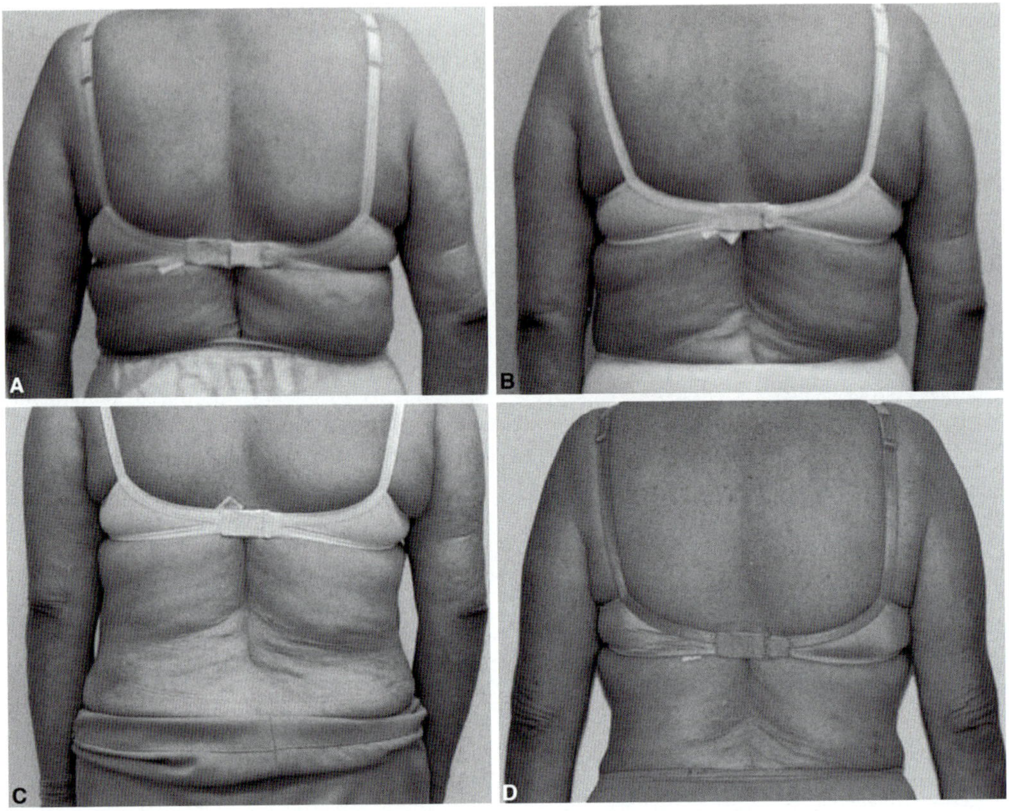

Fig. 7.5 A–D. A 57-year-old woman with local fat deposit because of cortisone use before procedure. B After two applications of phosphatidylcholine (PC; 30 days). C After four applications of phosphatidylcholine (60 days). D After eight applications of phosphatidylcholine (120 days). This figure was obtained with the permission of Springer-Verlag New York from Rittes (2003) [17]

plausible scientific mechanism to account for the medication's fat ablative effects [15]. PC, once assumed to be responsible for "fat dissolving," may prove to be at most an inactive bystander. The published basic science investigations reveal that DC in isolation, rather than PC, acts to lyse cell membranes (Fig. 7.6).

Deoxycholic acid (Fig. 7.7) has been used for decades as a basic laboratory detergent to isolate cell membrane components [26] and as a biocompatible solubilizing agent in several injectable formulations of amphotericin B, including Amphocin (Amphocin Prescribing Information, Pfizer) as well as Lipostabil [27]. DC is a secondary bile salt produced via the degradation of primary cholic bile salts by intestinal bacteria upon their release by the gall bladder into the intestinal tract [28]. Up to 90% of DC is reabsorbed into the intestinal wall, and thereafter recirculated back to the liver via the portal vein, and once again excreted after food consumption by the gall bladder back to the intestinal tract. Unabsorbed DC is excreted. Although it is speculated that exogenous DC administered in the form of subcutaneous injections would be compensated by natural feedback loops and is likely not a significant physiologic burden in the recommended doses, this is currently being evaluated in animal models [28].

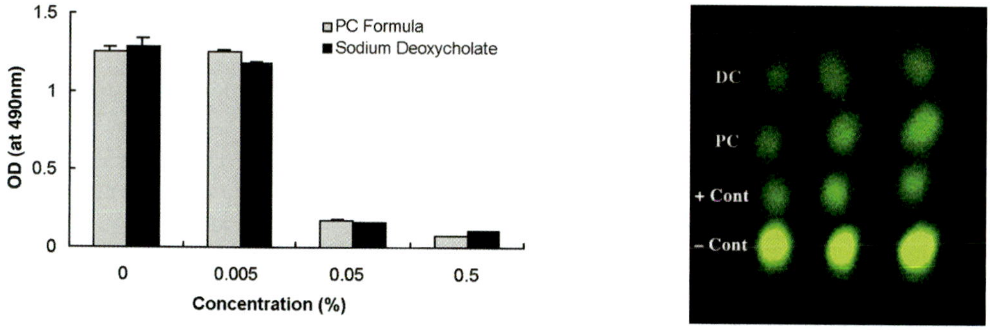

Fig. 7.6. A MTS assay measuring the viability of keratinocytes exposed to the PC formula (*gray*) and sodium deoxycholate (*black*). Absorbance (optical density, *OD*) is directly related to cell viability. Increasing the concentration of both compounds produces more cell death. B Calcein fluorescence in fat specimens (triplicates) treated with sodium deoxycholate (*DC*, 50 mg/ml); PC formula (50 mg/ml phosphatidylcholine and 47.5 mg/ml sodium deoxycholate); Triton detergent (positive control, *+Cont*); and phosphate buffered saline (negative control, *–Cont*). Loss of yellow-green fluorescence indicates cell lysis. These figures were obtained with the permission of Blackwell Publishing from Rotunda and Kolodney (2006) [1]

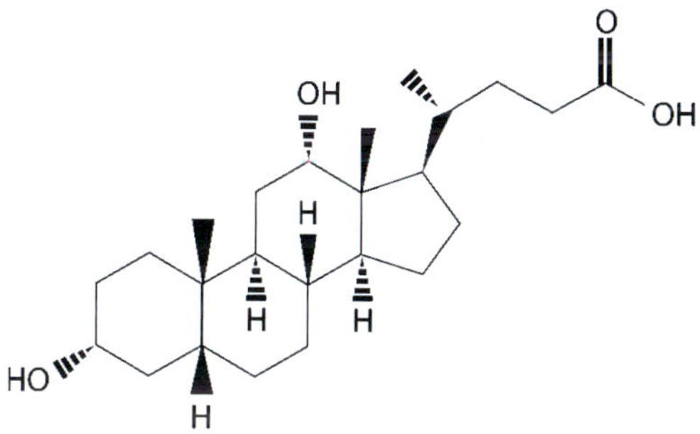

Fig. 7.7. Chemical structure of deoxycholic acid

Porcine, as well as human tissue, exposed to DC [1,15,29], as well as PC/DC combinations [15,18,29], reveals cell lysis, acute inflammation, and necrosis (Fig. 7.8). Despite these caustic effects, there are no reports suggesting long-term sequelae like focal contrac-

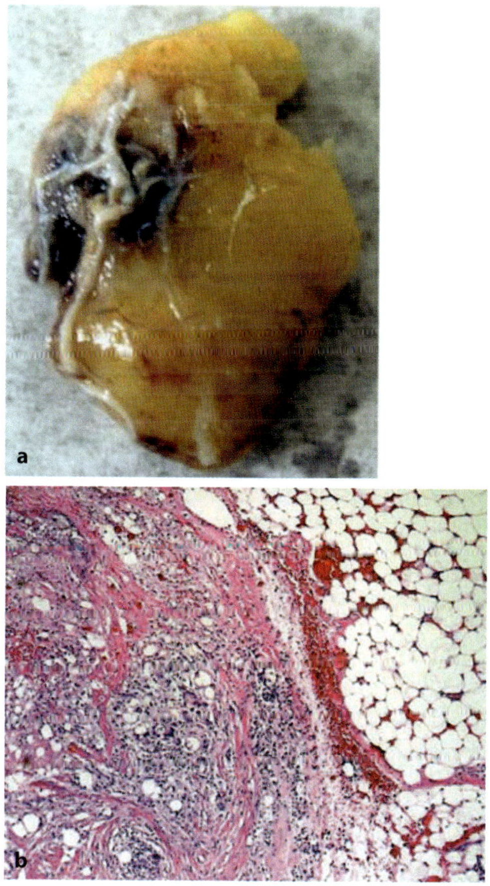

Fig. 7.8 a, b. a Excised lipoma 2 days after injection with sodium deoxycholate (10 mg/ml), revealing a well-demarcated area of necrosis. **b** Microscopic findings demonstrating acute inflammation and necrosis (hematoxylin and eosin stain, original magnification ×10). These figures were obtained with the permission of Blackwell Publishing from Rotunda and Kolodney (2006) [1]

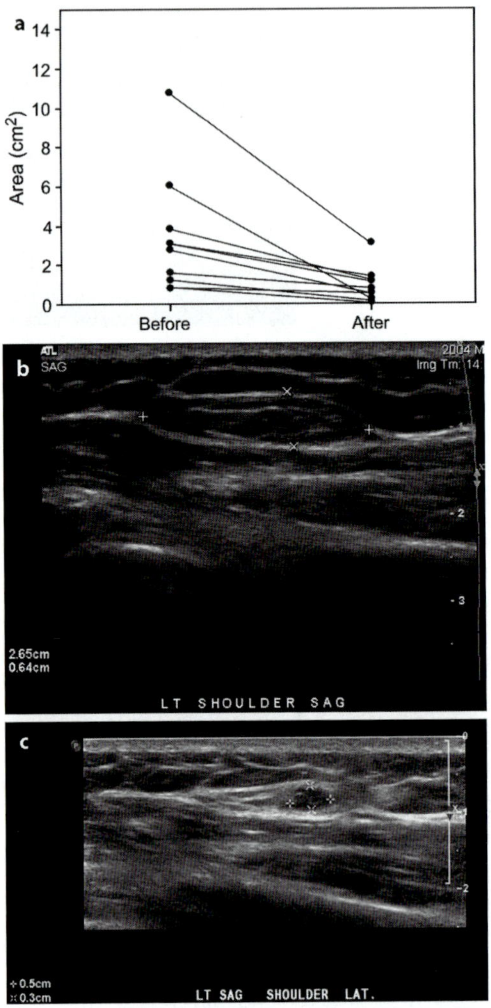

Fig. 7.9 a–c. **a** Area (cm^2) of 12 lipomas before and after an average of 2 subcutaneous deoxycholate injections. **b** Ultrasound of lipoma located on the shoulder, measuring 2.6–0.6 cm before treatment. **c** Same lipoma measuring 0.5×0.3 cm 4 months after the second and final injection. This Fig. 7.was obtained with the permission of Elsevier from Rotunda et al. (2005) [29]

ture, hardening, and skin dimpling or irregularity. Subcutaneous injections of DC alone into lipomas [29,30] and facial HIV lipoaccumulation has been proven effective without PC (Figs. 7.9 and 7.10), confirming the laboratory findings and suggesting that PC may not be necessary.

Available Technology

Mesotherapy

A wide number of medications and other ingredients (herbs, vitamins, minerals, enzymes) are available from compounding pharmacies for use in mesotherapy [1]. Only a limited number of these compounds are approved by the United States Food and Drug Administration (FDA) approved for intradermal use (i.e., hyaluronidase, collagenase). Even for those approved for use by another route of administration (i.e., intravenous or oral), the pharmacokinetics (absorption, distribution, and metabolism) after subcutaneous injection, are generally unknown. Most compounding pharmacies do not have the accreditation required by the FDA, or other international agencies, for large-scale production of pharmaceutical grade medications. While these pharmacies may be accountable for high sterility and purity standards, intralot variation and interpharmacy variations clearly exist [31]. Nevertheless, only United States physicians writing bona fide prescriptions for individual patients can legally have compounding pharmacies make non-FDA-approved medications [32].

Mesotherapy injections are made by syringe or mechanical-, electronic-, or pneumatic- powered hand-held injection guns (Fig. 7.8). Such guns standardize aliquots and relieves finger strain for some clinicians. The choice of syringe chosen may be 3, 5, or 10 ml in size (depending on the surface area injected), keeping in mind that the larger the syringe, the more difficult the force required per injection. Needles for facial treatments are typically 1–4 mm (Fig. 7.11).

Injectable Lipolysis

As of 2007, there are no approved, pharmaceutical-grade medications available in the United States for injectable lipolysis. Physi-

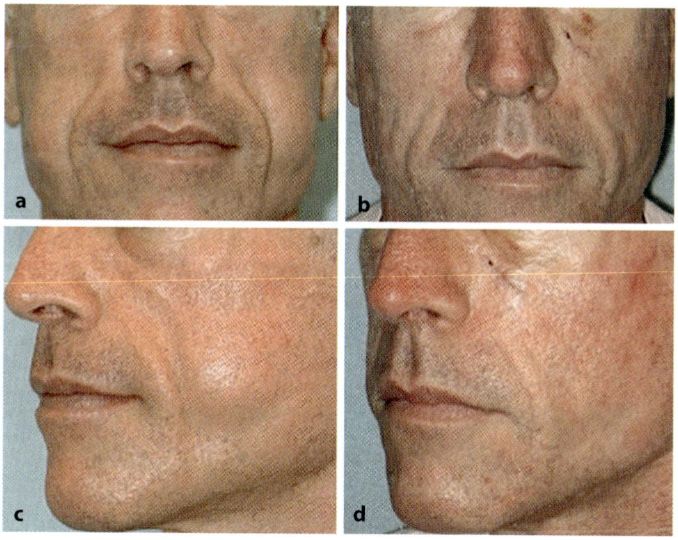

Fig. 7.10 a–d. HIV patient with localized, magnetic-resonance-imaging-confirmed fatty tumors on bilateral cheeks before (a, c) and after (b, d) three, monthly subcutaneous injections with 1% deoxycholate. Lesions decreased in size from approximately 4 cm to less than 2 cm in diameter (photographs courtesy of Derek Jones, MD)

cians obtain these ingredients at compounding pharmacies. As some clinicians prefer PC along with the DC, available concentrations of PC are 5% (50 mg/ml) or 10% (100 mg/ml) mixed with typically 4.2–4.75% DC. Higher-concentration (10%) PC solutions are usually diluted with sterile saline 1:1 as a more cost-effective means of obtaining the medication. It should be noted that PC has never been demonstrated to have lipolytic or detergent activity when isolated from DC; furthermore, there is no evidence suggesting that a specific concentration of PC is more effective than another. Rather, an increasing number of clinicians use DC alone (typically 1%, 10 mg/ml). This is subsequently mixed with lidocaine before injection (see below).

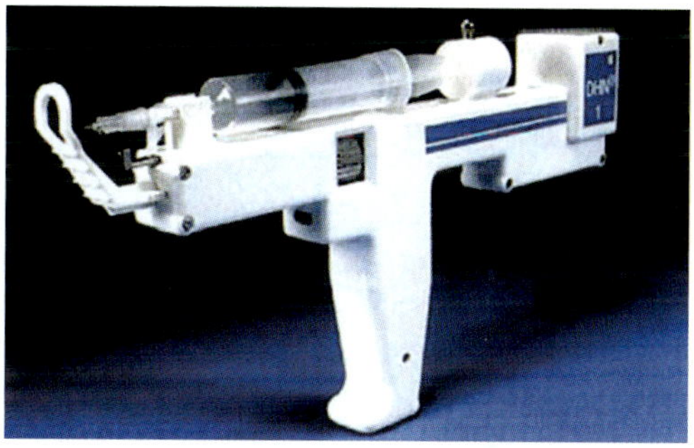

Fig. 7.11. Prototype hand-held syringe "gun," which allows rapid, standardized delivery of numerous mesotherapy ingredients (photograph courtesy of MesoUSA, New Jersey, USA)

Advantages, Disadvantages, and Indications

Relative to surgical approaches, other nonablative and noninvasive facial rejuvenation techniques described in this book, minimize disruption of work and social activity, and are relatively easily administered by physicians or supervised staff. Patients seeking cosmetic treatment are usually willing to trade some degree of efficacy from surgery for the convenience and relative comfort of these procedures.

Both mesotherapy and injectable lipolysis are not "lunch-time" procedures. While less invasive than blepharoplasty, liposuction, or barbed-thread surgical tightening techniques, facial injectable lipolysis is associated with significantly more downtime than photorejuvenation, facial peels, botulinum toxin, and dermal fillers. The advantages and disadvan-

Table 7.3. Advantages and disadvantages of using traditional mesotherapy

Issue	Advantages	Disadvantages
Technique	Administered by physician or health professional (supervision and licensure requirements vary by state) Technically simple and rapid to perform (by hand or specialized injection gun) Minimal equipment required, using syringes only Multiple visits are opportunities for the patient to receive complementary cosmetic procedures Mentorship/teaching courses effective for novice injectors	No standardized injection technique Protocols typically involve multiple weekly sessions delivered over months Injection guns expensive, cumbersome, and may be intimidating to patients
Indications	Multiple (purported): Dyspigmentation/melasma Improvements in skin tone and fine wrinkling	Studies limited to melasma and "facial rejuvenation"
Results	Insufficient peer review	Unpredictable outcomes Mixed clinical outcome using tranexamic acid for melasma No clinically significant outcome using nonconjugated hyaluronic acid and multivitamin mixture
Adverse events	Usually transient (hours to days)	Unpredictable and technique dependent Erythema, swelling, ecchymoses, abrasions, superficial infections, pin-point bleeding, atypical mycobacterial infections [33–35]

tages of using traditional mesotherapy and injectable lipolysis for facial rejuvenation are listed in Tables 7.3 and 7.4.

Contraindications

Both traditional mesotherapy and injectable lipolysis techniques are absolutely contraindicated in pregnant patients or those with known allergies against any of the ingredients. Other contraindications are relative and not based upon experimental or large-cohort clinical trials, but rather what has been recommended by others [18,21].

All patients should have a recent general physical examination, complete medical and drug history, and chemistries (including liver, renal, and lipid panels). Although the lit-

Table 7.4. Advantages and disadvantages of using traditional mesotherapy. *PC* Phosphatidylcholine

Issue	Advantages	Disadvantages
Technique	Easily learned, technically straightforward to performed No unique equipment or preparation required	Injector must be skilled at determining proper injection depth Technique effectively learned by direct observation Detergents potentially dangerous if injected directly into the orbit, muscle, or nerve
Indications	Infraorbital fat herniation, HIV-associated lipoaccumulation, submental and mandibular fat, jowls	Infraorbital swelling uncomfortable and cosmetically unacceptable to some patients
Results	Fat reduction localized to injection sites Treatments may complement liposuction (i.e., postsubmental liposuction irregularities)	Results may vary (dependent upon anatomic site treated, volumes of fat treated, and medication used) Proper patient selection and pretreatment counseling essential Multiple treatments required
Adverse events	Predictable Lidocaine significantly reduces immediate pain Prolonged effects resolve spontaneously, average 2–3 weeks No long-term effects (years) reported No systemic effects reported for facial indications (given limited volumes of <5 ml/session) No systemic effects thus far reported using deoxycholate alone	Immediate adverse events: edema, erythema, burning, itching, soreness Swelling may make patients self-conscious; significant reductions in swelling seen after 3–4 days Prolonged adverse events: ecchymoses, focal tenderness, nodularity, anesthesia Infraorbital injections significantly more risky (blindness) than other facial sites Potential systemic side effects reported if large quantities of PC solutions injected (typically around 2.5 g PC or 50 ml of 5% PC solution)

erature is limited to a small series of investigations, there have been no significant laboratory abnormalities in patients receiving injectable PC preparations [19]. Ongoing studies with DC alone by the author similarly reveal no resulting systemic alterations in serum chemistries, lipids, or blood counts. Avoid treating patients with liver and renal dysfunction, and those with autoimmune disease. Patients with hyperlipidemia are monitored before, once during, and again after treatment for potential changes in blood lipids, but injectable lipolysis appears to have no significant effect on cholesterol and triglycerides.

As with any trauma to the skin, darkly pigmented skin types (i.e., Fitzpatrick types IV–VI) are at increased risk for postinflammatory hyperpigmentation. Keloid or hypertrophic scar-prone patients should be forewarned.

Subcutaneous Deoxycholate Injections (Injectable Lipolysis) for the Nonsurgical Treatment of Fat

Sodium deoxycholate is one of the major active ingredients in a popular method of reducing fat on the neck, arms, waist, abdomen, hips, and knees. Deoxycholate is a natural component of bile that is released by the liver to emulsify and permit easy absorption of dietary fat and other lipids. The United States Food and Drug Administration (US FDA) has approved deoxycholate as a solvent for intravenous (IV) medication so that the medication can easily absorbed by the body. However, the FDA has not approved deoxycholate as a stand-alone medication, nor has the FDA approved deoxycholate for treatment of localized fat.

By signing this consent, you are agreeing to the following:

1. I understand that deoxycholate is approved by the US FDA as an IV medicine, but it is not approved to be used as an injection into fat, for the treatment of fat.
2. I understand the nature of the treatment and I understand that there are medically accepted alternative procedures (such as liposuction) to treat fat.
3. I understand that any risks or hazards inherent in the proposed procedure include but are not limited to: pain of the injection, burning, itching, swelling and redness at the site of injection (usually lasting 48–72 h, but may be up to 1 week), bleeding (hematoma formation), sensitivity (allergic response) to the injected material, bruising, firm inflammatory nodules, and parasthesias (change in sensation) in the overlying skin that may take up to several months to resolve. Furthermore, there may be risks or side effects that are unknown at this time.
4. Multiple treatments may be required to achieve results and there is no guarantee that the fat tissue deposits will soften, lessen, or disappear.
5. The treated fatty area may not get better after treatment and may become visibly larger while you are being treated.
6. I understand that deoxycholate injections will not be covered by my medical insurance carrier and therefore that I will be financially responsible for the treatments in full.
7. In the event of any injury or unusual reaction resulting from deoxycholate injections, treatment and all other costs resulting from such a reaction will be at my own expense.
8. I have been informed that the desired effect may require a series of injections at established intervals of time and up to five or more treatment sessions may be necessary.
9. I understand that aesthetic improvement may not be permanent.
10. I consent to the taking photographs, biopsy samples (only if you volunteer), and measurements in the course of this procedure or treatment for the purpose of assessing my progress, and/or advancing medical education.
11. I was given the opportunity to have the answers to my questions about this procedure adequately explained to me.
12. I understand that the results of my treatment may be published in the medical literature with no reference to my personal identity.

I hereby request, authorize, and give my consent for the performance of the treatment described above. My signature indicates that I have read and understand all of the 12 points, the information presented to me, and have had any questions answered. I hold Dr. ______________________ and the injecting physician (should they be different) harmless of any and all foreseen and unforeseen adverse events associated with the use of injectable deoxycholate.

____

Printed name of patient

______________________ ______________________

Signature of patient Date

____

Printed name of person conducting consent

______________________ ______________________

Signature of person conducting consent Date

Fig. 7.12. Sample patient consent for injectable lipolysis

Inflamed skin (i.e., rosacea, atopic dermatitis, inflammatory acne) should not be injected.

Informed Consent

Neither mesotherapy nor injectable lipolysis are regulated procedures, and may contain components unapproved for injection by the United States FDA and, in general, are considered unorthodox by the general medical community. Patients should be aware of the general results provided in the literature. A verbal understanding of the risks, benefits, and limitations and a signed consent should be documented in the patient's chart. Malpractice carriers may not be familiar with mesotherapy or injectable lipolysis. Therefore, physicians should forward proof of training and the published literature. See Fig. 7.12 for a sample patient consent form.

Personal Approach

I have limited my injectable lipolysis treatments of the face to submental contouring consisting of 1% DC mixed with lidocaine. Although the infraorbital fat pads are responsive to injectable lipolysis using PC/DC [16,21,22], I am not inclined to inject detergents adjacent to the conjunctiva, nor expose my patients to the swelling and discomfort. Because no significant cosmetic benefits are yet reported using traditional mesotherapy, I prefer conventional approaches like chemical peels, laser/light, botulinum toxin/fillers, and retinoid-based topical regimens.

Consultation with the patient focuses on safety, the published literature, and clinical experience. I will not commence treatment unless the patient understands the protocol, mechanism, anticipated events posttreatment, and frequency of treatments. The patient is then consented and photographed (left and right profiles, and straight views) using professional photographic equipment under standardized conditions.

The ideal submental region most responsive to DC injections has a mild-to-moderate amount of adipose tissue that is not enveloped with photodamaged or lax skin, but rather it is localized and not contiguous with fat on the jowls, lateral neck, mandible, or temperomandibular joint. Furthermore, it is ideal that patients have never had liposuction, although increasingly I am performing "touch-ups" for submental liposuction irregularities with satisfactory results. Aside from clinical studies, in everyday practice I will not measure the skinfold thickness, but rather rely on examination, photography, and the patient feedback to assess results. Photographs cannot capture the desired "firmer, tighter" sensation that most patients report after treatment. Comparing the photographs of pre- and posttreatment profiles with patients is a very gratifying process. It usually confirms changes that the patient may otherwise not observe in the mirror.

Patients are made comfortable sitting upright with the back-rest set slightly declined. The treated area is cleansed with cotton saturated with isopropyl alcohol. The patient may choose to have a topical anesthetic applied for 15–30 min; while the anesthetic decreases the pain of the needle, it does not appear to significantly affect the patient's reaction to the subcutaneous medication. The patient then rests her head back and raises the chin approximately 45°. A fine-tipped surgical marking pen or sharpened eyeliner pencil (more easily washed off) is used to mark the skin at 1.0- to 1.5-cm intervals (Fig. 7.13). The wider spacing is used when more medication is injected per site (see below). Adipose tissue will distribute itself along a wider area when the neck is raised slightly, making the treatment area wider. If jowls, lateral neck, or mandibular fat is treated, these sites are marked in a similar grid fashion, and injected directly (Fig. 7.14).

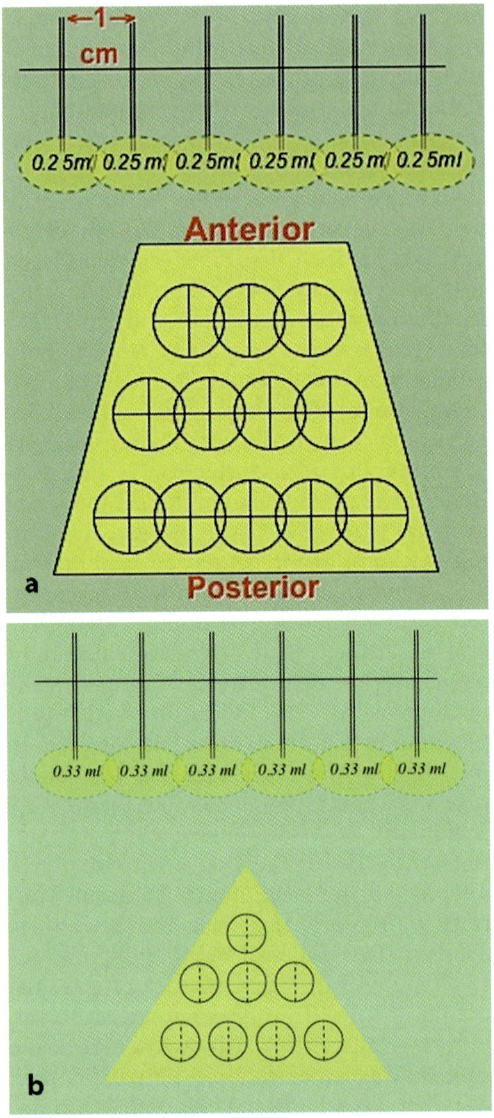

Fig. 7.13 a, b. Illustration of grid typically employed for injectable lipolysis of the submental region. The upper schematic demonstrates the anticipated minimal overlap of affected tissue when injections of 0.25 ml are spaced 1.0 cm apart. As described in the text, up to 0.4 ml injected 1.5 cm apart may be used for thicker (heavier) submental fat deposits. Volumes greater than 0.4 ml per site predisposes the patient to prolonged subcutaneous nodularity. The lower schematic represents the typical injection distribution pattern overlying submental fat ("anterior" represents anterior chin)

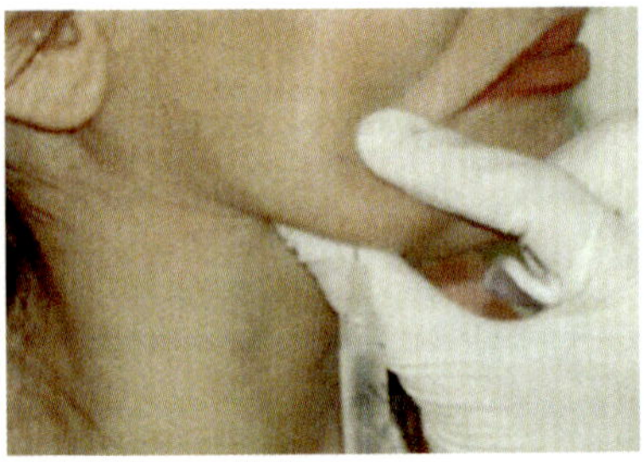

Fig. 7.14. Jowl injections performed in isolation or to complement treatment of the submental region (photograph courtesy of Hexsel et al. (2003) [19]

Injections are made with a 30-gauge, 0.5-inch needle. Depending on the total volume, a 3- or 5-ml syringe will suffice. The solution injected is a 3:1 ratio of preserved 1% DC (10 mg/ml) and 1% epinephrine-free lidocaine (i.e., 3.75 ml of DC is mixed with 1.25 ml lidocaine). Despite the added dilution with the anesthetic, the detergent is as effective as higher doses while avoiding the burning, itching, stinging, or tenderness encountered should the DC be used alone. The 0.9% benzyl alcohol acts like a preservative as well as an anesthetic. More often than not, a white precipitate forms upon mixing the medications extemporaneously before injection. A gentle shake of the syringe will resolubilize the precipitate. It is not advised to order premixed medication by the pharmacy because the stability of these solutions is not currently known and the precipitate may not resolubilize. Syringes can be kept at room temperature. Surplus medication is disposed of at the end of the day.

Once marked, the treated site is injected transdermally, infusing the medication directly into the subcutaneous fat. The proper depth of injection is essential as a general consideration, but in the submental region in particular, DC diffusion or direct injection into the platysma does not appear to have clinical significance. This may not hold true in other locations (e.g., arms and abdomen) since there is histologic evidence of muscle necrosis with high-concentration (5%) DC ex vivo [15]. The needle will "give" after it exits the dermis and enters the subcutaneous fat, where it should remain to infuse the medication. A range of 0.25–0.4 ml of solution is injected at 1.0- to 1.5-cm intervals, respectively. This technique should cause minimal medication overlap (Fig. 7.13). As a general rule, more volume is injected in thicker (heavier) collections of submental fat. Volumes greater than 0.4 ml per site predispose the patient to prolonged subcutaneous nodularity. After treatment, the patient is given a disposable icepack for several minutes of gentle application. The injected site should be monitored for minor injection-site bleeding, which can be cleaned with alcohol.

Postoperative Care and Complications

Immediate care consists of ice and gentle external manual compression. Immediate moderate erythema and localized swelling will be apparent. Despite the lidocaine, some patients experience breakthrough tenderness, and mild burning or itching. Most patients do not feel discomfort aside from mild-to-moderate focal tenderness once the anesthesia disappears (after about 1 h). At home the patients are instructed to ice the area on the hour for 10 min at a time, and if necessary, take extra-strength acetominephen (no nonsteroidal anti-inflammatory drugs) if there is any discomfort.

For the next 24–72 h, swelling will be moderate to significant (Fig. 7.15), as will focal tenderness. The swelling is best described as soft and unusually "jelly-like," unlike postoperative swelling. Cutaneous anesthesia may still be present and persist until most of the swelling subsides. Patients who are significantly concerned about having a "new double chin" may call the office if they are not forewarned. A majority of this swelling will subside after 3 days. Typically, first-time patients are scheduled prior to social inactivity (for several days, should they be concerned) or before the weekend, when they can better monitor their "social exposure." Most patients will experience less edema and tenderness after subsequent injections of similar volumes in the same location.

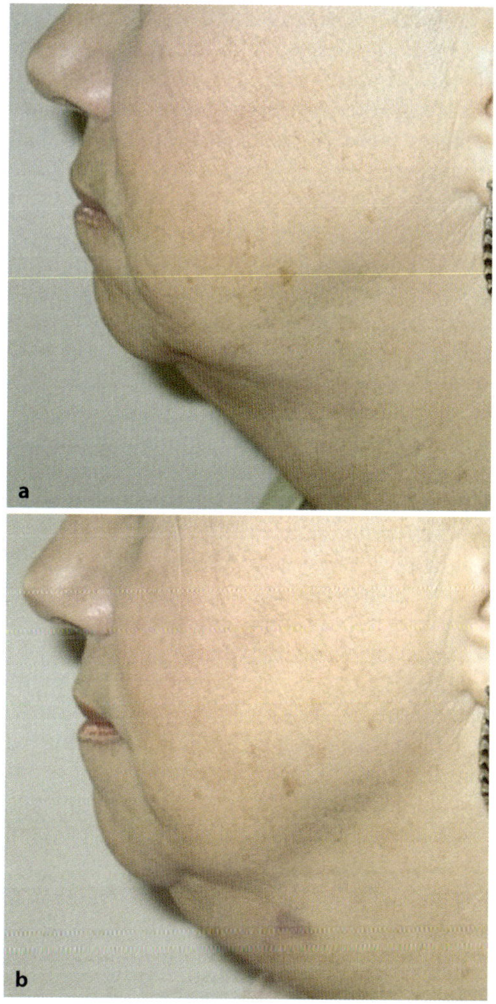

Fig. 7.15 a, b. Patient before (**a**) and 24 h after (**b**) 5.0 ml 1% deoxycholate injections into the submental region. Note the swelling and ecchymoses

Over the next week, the injected site will appear gradually less swollen and tender. The average duration of mild-to-moderate swelling, focal tenderness, and in some cases, superficial anesthesia, is about 10–14 days. Patients will notice that the poorly defined edema is replaced by relatively firm, small, round nodules at the injection sites. Patients are best forewarned and informed that nodules are welcome and expected – this is the focus of lysed fat that will no longer exist! Just as erythema and desquamation are expected after chemical peeling, tenderness, swelling and nodularity are anticipated after injectable lipolysis. Making this message clear will save innumerable visits and/or telephone calls from patients who did not expect otherwise.

Follow-up can be made at several days, or at a week or two to reassure the anxious patient (or novice injector!). Generally it is good practice to see a first-time patient back for a follow-up at least once before she is treated again. Injections are typically repeated at 4 weeks, although they can be delayed longer intervals with no detrimental outcome. At monthly follow-ups, patients injected with the above protocol should not have residual swelling. Nodularity may be present in more than half the cases, but this eventually resolves in 4–6 weeks. Rarely, I have seen nodularity persist for several months if the region is injected on multiple occasions with significant quantities of medication (i.e., 5 ml/session). It may have been that injection into areas of residual healing/inflammation prolonged the recovery, or rather, the subcutaneous fibrosis delays healing. Despite the postinflammatory fibrosis, I have not encountered cutaneous sclerosis or tactile hardening in any patient; without exception, the skin is just as it was beforehand. Hyperpigmentation is a very rare side-effect, but possible if too much solution is injected at too close an interval, in darkly pigmented patients.

Patients may question whether the results are "permanent." Just as aspirated fat is removed permanently in liposuction, "chemically ablated" adipocytes affected by DC are forever destroyed. Yet, similar to liposuction, local recurrence of fat as a result of unaffected adipocyte growth is possible should the patient gain weight.

There have been no reports of significant alterations in laboratory tests after injections of PC/DC or DC injections alone [19]. Nausea, diarrhea, and abdominal pain – all cholinergic symptoms associated with high quantities of oral PC – are common at high PC dosages (up to 2.5 g) [18]. DC dosages are at least half those of PC (given that most compounding pharmacies mix 2.5–4.75% DC per 5% PC). Injections of approximately 500 mg of DC (50 ml of 1% DC diluted with lidocaine) per treatment, in my experience, are not associated these symptoms.

Results

Photographic examples of the results treatment with injectable lypolytic agents can be seen in Figs. 7.16–7.19.

The Future

Although promising, subcutaneous PC and/or DC used in injectable lipolysis are not approved by the FDA for fat ablation. Currently, no standardized treatment regimens or formulations exist. Nevertheless, the studies cited, anecdotal experiences, and the availability of these ingredients from compounding pharmacies have paved the way for a potentially new, minimally invasive therapeutic treatment for adipose tissue.

Laboratory research is currently focusing on the attenuating effect of PC on the lytic activity of DC, the relative specificity of DC on adipocytes, and DC pharmacokinetics (absorption, distribution, metabolism, and elimination). As of 2007, a randomized, double-blind, Institutional-Review-Board-approved study evaluating the safety and efficacy of a PC/DC combination versus DC alone for the submental region is under way. Data from clinical studies like this are necessary to evaluate whether DC may be used alone with results comparable to PC/DC

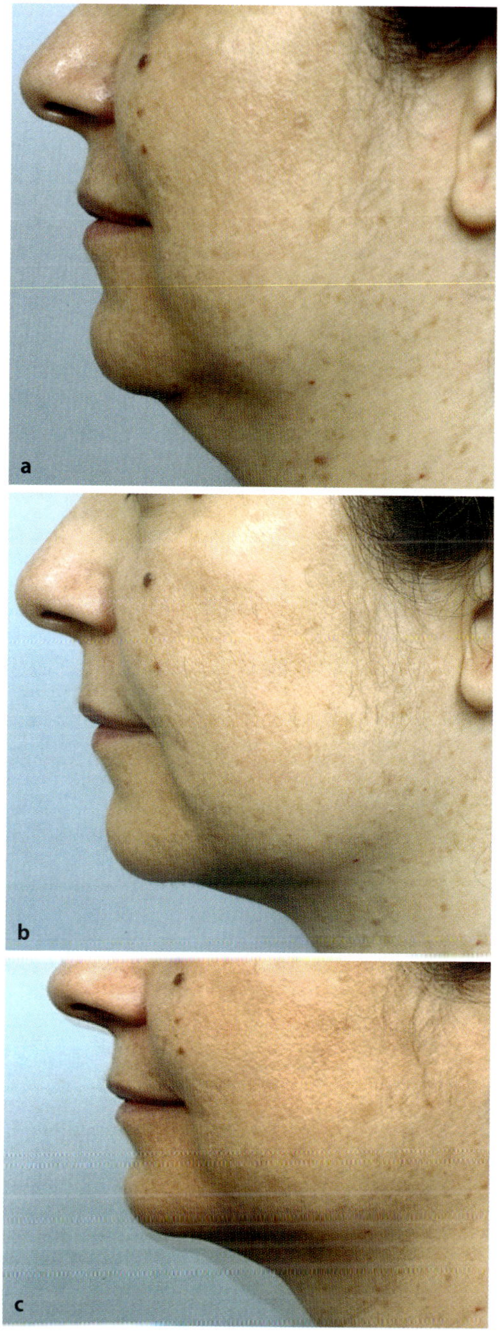

Fig. 7.16 a–c. Patient (**a**) before and (**b**) 2 months after five, monthly 1.0-ml injectable lipolysis treatments using 1% deoxycholate. **c** A "before" image taken prior to treatment is superimposed as a shadow on the "after" image taken after treatment

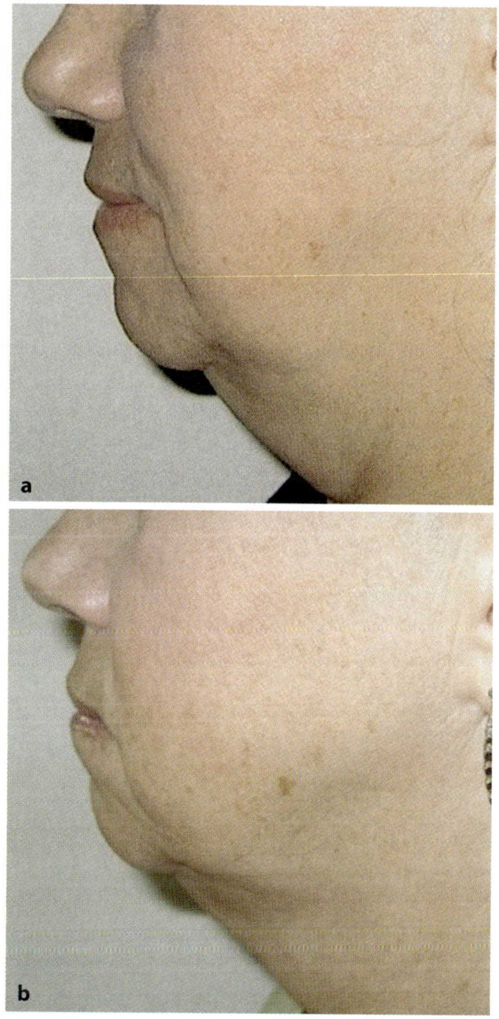

Fig. 7.17 a, b. Patient (**a**) before and (**b**) 1 month after three, monthly treatments totaling 10 ml 1% deoxycholate (premixed with lidocaine, as described)

combinations, thus avoiding exposing the patient to a potentially redundant substance and unnecessary expense. There is currently a pharmaceutical sponsor willing to take the action necessary for FDA drug approval. Thus, looking further, it is hoped that injectable lipolysis may one day become a regulated, minimally invasive technique designed to safely treat small quantities of unwanted adipose tissue.

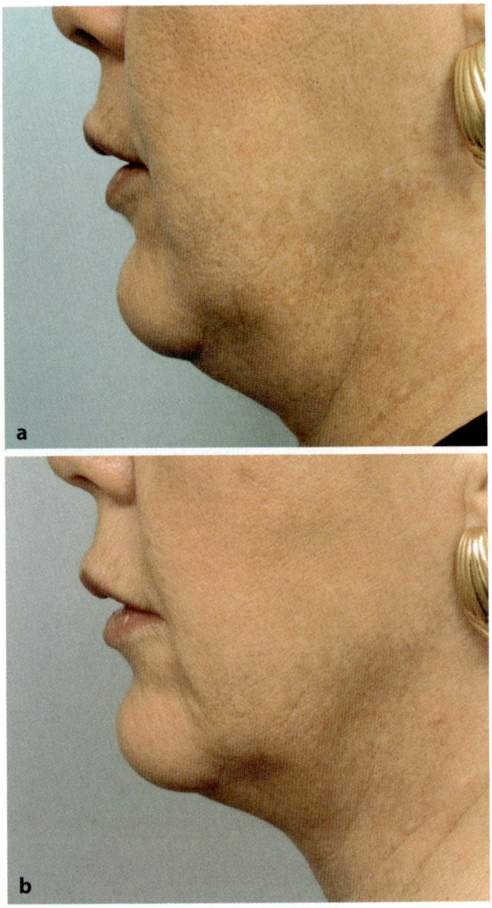

Fig. 7.18 a, b. Patient (**a**) before and (**b**) 2 months after five monthly 1.0-ml injectable lipolysis treatments using 1.0 ml solution to the submental region

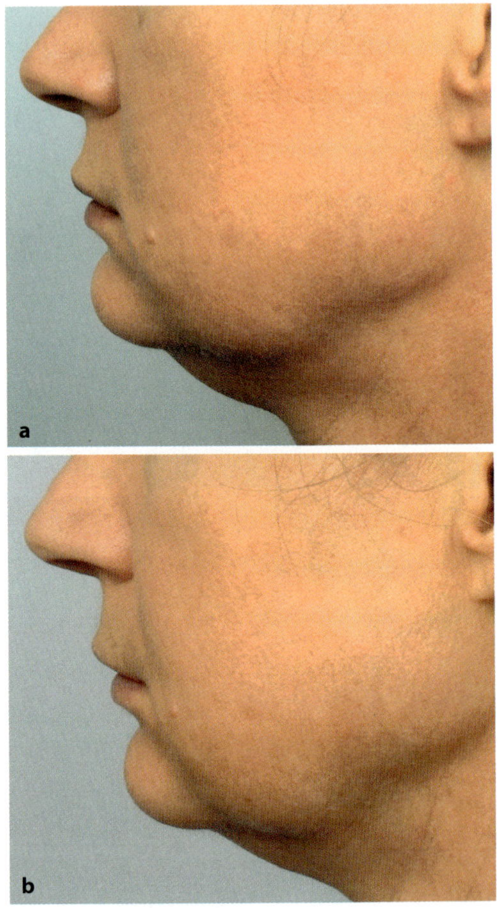

Fig. 7.19 a, b. Patient (**a**) before and (**b**) 2 months after five, monthly 1.0-ml injectable lipolysis treatments using 1.0 ml solution to the submental region

References

1. Rotunda AM, Kolodney MS (2006) Mesotherapy and phosphatidylcholine injections: historical clarification and review. Dermatol Surg 32:465–480
2. Rohrich RJ (2005) Mesotherapy: what is it? Does it work? Plast Reconstr Surg 115:1425
3. Matarasso A, Pfeifer TM, et al (2005) Mesotherapy for body contouring. Am Soc Plast Surg 115:1420–1424
4. Pistor M (1976) What is mesotherapy? Chir Dent Fr 46:59–60
5. Medioni G (1980) Results of 6 years of treatment of painful periodontal episodes by mesotherapy. Chir Dent Fr 50:35–37
6. Rotunda AM, Avram M.M, Avram A (2005) Cellulite: is there a role for injectables? J Cosmet Laser Ther 7:147–154
7. American Society for Dermatologic Surgery (ASDS) Emerging technology report: Mesotherapy. Available at http://www.asds.net/Media/PositionStatements/emerging_technology-mesotherapy.html
8. Lee JH, Park JG, Lim SH, et al (2006) Localized intradermal microinjection of tranexamic acid for treatment of melasma in Asian patients: a

preliminary clinical trial. Dermatol Surg 32:626–631
9. Amin SP, Phelph RG, Goldberg DJ (2006) Meostherapy for facial skin rejuvenation: a clinical, histologic, and electron microscopic evaluation. Dermatol Surg 32:1467–1472
10. Maggio S (1988) Treatment of xanthelasma with phosphatidylcholine. Presented at the Fifth International Meeting of Mesotherapy, Paris, France
11. Stryer L (1995) Biosynthesis of membrane lipids and steroids. In: Berg JM, Tymoczko JL, Stryer L (eds) Biochemistry. WH Freeman and Co, New York, pp 691–707
12. Klimov AM, Konstantinov VO, Lipovetsky BM, et al (1995) Essential phospholipids versus nicotinic acid in the treatment of patients with type IIb hyperlipoproteinemia and ischemic heart disease. Cardiovasc Drugs Ther 9:779–784
13. Lieber CS, Weiss DG, Groszmann R, et al (2003) Veteran Affairs Cooperative Study of the polyenylphosphatidylcholine in alcoholic liver disease. Alcohol Clin Exp Res 27:1765–1772
14. Schroder D, Buttenschon K, Herrmann F, Brede S (1991) Is there a drug treatment approach for prevention and therapy of fat embolism syndrome? Klin Wochenscr 69:229–233
15. Rotunda AM, Suzuki H, Moy RL, Kolodney MS (2004) Detergent effects of sodium deoxycholate are a major feature of an injectable phosphatidylcholine formulation used for localized fat dissolution. Dermatol Surg 30:1001–1008
16. Rittes PG (2001) The use of phosphatidylcholine for correction of lower lid bulging due to prominent fat pads. Dermatol Surg 27:391–392
17. Rittes PG (2003) The use of phosphatidylcholine for correction of localized fat deposits. Aesthetic Plast Surg 27:315–318
18. Duncan DI, Hasengschwandtner F (2005) Lipodissolve for subcutaneous fat reduction and skin retraction. Aesthetic Surg J 25:530–543
19. Hexsel D, Serra M, Mazzuco R, Dal'Forno T, Zechmeister D (2003) Phosphatidylcholine in the treatment of localized fat. J Drugs Dermatol 2:511–518
20. Myers P (2006) The cosmetic use of phosphatidylcholine in the treatment of localized fat. J Cosmet Dermatol 19:416–420
21. Ablon G, Rotunda AM (2004) Treatment of lower eyelid fat pads using phosphatidylcholine: clinical trial and review. Dermatol Surg 30:422–428
22. Treacy PJ, Goldberg DJ (2006) The use of phosphatidylcholine for correction of lower lid bulging due to prominent fat pads. J Cosmet Laser Ther 8:129–132
23. Carruthers A, Carruthers J (2004) Counterpoint. Dermatol Surg 30:428
24. Walsh N (2004) Some would halt lipolysis Tx pending safety data. Skin Allergy News 35:26
25. Kopera D, Binder B, Toplak H (2006) Intralesional lipolysis with phosphatidylcholine for the treatment of lipomas: pilot study. Arch Dermatol 142:395–396
26. Jones MN (1999) Surfactants in membrane solubilisation. Int J Pharm 177:137–159
27. Wiedmann TS, Kamel L (2002) Examination of the solubilization of drugs by bile salt micelles. J Pharm Sci 91:1743–1764
28. Bahar RJ (1999) Bile acid transport. Gastroenterol Clin North Am 28:27–58
29. Rotunda AM, Ablon G, Kolodney MS (2005) Lipomas treated with subcutaneous deoxycholate injections. J Am Acad Dermatol 53:973–978
30. Rose PT, Morgan M (2005) Histological changes associated with mesotherapy for fat dissolution. J Cosmet Laser Ther 7:17–19
31. Spenver J, Matthews AW (2004) Stirring debate: as druggists mix customized brews, FDA raises alarm. Wall Street Journal, Feb 27
32. International Academy of Compounding Pharmacists (IACP) August 31, 2006. Press release. Available at: http://www.iacprx.org/site/PageServer?pagename=Press_Releases#083106
33. Lee DP, Chang SE (2005) Subcutaneous nodules showing fat necrosis owing to mesotherapy. Dermatol Surg 31:250–251
34. Centers for Disease Control and Prevention (CDC) (2005) Outbreak of Mesotherapy-Associated Skin Reactions – District of Columbia Area, January–February 2005. MMWR Morb Mortal Wkly Rep 54:1127–1130
35. Nagore E, Ramos P, Botella-Estrada R, Ramos-Niguez JA, Sanmartin O, Castejon P (2001) Cutaneous infection with *Mycobacterium fortuitum* after localized microinjections (mesotherapy) treated successfully with a triple drug regimen. Acta Derm Venereol 81:291–293

Chapter 8

Cosmeceuticals

8

Zoe Diana Draelos

Core Messages

- Cosmeceuticals represent functional cosmetics and skincare products.
- The cutaneous effect of a cosmeceutical is the combined action of the moisturizing abilities of the vehicle combined with the intent of the active ingredients.
- The most common antiaging effect of cosmeceuticals on the skin is to enhance barrier function and provide photoprotection.
- Areas of research in cosmeceutical ingredients include substances intended to improve skin function by activating a receptor, altering an enzyme, functioning as a cellular messenger, acting as an antioxidant, or providing anti-inflammatory capabilities.
- Cosmeceuticals are considered cosmetics and, because of their unregulated status, their manufacturers can only make appearance-related claims.

History

The Concept of Functional Cosmetics

The over-the-counter (OTC) world of beauty and well-being is expanding due to new raw materials, advanced technology, and a growing consumer-market willingness to purchase promises. This need for cosmetics that do something other than adorn the skin has led to a new category of functional cosmetics. Functional cosmetics encompass the realms of colored cosmetics, cosmeceuticals, neurocosmeceuticals, and nutraceuticals. All of these categories have the same goal, namely improving senescence of the skin, body, and/or mind. Before proceeding with an analysis of the world of functional cosmetics, it is necessary to distinguish the subtle differences between each of the categories. Colored cosmetics traditionally have been identified as products designed to color and scent the body. Lipstick, eye shadow, mascara, eyeliner, blush, and perfume are the cosmetic mainstays; however, these products do cross over into the cosmeceutical category. For example, moisturizing lipsticks, hair-growth-enhancing mascaras, and sunscreen-containing blushes combine body adornment with an improvement in functionality.

Cosmeceuticals extend beyond cosmetics to enhance functioning, usually returning the structure to a more youthful state. For example, wrinkle-reducing moisturizers, nail growth serums, and skin lightening creams all fall into this category. Cosmeceuticals are somewhat confusing, however, as both prescription and OTC products have been labeled by this term. Drug cosmeceuticals include topical retinoids for improving dermal collagen production, topical minoxidil for enhanced scalp hair growth, and eflornithine for facial hair growth reduction. These products will not be discussed, as they are not available to the consumer except by prescription. The second category of cosmeceuticals includes OTC drugs, such as sunscreens and antiperspirants. Sunscreens are some of the most important functional cosmetics currently available and will be discussed at length.

A subgroup of functional cosmetics has been recently termed neurocosmeceuticals. These are topical agents applied to the skin to induce a feeling of well being, playing into the philosophical concept of the mind/body connection. There are those who believe that the skin cannot appear healthy unless the mind is content. Furthermore, the health of the mind can be improved through the skin. Neurocosmeceuticals claim to improve well-being by altering neurotransmitters through topical applications. Indeed, ingredients have been identified that inhibit the release of substance P and enhance the release of beta-endorphins.

Nutrition is also considered to be part of the mind/body connection in the form of nutraceuticals. Nutraceuticals have been billed as the oral equivalent of cosmeceuticals, since most dermatologists agree that the best way of improving skin appearance is through improved overall general health. Both neurocosmeceuticals and nutraceuticals are beyond the scope of this discussion, which will mainly focus on topical agents designed to improve the functioning and appearance of the skin, known as cosmeceuticals.

Currently Available Products

Cosmeceutical Development

The world of cosmeceuticals is rapidly changing, since it is driven to a large extent by new product introductions designed to capture consumer attention and fads. This accounts for the dizzying array of ingredients with an even more amazing number of appearance claims. However, it is possible to make some generalizations regarding cosmeceutical development that might be useful to the reader.

Table 8.1. Steps in Cosmeceutical Ingredient Development

1	New botanical material received in the laboratory
2	Various fractions of the botanical material extracted
3	Fractions analyzed for relationship to known chemical compounds
4	Purified fraction exposed to gene array chip
5	Analysis completed for upregulation or downregulation of key events in cellular oxidation, inflammation, or irritation
6	New isolate studied in an in vitro model of cell culture for confirmation of gene array results
7	Positive in vitro findings lead to isolate analysis in mouse model focusing on markers of possible cutaneous benefit
8	Positive mouse findings lead to formulation in a vehicle suitable for human use
9	Human model testing conducted to determine if active has any cutaneous value
10	Formulation fine-tuned and patented
11	New ingredient licensed to cosmetic manufacturer
12	New technology enters the marketplace

First, cosmeceuticals are basically cosmetics and as such must be safe. This means that the best source of new materials for formulation would be substances derived from either plants or food components. Second, cosmeceutical additives must be available as a powder or liquid, since the majority of cosmeceuticals must be elegantly applied to the external body. Third, cosmeceuticals must have some easily identifiable benefit upon which to base a functional claim. For all of these reasons, the majority of cosmeceutical ingredients have their origin in the botanical realm or in foods.

New cosmeceuticals ingredients in the botanical realm are identified based on the algorithm presented in Table 8.1. Once the botanical active ingredient (active) is identified and synthesized, it is typically applied to a fibroblast gene chip to determine if it affects any key cellular event. After demonstration of a presumed physiologic effect, the active is tested in vitro to determine an effect on cultured fibroblasts. If positive data is obtained, the active is studied in a mouse model for confirmation. The active is then placed in a vehicle suitable for human application and clinical studies are undertaken. Successful human clinical studies pave the way for successful introduction into the marketplace via ingredient licensing arrangements.

The search for botanicals suitable for formulation into cosmeceuticals has led to the gathering of flowers, seeds, roots, leaves, twigs, and berries from plants all over the world. It important to remember, however, that the constituents of a plant component are influenced by the season in which the plant material was picked, the growing conditions, and the processing of the agent. These variables are summarized in Table 8.2.

Table 8.2. Sources of cosmeceutical actives

1	**Plant source:** leaves, roots, fruits, berries, stems, twigs, barks, flower
2	**Growing conditions:** soil composition, amount of available water, climate variations, plant stress
3	**Harvesting conditions:** time from harvest to transport, care of plant materials during shipping, storage conditions prior to manufacture
4	**Preparation method:** crushing, grinding, boiling, distilling, pressing, drying
5	**Final extract status:** liquid, powder, paste, syrup, crystal
6	**Concentration:** sufficient amount of active to produce biologic effect

Table 8.3. Mechanisms of action for cosmeceuticals

1	Enhance barrier function
2	Provide a sunscreen
3	Decrease pigmentation
4	Activate a receptor
5	Cellular messenger
6	Antioxidant
7	Anti-inflammatory

Mechanism of Action for Cosmeceuticals

While the cosmeceutical market may be vast and confusing, it is possible to simplify the discussion by organizing cosmeceutical ingredients in terms of their functionality. There are only so many identified scientifically valid methods of improving the skin. The major mechanisms of action for cosmeceuticals for discussion in this chapter are listed in Table 8.3. Note that the main antiaging mechanism of action for cosmeceuticals is enhancing the barrier and providing photoprotection. These are activities that modify the stratum corneum, which is nonliving, and clearly fall within the intended cosmetic realm. The remainder of the cosmeceutical functional categories actually alters the structure and function of the skin, making them drugs and not cosmetics. Herein lies the cosmeceutical controversy.

Barrier Function

The main cutaneous function of cosmeceuticals is to enhance the barrier function of the skin. Enhancing the barrier decreases stinging and burning from a sensory standpoint and improves the look and feel of the skin. Moisturizers can smooth down desquamating corneocytes and fill in the gaps between the remaining corneocytes to create the impression of tactile smoothness. This effect is temporary, of course, until the moisturizer is removed from the skin surface by wiping or cleansing. From a functional standpoint, moisturizers can create an optimal environment for healing and minimize the appearance of lines of dehydration by decreasing transepidermal water loss. Transepidermal water loss increases when the brick and mortar organization of the protein-rich corneocytes held together by intercellular lipids is damaged. A well-formulated cosmeceutical moisturizer can decrease the water loss until healing occurs.

There are three cosmeceutical ingredient categories that can reduce transepidermal water loss: occlusives, humectants, and hydrophilic matrices [1]. The most common method for reducing transepidermal water loss is the application of an occlusive ingredient to the skin surface. These are basically oily substances that create a barrier to water evaporation. The more commonly used occlusive ingredients in current formulations and their chemical category are listed in Table 8.4 [2].

Table 8.4. Moisturizing ingredients for barrier enhancement

1	Hydrocarbon oils and waxes: petrolatum, mineral oil, paraffin, squalene
2	Silicone oils
3	Vegetable and animal fats
4	Fatty acids: lanolin acid, stearic acid
5	Fatty alcohol: lanolin alcohol, cetyl alcohol
6	Polyhydric alcohols: propylene glycol
7	Wax esters: lanolin, beeswax, stearyl stearate
8	Vegetable waxes: carnauba, candelilla
9	Phospholipids: lecithin
10	Sterols: cholesterol

Occlusive Moisturizers

The most popular and effective occlusive ingredient is time-tested petrolatum, which blocks 99% of water loss from the skin surface [3]. This remaining 1% transepidermal water loss is necessary to provide the cellular message for barrier repair initiation. If the transepidermal water loss is completely halted, the removal of the occlusion results in failure to repair the barrier and water loss quickly resumes at its preapplication level. Thus, the occlusion does not initiate barrier repair [4]. Petrolatum does not function as an impermeable barrier, rather it permeates throughout the interstices of the stratum corneum allowing barrier function to be reestablished [5].

Humectant Moisturizers

Another concept in rehydrating the stratum corneum is the use of humectants. Humectants have been used in cosmetics for many years to increase shelf life by preventing product evaporation and subsequent thickening due to variations in temperature and humidity. Humectants are a necessary in all oil-in-water creams to maintain the required water content. Substances that function as humectants include glycerin, honey, sodium lactate, urea, propylene glycol, sorbitol, pyrrolidone carboxylic acid, gelatin, hyaluronic acid, vitamins, and some proteins [2,6].

Some cosmeceuticals claim to hydrate the skin by drawing water from the environment. For all practical purposes, this is not the case. Humectants only draw water from the environment when the ambient humidity exceeds 70%. In environmentally controlled spaces, this does not occur; thus, humectants pull water from the deeper epidermal and dermal tissues to rehydrate the stratum corneum. This water is then trapped by an occlusive film placed on top of the stratum corneum [7]. Humectants may also allow the skin to feel smoother by filling holes in the stratum corneum through swelling [8,9]. Therefore, a good moisturizer should combine both occlusive and humectant ingredients.

Hydrophilic Matrix Moisturizers

The final method employed by cosmeceuticals to moisturize the skin is through hydrophilic matrices. These are large-molecular-weight substances that create a film over the skin surface, thereby retarding water evaporation. The first hydrophilic matrix developed was an oatmeal bath. The colloidal oatmeal created a film that prevented water from leaving the skin to enter the bath water. A newer hydrophilic matrix is a peptide film that also retards water loss while functioning as a humectant. Peptides will be discussed in detail later in this chapter.

There can be no doubt that most antiaging cosmeceuticals are primarily well-constructed moisturizers. Furthermore, most of the claims associated with cosmeceuticals are moisturizer claims. Keep in mind that the moisturizer is really the vehicle for transporting the special ingredient to the skin surface, but the vehicle may actually be the active in many products.

Photoprotection

In addition to providing moisturization benefits, many cosmeceuticals make antiaging claims based on the presence of a sunscreen ingredient. The moisturization effects of the cosmeceutical are perceived within a matter of hours as the skin feels softer and looks shinier, but the antiaging claims related to photoprotection take years to manifest. Yet, promoting younger-looking skin is definitely scientifically supported by sunscreens.

Many new developments have occurred in the photoprotection cosmeceutical market to increase both efficacy and cosmetic acceptability. Higher sun protection factor (SPF) formulations are more popular as new sunscreen combinations arise that provide better UVB protection. New methods of increasing the longevity of UVA photoprotectants provide better broad-spectrum protection. Dry-touch sunscreens have even been developed that dry quickly in place on the skin surface, preventing rub-off and a sticky feel. All of these advances make sunscreens able to provide superior photoprotection. This section examines some of the major active ingredients in cosmeceutical sunscreens.

Sunscreen Ingredient Categories

Sunscreen actives can be classified into two major categories, chemical and physical. Chemical sunscreens, also known as organic filters, undergo a chemical transformation, known as resonance delocalization, to absorb UV radiation and transform it to heat. This reaction occurs within the phenol ring, which contains an electron-releasing group in the ortho and/or para position, and is irreversible, rendering the sunscreen inactive once it has absorbed the UV radiation. Physical sunscreens, also known as inorganic filters, are usually ground particulates that reflect or scatter UV radiation, absorbing relatively little of the energy. For this reason they have longer activity on the skin surface.

Sunscreen ingredients can be divided into the following three groups:

1. UVA absorbers: 320–360 nm (benzophenones, anthranilates, avobenzone)
2. UVB absorbers: 290–320 nm (para-aminobenzoic acid, PABA, derivatives, salicylates, cinnamates)
3. UVB/UVA blocks: reflect or scatter UVA and UVB (titanium dioxide, zinc oxide)

Each of these filters is discussed separately to highlight advantages and disadvantages in cosmeceutical formulations. Most cosmeceutical sunscreen formulations are a blend of two to three filters carefully selected to compliment one another and enhance product performance.

UVA Organic Filters

Benzophenones

There are three sunscreens in the benzophenone family: oxybenzone, dioxybenzone, and sulisobenzone. Oxybenzone is used in the United States and provides weak UVA photoprotection below 320 nm. There have been some reports of allergic contact dermatitis to benzophenone, but they are rare. Benzophenone is commonly used as a secondary sunscreen to increase the broad-spectrum protection of the formulation. It is an oil-soluble ingredient that can add to the sticky feel of a sunscreen, if used in too high a concentration. Benzophenone has found a new importance in the sunscreen industry for its ability to stabilize avobenzone, an important UVA photoprotectant discussed next.

Avobenzone

Avobenzone, also known as Parsol 1789, was an important step forward in UVA photoprotection. Unfortunately, it is highly photounstable with 36% of the avobenzone is destroyed shortly after sun exposure. It is estimated that all of the avobenzone is gone from a sunscreen after 5 h or 50 J of UVA exposure, necessitating frequent reapplication. Avobenzone is also chemically incompatible with other commonly used inorganic filters, such as zinc oxide and titanium dioxide. However, avobenzone has assumed new importance as a proprietary sunscreen complex, known as Helioplex (Neutrogena), has been introduced that combines avobenzone with oxybenzone and Hallbrite TQ to create a photostable avobenzone with long-lasting UVA photoprotectant qualities. Hallbrite TQ is chemically known as 2-6-diethylhexylnaphthalate. Photostable UVA organic filters are finding their way into many antiaging cosmeceuticals.

Ecamsule

The newest sunscreen ingredient to be added to the monograph is ecamsule, better known as Mexoryl. Mexoryl (L'Oreal) was originally developed to stabilize avobenzone, much like Helioplex (Neutrogena) discussed earlier. It is available in two forms: Mexoryl SX and Mexoryl XL. Mexoryl SX is a water-soluble form that is suitable for daywear sunscreen formulations. This would include sunscreen-containing moisturizers, sunscreens, and cosmeceuticals. Mexoryl XL is an oil soluble form that is suitable for water-resistant sunscreen formulations, including those worn on the beach and during vigorous physical exercise. Only Mexoryl SX has been approved for use in the United States.

Menthyl Anthranilate

Menthyl anthranilate is the only sunscreen of the anthranilate filter family approved in the United States, where it is also known as Meradimate. Its peak absorption is at 336 nm, but it is a clear, thick, sticky oil that can only be used in low concentrations in for aesthetic reasons. It has an excellent safety profile and low allergenicity. It is very stable in formulation without photoinstability issues, and is commonly used as a secondary UVA photoprotectant in antiaging cosmeceuticals.

UVB Organic Filters

PABA Derivatives

For all practical purposes, the PABA derivatives are rarely used in modern cosmeceutical sunscreen formulations. A recent review of the marketplace showed that less than 2% of sunscreens use PABA derivatives due to allergenicity concerns. Octyldimethyl PABA, also known as Padimate O, is the most commonly used PABA substance, with a maximal absorption at 296 nm. It has average photostability with about 15.5% of this lost after photoexposure.

Salicylates

The salicylates are an important class of UVB photoprotectants. This class includes octyl salicylate (Octisalate) and homomenthyl salicylate (Homosalate). It is the internal hydrogen bonding of the salicylates that provides for maximal UVB absorption at 300–310 nm. Approximately 56% of the sunscreens in the current United States marketplace use the salicylates as a secondary sunscreen active, since they have an excellent safety record with minimal allergenicity.

Cinnamates

The cinnamates are the most popular sunscreen category currently used in antiaging cosmeceuticals. 86% of products with an SPF rating contain octyl methoxycinnamate, also known as Octinoxate, which has maximal absorption at 305 nm. Octyl methoxycinnamate has excellent photostability, with only 4.5% degradation after UVB exposure.

Inorganic UVA/UVB Filters

The inorganic UVA/UVB filters are titanium dioxide and zinc oxide. Titanium dioxide is usually micronized to contain particles of many sizes to provide optimal UV scattering abilities. Unfortunately, it leaves a white film on the skin and is used mainly for beachwear sunscreens and not cosmeceuticals. Zinc oxide is usually available in a microfine form, meaning it contains small particles of one size making it appropriate for day wear. A newly introduced colorless zinc oxide with extremely small particles is finding its way into many cosmeceuticals; however, there is concern that the nanoparticles may enter the skin through appendageal structures, creating a permanent reservoir. The cosmeceutical industry has placed a voluntary hold on nanoparticle inorganic filters and pigments until the penetration issues are better understood.

The aforementioned paragraphs have described two mechanisms by which cosmeceuticals function, barrier enhancement and photoprotection. These lead to functional modifications of the stratum corneum. Such products do not alter skin physiology. There are, in fact, cosmeceutical ingredients that do alter skin physiology. The most obvious, among this group, are those that promote pigment lightening.

Pigment Lightening

Facial hyperpigmentation is one of the most common signs of photoaging. It is something for which many patients seek facial rejuvenation. Many different patterns of facial hyperpigmentation can be seen. Focal hyperpigmentation in the form of small lentigenes across the lateral cheeks usually begins about age 25–30 years, depending on cumulative sun exposure, with continued accumulation of lesions throughout life. Pigmentation can also present in the form of melasma with reticulated pigment over the sides of the fore head lateral jawline and upper lip. Finally, hyperpigmentation can present as overall darkening of the skin from a combination of melanin pigment, fragmented elastin fibers, and residual hemosiderin. Cosmeceutical treatments for hyperpigmentation are problematic. A successful treatment must remove existing pigment from the skin, shut down the manufacture of melanin, and prevent the transfer of existing melanin to the melanosomes. This section examines the ingredients currently used in cosmeceutical preparations to lighten pigment.

Hydroquinone

The gold standard for hyperpigmentation therapy in the United States remains hydroquinone. This substance is actually quite controversial, having been removed from the OTC markets in Europe and Asia. Concern arose because oral hydroquinone has been reported to cause cancer in mice fed large amounts of the substance. While oral consumption probably is not related to topical application, hydroquinone remains controversial because it actually is toxic to melanocytes. Hydroquinone, a phenolic compound chemically known as 1,4 dihydroxybenzene, functions by inhibiting the enzymatic oxidation of tyrosine and phenol oxidases. It covalently binds to histidine or interacts with copper at the active site of tyrosinase. It also inhibits RNA and DNA synthesis and may alter melanosome formation, thus selectively damaging melanocytes. These activities suppress the melanocyte metabolic processes inducing gradual decrease of melanin pigment production [10].

Hydroquinone is currently undergoing investigation in the United States OTC market. As of 2007, OTC hydroquinone in concentrations of 2% or less has been removed from the list of ingredients considered safe by the United States Food and Drug Administration (FDA). This means that all companies manufacturing hydroquinone products sold without a prescription can produce no more once the current stock is exhausted. It is felt that this is the first step in removing hydroquinone from all cosmeceuticals sold in the United States for pigment-lightening purposes.

Azelaic Acid

Azelaic acid is one of the ingredients that may take the place of hydroquinone in pigment lightening cosmeceuticals. It is a 9-carbon dicarboxylic acid obtained from cultures of Pityrosporum ovale. Although its pigment lightening effects are mild, several large studies done with a diverse ethnic background population have compared its efficacy to that of hydroquinone [11,12]. It also interferes with tyrosinase activity, but additionally interferes with DNA synthesis. It appears to have specificity for abnormal melanocytes and for this reason it may be able to prevent lentigo maligna, but this claim would not be appropriate in the cosmeceutical realm.

Ascorbic Acid

Ascorbic acid, also known as vitamin C, is used in cosmeceuticals for hyperpigmentation because it interrupts melanogenesis by interacting with copper ions to reduce dopaquinone and blocks dihydrochinindol-2-carboxyl acid oxidation [13]. Ascorbic acid, an antioxidant, is rapidly oxidized when exposed to air, which limits the stability of this product. For this reason, many cosmeceuticals are using the more stable magnesium ascorbyl phosphate, which is metabolized to ascorbic acid in the skin. High concentrations of ascorbic acid must be used with caution, however, as the low pH can be irritating to the skin. Pigment-lightening cosmeceuticals may contain ascorbic acid as a pH adjustor or to function as an antioxidant preservative. It is important to recognize that ascorbic acid is a multifunctional ingredient with very minimal pigment-lightening capabilities.

Licorice Extract

Licorice extracts are placed in cosmeceuticals to decrease facial redness and reduce pigmentation. The extract contains liquiritin and isoliquertin, which are glycosides containing flavonoids [14], that induce skin lightening by dispersing melanin. To see clinical results, the liquiritin must be applied in the dose of 1 g/day for 4 weeks. Irritation, so frequently observed with hydroquinone and ascorbic acid products, is rare from licorice extract; however, the efficacy of licorice extract appears to be minimal.

Alpha Lipoic Acid

Alpha lipoic acid is found in a variety of antiaging cosmeceuticals and functions as an antioxidant. It may also have very limited pigment-lightening properties. It is a disulfide derivative of octanoic acid that is able to inhibit tyrosinase. However, it is a large molecule and cutaneous penetration to the level of the melanocyte is challenging, significantly reducing its efficacy.

Kojic Acid

Kojic acid, chemically known as 5-hydroxymethyl-4H-pyrane-4-one, is one of the most popular cosmeceutical skin-lightening agents found in cosmetic OTC skin-lightening cream distributed worldwide. It is a hydrophilic fungal derivative obtained from *Aspergillus* and *Penicillium* species. It is the most popular agent employed in the Orient for the treatment of melasma [15]. Some studies indicate that kojic acid is equivalent to hydroquinone in its pigment-lightening ability [16]. The activity of kojic acid is attributed to its ability to prevent tyrosinase activity by binding to copper.

Aleosin

Aleosin is a low-molecular-weight glycoprotein obtained from the aloe vera plant. It is a natural hydroxymethylchromone that inhibits tyrosinase by competitive inhibition at the DOPA oxidation site [17,18]. In contrast to hydroquinone, it shows no cell cytotoxicity. However it has a limited ability to penetrate the skin due to its hydrophilic nature. It is sometimes mixed with arbutin, as described below, to enhance its skin-lightening abilities.

Arbutin

Arbutin is obtained from the leaves of the *Vaccinicum vitis-idaca* and other related plants. It is a naturally occurring gluconopyranoside that causes decreased tyrosinase activity without affecting messenger RNA expression [19]. It also inhibits melanosome maturation. Arbutin is not toxic to melanocytes and is used in a variety of pigment-lightening preparations in Japan at concentrations of 3%. Higher concentrations are more efficacious than lower concentrations, but a paradoxical pigment darkening may occur.

With the recent loss of hydroquinone as a cosmeceutical pigment-lightening agent, botanicals are sure to assume a more important role. Pigment lightening is the most important function of antiaging cosmeceuticals in individuals with Fitzpatrick skin type III and higher. Thus, more research into pigment-lightening cosmeceuticals is assured.

Receptor Activation

The next important mechanism of action for cosmeceuticals is receptor activation. There is only one skin receptor that has been well characterized, the retinoid receptor [20]. Prescription retinoids, such as tazarotene and treti-

Table 8.5. Cutaneous effects of topical retinoids

Gross dermatologic effects	
1	Improvement in fine and coarse facial wrinkling
2	Decreased tactile roughness
3	Reduction of actinic keratoses
4	Lightening of solar lentigenes
Histologic dermatologic effects	
1	Reduction in stratum corneum cohesion
2	Decreased epidermal hyperplasia
3	Increased production of collagen, elastin, and fibronectin
4	Reduction in tonofilaments, desmosomes, melanosomes
5	More numerous Langerhans cells
6	Angiogenesis
7	Decreased glycosaminoglycans
8	Reduced activity of collagenase and gelatinase
9	Normalization of keratinization of the pilosebaceous unit

noin, are well studied for their ability to induce the skin changes noted in Table 8.5; however, OTC retinoids may demonstrate some of the same effects, if to a lesser degree [21,22]. It is theoretically possible to interconvert the retinoids from one form to another. For example, retinyl palmitate and retinyl propionate, chemically known as retinyl esters, can become biologically active following cutaneous enzymatic cleavage of the ester bond and subsequent conversion to retinol. Retinol is the naturally occurring vitamin A form found in red, yellow, and orange fruits and vegetables. It is the pigment responsible for vision, but it is highly unstable. Retinol can be oxidized to retinaldehyde and then oxidized to retinoic acid, also known as prescription tretinoin. It is this cutaneous conversion of retinol to retinoic acid that is responsible for the biologic activity of some of the new stabilized OTC vitamin A preparations designed to improve the appearance of benign photodamaged skin [23]. Unfortunately, only small amounts of retinyl palmitate and retinol can be converted by the skin, accounting for the increased efficacy seen with prescription preparations containing retinoic acid.

The main problem with prescription retinoids is their irritancy. Unfortunately, as the biological efficacy of the retinoid increases, so does its irritancy. This is also the case with the OTC retinoids. Retinol is more irritating than the retinyl esters and also more unstable. It is for this reason that cosmeceutical formulations, which may not be manufactured under strict oxygen-devoid conditions, prefer to add retinyl palmitate to moisturizing creams. However, the retinyl palmitate may not be added for its activation of the retinoid receptor. Retinyl plamitate is a potent antioxidant and humectant. It is this multifunctionality that may conceal its true use in cosmeceutical formulations.

Peptide Cellular Messengers

Peptides are not new to the world of cosmetics, but their purported role as cellular messengers in cosmeceuticals is a recent concept. Proteins, historically, were produced by boiling cow skin and then added as thickeners to moisturizers. Proteins have also functioned as humectants to increase the amount of water present in the stratum corneum and viable epidermis. This enhanced water content decreased wrinkles of dehydration and created a moist environment optimal for barrier repair, as discussed previously.

As cosmetic science has evolved, more and more complex uses for peptides, which form the building blocks of proteins, have appeared. One cosmeceutical use of peptides is as a carrier for larger-molecular-weight molecules to enhance penetration. For example, copper, a known cofactor in the production of collagen during wound healing, has been linked to a peptide to enhance penetration in wounded skin. This copper peptide technology was then adapted to general skin care, as an antiaging moisturizer, in both the physician-dispensed and mass markets.

Probably the newest use of peptides are as regulators of cellular function. Since the body uses peptides to communicate between cells, it was theorized that perhaps engineered peptides might be able to upregulate or downregulate cutaneous functions that had decayed with time due to the cumulative effects of aging. This theory was investigated more thoroughly by chemists under the direction of Dr. Karl Lintner at Sederma in France. They developed a variety of peptides and tested them in cell culture to determine their biologic effects. The most interesting peptide was found to be a pentapeptide composed of lysine, threonine, threonine, lysine, and serine. This pentapeptide is abbreviated as KTTKS.

One of the challenges of peptide chemistry is to achieve penetration into the skin. This is essential if the peptide is to exert cellular effects. In order to enhance penetration, the KTTKS peptide was linked to palmitic acid. Thus, the commercialized pentapeptide is termed Pal-KTTKS with the trade name Matrixyl. Matrixyl contains 800 parts per million of Pal-KTTKS, which is typically used at a concentration of 1–4 parts per million in currently marketed cosmeceutical moisturizers.

The exact mechanism of action of Pal-KTTKS has not been fully elucidated, but it is known that this pentapeptide is a fragment of collagen type I. Many different fragments of collagen type I have been studied, but Pal-KTTKS has demonstrated the best in vitro biologic response in fibroblast subconfluent monolayer cultures. It is thought that the exposure of the fibroblasts to high levels of collagen type I breakdown products triggers a cellular recognition that too much collagen has been destroyed. This in turn downregulates the activity of collagenase, resulting in less collagen destruction and enhanced collagen synthesis. Further research is ongoing in this area.

The science of peptides as topically applied cellular messengers is in its infancy. The peptide-containing moisturizers are currently quite popular. This popularity may be due to the fact that the peptides are used as film-forming agents to alter the optical characteristics of the skin and possibly may function as hydrophilic matrices, a method of moisturization described above. Peptide moisturizers also contain additional substances that may enhance the skin, in addition to the moisturizing effect of the vehicle. For example, a currently marketed product with three parts per million of Matrixyl also contains panthenol as a humectant, niacinamide as an enhancer of cell turnover, vitamin E as a skin-soothing agent, allantoin as an anti-inflammatory, and four green tea polyphenols to function as cutaneous antioxidants (Regenerist, Olay, Procter and Gamble). Thus, all the ingredients work together to create an antiaging cosmeceutical.

Antioxidants

Antioxidants form one of the most popular categories of cosmeceutical ingredients. This is due to the fact that the major cause of cutaneous aging is oxidation of skin structures from highly reactive oxygen molecules present in our oxygen-rich environment. It is quite remarkable to note that the life-giving oxygen required to survive is also the same oxygen responsible for aging the human body. The primary source of cosmeceutical antioxidant ingredients is botanical extracts, since all plants must protect themselves from oxidation following UV exposure in the outdoor environment in which they grow.

Antioxidant botanicals function by quenching singlet oxygen and reactive oxygen species, such as superoxide anions, hydroxyl radicals, fatty peroxy radicals, and hydroperoxides. There are many botanical antioxidants

Table 8.6. Botanical antioxidants classified by chemical class

Common botanical name	Chemical class
Rutin (apples, blueberries)	Flavone
Quercetin (apples, blueberries)	Flavone
Hesperedin (lemons, oranges)	Flavone
Diosmin (lemons, oranges)	Flavone
Mangiferin (mango plant)	Xanthone
Mangostin (bilberry plant)	Xanthone
Astaxanthin (tomatoes)	Carotenoid
Lutein (tomatoes)	Carotenoid
Lycopene (tomatoes)	Carotenoid
Rosmarinic acid (rosemary)	Polyphenol
Hypericin (St. John's wort)	Polyphenol
Ellagic acid (pomegranate fruit)	Polyphenol
Chlorogenic acid (blueberry leaf)	Polyphenol
Oleuropein (olive leaf)	Polyphenol

available from raw material suppliers to the cosmeceutical industry, which can be classified into one of three categories as flavonoids, carotenoids, and polyphenols. Flavonoids possess a polyphenolic structure that accounts for their antioxidant, UV protectant, and metal chelation abilities. Carotenoids are chemically related to retinoids, previously discussed. Finally, polyphenols compose the largest category of botanical antioxidants. Table 8.6 lists currently popular botanical antioxidants and their corresponding chemical class. Soy, kinetin, curcumin, silymarin and pycnogenol all represent examples of each class.

Soy

Soybeans are a rich source of flavonoids called isoflavones, such as genistein and daidzein. These isoflavones function as phytoestrogens when consumed orally and have been credited with the decrease in cardiovascular disease and breast cancer seen in Asian women [24]. Some of the cutaneous effects of soy have been linked to its estrogenic effect in postmenopausal women. Topical estrogens have been shown to increase skin thickness and promote collagen synthesis [25]. It is interesting to note that genistein increases collagen gene expression in cell culture. However, there are no published reports of this collagen-stimulating effect in topical human trials. Genestein has also been reported to function as a potent antioxidant scavenging peroxyl radicals and protecting against lipid peroxidation in vivo [26].

Curcumin

Curcumin is a polyphenol antioxidant derived from the turmeric root. Tumeric is a popular natural yellow food coloring used in everything from prepackaged snack foods to meats. It is sometimes used in skincare products as a natural yellow coloring in products that claim to be free of artificial ingredients. Curcumin is consumed orally as an Asian spice, frequently found in rice dishes to color the otherwise white rice yellow. However, this yellow color is undesirable in cosmetic preparations, since yellowing of products is typically associated with oxidative spoilage. Tetrahydrocurcumin, a hydrogenated form of curcumin, is off-white in color and can be added to skincare products not only to function as a skin antioxidant, but also to prevent the lipids in the moisturizer from becoming rancid. The antioxidant effect of tetrahydrocurcumin is said, by cosmetic chemists, to be greater than vitamin E. Resveratrol, a related chemical to curcumin, is found in red wine, accounting for the antioxidant effect of this beverage.

Silymarin

Silymarin is an extract of the milk thistle plant (*Silbum marianum*), which belongs to the aster family of plants including daisies, thistles, and artichokes. The extract consists of three flavonoids derived from the fruit, seeds, and leaves of the plant. These flavonoids are silybin, silydianin, and silychristine. Homeopathically, silymarin is used to treat liver disease, but it is a strong antioxidant preventing lipid peroxidation by scavenging free radical species. Its antioxidant effects have been demonstrated topically in hairline mice by the 92% reduction of skin tumors following UVB exposure [27]. The mechanism for this decrease in tumor production is unknown, but topical silymarin has been shown to decrease the formation of pyrimidine dimers in a mouse model [28]. Silymarin is found in several high-end moisturizers for benign photoaging to prevent cutaneous oxidative damage.

Pycnogenol

Pycnogenol is an extract of French marine pine bark (*Pinus pinaster*), which is said to function as a plant-derived antioxidant. It is a water-soluble liquid that contains several phenolic constituents, including taxifolin, catechin, procyanidins. It also contains several phenolic acids, including p-hydroxybenzoic, protocatechuic, gallic, vanillic, p-couric, catfeic, and ferulic. It is a trademarked ingredient that is sold for oral consumption as a preventative for cardiovascular disease and as a topical skin antioxidant [29]. It is a potent free-radical scavenger that can reduce the vitamin C radical, returning the vitamin C to its active form [30]. The active vitamin C in turn regenerates vitamin E to its active form, maintaining the natural oxygen scavenging mechanisms of the skin intact.

Pycnogenol is the ideal antiaging additive since it demonstrates no chronic toxicity, no mutagenicity, no teratogenicity, and no allergenicity [31]. It is also consumed orally to enhance the production of nitric oxide, which inhibits platelet aggregation in coronary artery disease, thus it is also deemed safe for topical use. In short, pycnogenol is one of the new breed of oral supplements sold for improving the appearance of benign photoaged skin from the inside, while topical application is said to augment this effect. As with many trademarked dietary supplements, it is difficult to validate the purported benefits.

Kinetin

Kinetin is a member of the N6-substituted adenine derivatives, known as cytokinins. In plants, this hormone has been shown to stimulate transcription and influence the cell cycle by stimulating growth. It is also a plant antioxidant. The specific cytokinin that is used in the commercial moisturizers currently marketed is N6-furfuryladenine. Kinetin is said to improve benign photoaging by decreasing fine wrinkles, improving pigmentation, and increasing skin smoothness. It is typically compared to the retinoids, but human cells do not contain kinetin receptors, while they do contain retinoid receptors. It is currently unknown whether moisturizers containing this active agent provide benefits above and beyond those attributed to moisturization alone.

Anti-inflammatories

Oxidation of the human body leads to chronic low-level inflammation. Thus, anti-inflammatories play an important role in cosmeceuticals. Much like many antioxidants, most anti-inflammatory extracts are botanically derived. These include ginkgo biloba, green tea, aloe vera, and allantoin (see Table 8.7). Some of these substances, such as green tea, are also felt to be antioxidants, thus the distinction between anti-inflammatories and antioxidants is somewhat blurred.

Table 8.7. Cosmeceutical anti-inflammatory ingredients

Anti-inflammatory	Chemical classification of anti-inflammatory	Cosmeceutical active
Gingko biloba	Polyphenol fraction	Ginkgolides, bilobalides
Gingko biloba	Flavonoid fraction	Quercetin, kaempferol, sciadopitysin, ginkgetin, isoginkgetin
Aloe vera	Mucilage containing 99.5% water and a mixture of mucopolysaccharides, amino acids, hydroxy quinone glycosides, and minerals	Aloin, aloe emodin, aletinic acid, choline, and choline salicylate
Allantoin	Comfrey root	Alkaline oxidation of uric acid in a cold environment

Ginkgo Biloba

Ginkgo biloba is a plant with numerous purported benefits that is a common part of homeopathic medicine in the Orient. The plant leaves are said to contain unique polyphenols such as terpenoids (ginkgolides, bilobalides), flavonoids, and flavonol glycosides that have anti-inflammatory effects. These anti-inflammatory effects have been linked to antiradical and antilipoperoxidant effects in experimental fibroblast models [32]. Ginkgo flavonoid fractions containing quercetin, kaempferol, sciadopitysin, ginkgetin, and isoginkgetin have been demonstrated to induce human skin fibroblast proliferation in vitro. Increased collagen and extracellular fibronectin were also demonstrated by radioisotope assay [33]. Thus, ginkgo biloba extracts are added to many cosmeceuticals to function as antioxidants and promoters of collagen synthesis.

Green Tea

Green tea, also known as *Camellia sinensis*, is another botanical popular in the Orient for both topical application and oral ingestion manufactured from both the leaf and the bud of the plant. Orally, green tea is said to contain beneficial polyphenols, such as epicatechin, epicatechin-3-gallate, epigllocatechin, and eigallocatechin-3-gallate, which function as potent antioxidants [34]. The term "green tea" refers to the manufacture of the botanical extract from fresh leaves of the tea plant by steaming and drying them at elevated temperatures, being careful to avoid oxidation and polymerization of the polyphenolic components. Green tea can be easily added to topical creams and lotions designed to combat the signs of photoaging, but it must be stabilized itself with an antioxidant, such as butylated hydroxytoluene.

A study by Katiyar et al. demonstrated the anti-inflammatory effects of topical green tea application on C3H mice. A topically applied green tea extract containing GTP [(-)-epigallocatechin-3-gallate] was found to reduce UVB-induced inflammation as measured by double skin-fold swelling [35]. They also found protection against UV-induced edema, erythema, and antioxidant depletion in the epidermis. This work was further investigated by applying GTP to the back of humans 30 min prior to UV irradiation, which resulted in decreased myeloperoxidase activity and decreased infiltration of leukocytes as compared to untreated skin [36].

The application of topical green tea polyphenols prior to UV exposure has also been shown to decrease the formation of cyclobutane pyrimidine dimers [37]. These dimers are critical in initiating UV-induced mutagenesis and carcinogenesis, which represent the end stage of the aging process. Thus, green tea polyphenols can function topically as antioxidants, anti-inflammatories, and anticarcinogens, making them a popular cosmeceutical additive.

Aloe Vera

Probably the most widely used cutaneous botanical anti-inflammatory is aloe vera. The mucilage that is released from the aloe vera plant leaves as a colorless gel and contains 99.5% water and a complex mixture of mucopolysaccharides, amino acids, hydroxy quinone glycosides, and minerals. Compounds isolated from aloe vera juice include aloin, aloe emodin, aletinic acid, choline, and choline salicylate [38]. The reported cutaneous effects of aloe vera include increased blood flow, reduced inflammation, decreased skin bacterial colonization, and enhanced wound healing [39]. The anti-inflammatory effects of aloe vera may result from its ability to inhibit cyclooxygenase as part of the arachidonic acid pathway.

Allantoin

Allantoin is one of the oldest botanical anti-inflammatory extracts in the cosmeceutical marketplace. It is obtained from the common comfrey root. Allantoin is the basis for sensitive skin and antiaging claims made for several moisturizers. Most allantoin currently used in skincare products is not botanically derived, but manufactured by the alkaline oxidation of uric acid in a cold environment. It is a white crystalline powder that is readily soluble in hot water, making it easy to formulate in cream and lotion moisturizers. Allantoin is felt to induce cell proliferation, promoting the repair of photodamaged skin, and reducing UV-induced inflammation.

The Future

Cosmeceuticals form an important part of the OTC skin treatment market. There are some industry forecasters who feel that the cosmetics industry has hit a glass ceiling in new cosmeceutical development, largely due to the failure of the FDA to develop a new classification system. It is thought that a new "quasi-drug" category, similar to the Japanese designation, would allow the introduction of more robust active ingredients into cosmeceuticals. These more robust ingredients would provide enhanced consumer-perceived skin benefits, supporting stronger claims. Physicians may wonder why cosmeceuticals are not more thoroughly studied and tested. This is in part because it may be in the manufacturer's best interest not to fully understand exactly what a cosmeceutical active can accomplish. Cosmeceuticals that function too well would alter the structure and function of the skin and become drugs. The current state of the cosmeceutical marketplace is not due to the industry's lack of desire to perform thoughtful research and develop quality products, but rather due to limitations imposed by the present regulatory climate. This chapter has discussed cosmeceuticals in such a way to help the physician obtain greater respect for this skincare category and its role in facial rejuvenation.

References

1. Baker CG (1987) Moisturization: new methods to support time proven ingredients. Cosmet Toilet 102:99–102
2. De Groot AC, Weyland JW, Nater JP (1994) Unwanted Effects of Cosmetics and Drugs Used in Dermatology, 3rd edn. Elsevier, Amsterdam, pp 498–500
3. Friberg SE, Ma Z (1993) Stratum corneum lipids, petrolatum and white oils. Cosmet Toilet 107:55–59
4. Grubauer G, Feingold KR, Elias PM (1987) Relationship of epidermal lipogenesis to cutaneous barrier function. J Lipid Res 28:746–752

5. Ghadially R, Halkier-Sorensen L, Elias PM (1992) Effects of petrolatum on stratum corneum structure and function. J Am Acad Dermatol 26:387–396
6. Spencer TS (1988) Dry skin and skin moisturizers. Clin Dermatol 6:24–28
7. Rieger MM, Deem DE (1974) Skin moisturizers II The effects of cosmetic ingredients on human stratum corneum. J Soc Cosmet Chem 25:253–262
8. Robbins CR, Fernee KM (1983) Some observations on the swelling of human epidermal membrane. J Soc Cosmet Chem 37:21–34
9. Idson B (1992) Dry skin: moisturizing and emolliency. Cosmet Toilet 107:69–78
10. Halder RM, Richards GM (2004) Management of dischromias in ethnic skin. Dermatol Ther 17:151–157
11. Fitton A, Goa KL (1991) Azelaic acid: a review of its pharmacological properties and therapeutic efficacy in acne and hyperpigmentary skin disorders. Drugs 5:780–798
12. Balina LM, Graupe K (1991) The treatment of melasma. 20% azelaic acid versus 4% hydroquinone cream. Int J Dermatol 30:893–895
13. Espinal-Perez LE, Moncada B, Castanedo-Cazares JP (2004) A double blind randomized trial of 5% ascorbic acid vs 4% hydroquinone in melasma. Int J Dermatol 43:604–607
14. Amer M, Metwalli M (2000) Topical Liquiritin improves melasma. Int J Dermatol 39:299–301
15. Lim JT (1999) Treatment of melasma using kojic acid in a gel containing hydroquinone and glycolic acid. Dermatol Surg 25:282–284
16. Garcia A, Fulton JE Jr (1996) The combination of glycolic acid and hydroquinone or kojic acid for the treatment of melasma and related conditions. Dermatol Surg 22:443–447
17. Choi S, Lee SK, Kim JE, et al (2002) Aloesin inhibits hyperpigmentation induced by UV radiation. Clin Exp Dermatol 27:513–515
18. Jones K, Hughes J, Hong M, et al (2002) Modulation of melanogenesis by aloesin: a competitive inhibitor of tyrosinase. Pigment Cell Res 15:335–340
19. Hori I, Nihei K, Kubo I (2004) Structural criteria for depigmenting mechanism of arbutin. Phytother Res 18:475–469
20. Kligman LH, Do CH, Kligman AM (1984) Topical retinoic acid enhances the repair of ultraviolet damaged dermal connective tissue. Connect Tissue Res 12:139–150
21. Goodman DS (1984) Vitamin A and retinoids in health and disease. N Engl J Med 310:1023–1031
22. Noy N (1993) Interactions of retinoids with lipid bilayers and with membranes. In: Livrea MA, Packer L (eds) Retinoids. Marcel Dekker, New York, pp 17–27
23. Duell EA, Derguini F, Kang S, Elder JT, Voorhees JJ (1996) Extraction of human epidermis treated with retinol yields retro-retinoids in addition to free retinol and retinyl esters. J Invest Dermatol 107:178–182
24. Glazier MG, Bowman MA (2001) A review of the evidence for the use of phytoestrogens as a replacement for traditional estrogen replacement therapy. Arch Intern Med 161:1161–1172
25. Maheux R, Naud F, Rioux M, Grenier R, Lemay A, Guy J, et al (1994) A randomized, double-blind, placebo-controlled study on the effect of conjugated estrogens on skin thickness. Am J Obset Gynecol 170:642–649
26. Wiseman H, O'Reilly JD, Adlercreutz H, Mallet AL, Bowey EA, Rowland IR, et al (2000) Isoflavone phytoestrogens consumed in soy decrease F-2-isoprostane concentrations and increase resistance of low-density lipoprotein to oxidation in humans. Am J Clin Nutr 72:395–400
27. Katiyar SK, Korman NJ, Mukhtar H, Agarwal R (1997) Protective effects of silyarin against photocarcinogenesis in a mouse skin model. J Natl Cancer Inst 89:556–566
28. Chatterjee L, Agarwal R, Mukhtar H (1996) Ultraviolet B radiation-induced DNA lesions in mouse epidermis: an assessment sing a novel 32P-postlabeling technique. Biochem Biophys Res Commun 229:590–595
29. Devaraj S, Vega-Lopez S, Kaul N, Schonlau F, Rohdewald P, Jialal I (2002) Supplementation with a pine bark extract rich in polyphenols increases plasma antioxidant capacity and alters the plasma lipoprotein profile. Lipids 37:931–934
30. Cossins E, Lee R, Packer L (1998) ESR studies of vitamin C regeneration, order of reactivity of natural source phytochemical preparations. Biochem Mol Biol Int 45:583–598
31. Schonlau F (2002) The cosmetic Pycnogenol. J Appl Cosmetol 20:241–246
32. Joyeux M, Lobstein A, Anton R, Mortier F (1995) Comparative antilipoperoxidant, antinecrotic and scavenging properties of terpenes and biflavones from Ginkgo and some flavonoids. Plant Med 61:126–129
33. Kim SJ, Lim MH, Chun IK, Won YH (1997) Effects of flavonoids of Ginkgo biloba on proliferation of human skin fibroblast. Skin Pharmacol 10:200–205
34. Katiyar SK, Elmets CA (2000) Green tea and skin. Arch Dermatol 136:989–994
35. Katiyar SK, Elmets CA, Agarwal R, et al (1995) Protection against ultraviolet-B radiation-induced local and systemic suppression of contact

hypersensitivity and edema responses in C3H/HeN mice by green tea polyphenols. Photochem Photobiol 62:855–861

36. Elmets CA, Singh D, Tubesing K, Matsui MS, Katiyar SK, Mukhtar H (2001) Green tea polyphenols as chemopreventive agents against cutaneous photodamage. J Am Acad Dermatol 44:425–432
37. Katiyar SK, Afaq F, Perez A, Mukhtar H (2000) Green tea polyphenol treatment to human skin prevents formation of ultraviolet light B-induced pyrimidine dimers in DNA. Clin Cancer Res 6:3864–3869
38. McKeown E (1987) Aloe vera. Cosmet Toilet 102:64–65
39. Waller T (1992) Aloe vera. Cosmet Toilet 107:53–54

Subject Index

Printed in the United States of America